# Bioinformatics for Vaccinology

# Bioinformatics for Vaccinology

**Darren R Flower**
*Edward Jenner Institute for Vaccine Research, Compton, Berkshire, UK*

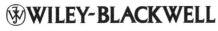

A John Wiley & Sons, Ltd., Publication

*Library of Congress Cataloguing-in-Publication Data*

Flower, Darren R.
  Bioinformatics for vaccinology / Darren R. Flower.
      p. ; cm.
  Includes bibliographical references and index.
  ISBN 978-0-470-02711-0 (pbk. : alk. paper)   1. Immunoinformatics.   2. Vaccines–Design–Data processing.   I. Title.
  [DNLM:   1. Computational Biology–methods.   2. Vaccines.   3. Vaccination–methods.
4. Vaccination–trends.   QW 805 F644b 2008]
  QR182.2.I46F56 2008
  615'.3720285–dc22

                                                                                        2008032154

A catalogue record for this book is available from the British Library.

ISBN 978 0 470 02711 0

Set in 10.5/12.5 pt Times by Aptara, New Delhi, India

First printing   2008

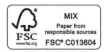

*This work is dedicated to my wife Christine Jennifer
and to my daughter Isobel Emily Rebecca*

# Contents

## 4   Vaccines: Data and databases     113

# Preface

This book is a gentle but useful introduction to a seemingly recondite subject, but a subject of unrivalled importance nonetheless. It provides an informative overview and places computational vaccinology into context. It also seeks to proselytise the potential, and I believe growing importance, of *in silico* vaccinology.

This book is divided into seven chapters. Chapter One will serve as a historical introduction to the remainder of the book. While it must, of necessity, be somewhat superficial, Chapter One tries to outline some of key discoveries in, and discoverers of, vaccinology. Chapter Two deals with the threats addressed, and opportunities offered, by vaccine research to a world beset by climate change and bioterrorism. Chapter Three addresses in a more technical manner the immunological background to vaccines, with a special emphasis on problems which bioinformatics can tackle. Chapter Four deals with databases and their role within bioinformatics, albeit slanted towards immunology. Chapter Five explores the role for prediction methods in bioinformatic applications in vaccinology. Chapter Six deals with structural bioinformatics albeit within an immunological context. Chapter Seven addresses real world applications and draws together some of the dangling threads. The book will largely forego the worst excesses of the academic text, and thus avoid an overabundance of citations and foot-notes.

It is not my intention that this should necessarily be a book which anyone would sit down and read from cover to cover. It would be wonderful to think that someone might. If they did, it would be even more wonderful to think that by doing so they would find the book edifying and enjoyable. I hope that those who try, find at least some of it useful. Readers should feel free to choose appropriate chapters for themselves or to dip in and out of the book, selecting sections at will.

**Darren R. Flower**

# Acknowledgements

In scientific papers, acknowledgements often come at or near the end of an article. In writing a book like this, I feel it appropriate to recognize the contributions made by a whole plethora of people, and acknowledge their help earlier rather than later.

First, I should like to express my heartfelt thanks to my group at the Edward Jenner Institute and, latterly, the Jenner Institute for Vaccine Research, University of Oxford. My group has, over the years, included a host of outrageously gifted and remarkably insightful researchers; they include, in no particular order: Matthew Davies, Channa Hattotuwagama, Pingping Guan, Paul Taylor, Helen Cattan, Valerie Walshe, Helen McSparron, Shunzhou Wan, Martin Blythe, Hannah Tipney, Keiran Raine, Sarah Thompson, Karma Dorje Tarap, Kamna Ramakrishnan, Christopher Toseland, Shelley Hemsley, Debra Clayton, Christianna Zygouri, Kelly Paine and Isabel McDonald.

I should also like to single out one colleague for special mention: Dr Irini A Doytchinova, for her inestimable contribution to the group and to the work I mention in this text. I do not suppose I would have done nearly so much without her help.

I should also thank my many colleagues for their enlightening and nurturing comments. Most notable are: Professor Peter Beverley, Dr Persephone Borrow, Dr David Tough, Dr Tongbin Li, Professor Vladimir Brusic, Professor Terri Attwood, Dr Jon Timmis and Professor Peter Coveney.

There are, of course, a vast number of others particularly, but in no way limited to, my friends from the pharmaceutical industry and the Royal Society of Chemistry, to whom I also owe thanks. These people are too numerous to mention by name but I happily extend a generic thankyou to them all.

Lastly, I should thank everyone at John Wiley & Sons, Ltd, for their efforts in publishing this work.

**Darren R. Flower**

# Exordium

## Vaccines: A Very, Very Short Introduction

*Bioinformatics for Vaccinology* addresses the newly emergent discipline of immunoinformatics, specifically in the context of high-throughput immunology, or immunomics, and the design and discovery of vaccines. As the science of bioinformatics, the application of informatics techniques to biological macromolecules, has grown, matured and deepened, so novel subdisciplines have begun to emerge within it. Immunoinformatics, the application of informatics techniques to molecules of the immune system, is one of the most exciting of these newly emergent disciplines.

One of the principal goals of immunoinformatics is to help develop computer-aided vaccine design, or computational vaccinology, and to apply it to the search for new or enhanced vaccines. The identification of novel vaccine targets through *in silico* genomic analysis has great potential in the fight against disease. The pivotal challenge for immunoinformatics, at least as applied to vaccines, is the prediction of immunogenicity, be that at the level of epitope, subunit vaccine or attenuated pathogen. As the veracity of *in silico* predictions improves, so subsequent experimental work will become ever faster, ever more efficient and, ultimately, ever more successful; and that, in a nutshell, is what this book is about.

Vaccines are a good idea; a really, really good idea. The great French philosopher Voltaire (1694–1778) said: 'If God did not exist, it would be necessary to invent him.' We could say something similar about vaccines: they are such a good thing that if they did not exist we would have to create them. The vaccine-mediated abrogation of childhood mortality is often considered to be the greatest historical success of public health. In many developed countries, the annual mortality for a variety of diseases – smallpox, polio, measles and diphtheria – has fallen to truly nugatory levels of no more than 0.1%. It is now generally accepted that mass vaccination – taking account, as it does, of the principle of herd immunity – is one of the most effective prophylactic means of controlling and preventing infectious disease. It also offers the best chance of offsetting the burgeoning problem of antibiotic resistance, since resistance to vaccines has never been observed. Very successful vaccines can empty ecological niches, allowing related microorganisms not tackled by the vaccine to occupy them. Many vaccines are also suboptimal requiring clever strategies, such as prime/boost approaches, to maximize their efficacy for diseases threatening human health, such as tuberculosis or malaria.

In developed countries in particular, vaccines have proved exceptionally effective in preventing death from diseases which were hitherto major killers. In developing countries, the efficacy of vaccines is unrivalled and offers the prize of eradicating endemic diseases of high incidence, morbidity and mortality. The example par excellence is smallpox, followed by polio. Smallpox eradication prevented over 300 million infections and saved perhaps 100 million lives. In the developed world, it is possible to compare systematically the prevalence of a certain infection prior to the introduction of a vaccine with its occurrence now, long after the advent of vaccination. In such a comparison, we see that the incidence of many diseases has fallen to virtually zero: a 100% reduction for polio, a reduction of over 99% for diphtheria and measles, mumps and rubella (MMR), and a greater than 97% reduction for tetanus.

Thus in the developed world, economic assessments of vaccination focus on the societal impact of paediatric vaccines. However, disentangling the benefits of new vaccine treatments in a paediatric environment must account for the effect of herd immunity, the different operational logistics of vaccination schedules and for any decrease of efficacy over time. Health economists tend to concur that if a medical intervention saves a year of life for less than $50 000, it is cost effective. On this basis, most studies agree that virtually all vaccinations will be both cost effective and cost saving, except where disease incidence is atypically low, and that most societies would benefit from blanket immunization. When compared with other health interventions, vaccines are among the best health investments a government can make. This should be particularly true for developing countries where the cost of mortality and morbidity is such that potential benefits will easily outweigh extra financial cost.

Despite the initial success of antibiotics and early vaccines, threats from infectious diseases remain: if not in the developed world then certainly in developing countries. There are 35 infectious diseases – HIV, SARS and West Nile amongst them – which have been recognized during the past 25 years. During the coming century, many believe new contagious diseases will surface with escalating frequency. A number of causes – a growing global population, an increasing disparity between the richest and the poorest, burgeoning urbanization, increased ease of travel, alterations to food production and the inexorable effects of climate change on the biogeography of disease – will conspire together to foment and foster the rise of a whole raft of new threats to human health.

Thus this is a book about how modern computational methods can encourage the discovery of vaccines; how such methods can help and encourage humanity's continuing quest to master disease. The book begins with an introduction to immunology, progresses to a description of the threats which vaccinology must deal with today, primarily (but not exclusively) infectious disease, and finally elaborates on how a combination of bioinformatics and postgenomic techniques can help realize the great potential of vaccines. The intention of *Bioinformatics for Vaccinology* may therefore seem prosaic, but it has a hidden subtext. This book is as much about presenting this concept as a principal way forward for vaccinology, as it is about explaining the hows and the whys of immunoinformatics.

# 1

# Vaccines:
# Their Place in History

*There is nothing new except what has been forgotten.*

—Marie Antoinette (1755–1793)

## Smallpox in history

For the first hundred years or so, the story of vaccination was the story of smallpox. Smallpox first appeared in remote antiquity, perhaps 10 thousand years ago when humankind first embraced settled farming in preference to transhumance. It was, many say, the most feared of all ancient diseases: smallpox killed 20–30% of those who contracted it, disfiguring or blinding those that survived.

It has been suggested, primarily on the basis of extant historical evidence, that virulent smallpox did not appear in Europe until the early modern era – most probably during the seventeenth century – and gradually replaced an endemic and much less virulent form of the disease. This transition seems to have occurred during a series of erratic smallpox outbreaks during the fifteenth and sixteenth centuries. With more certainty we can say that smallpox's case fatality – the proportion of the infected population that dies – escalated over the centuries, peaking during the eighteenth century.

*Homo sapiens* is the only species susceptible to smallpox; there is no known animal reservoir for the disease. Smallpox is contagious – it is transmitted from person to person. The smallpox virus is usually transmitted via the respiratory tract, primarily by inhaling respiratory droplets. While contagious, smallpox is not highly transmissible; dense populations are necessary to maintain transmission. Prolonged close contact foments infection. After a 10 to 14 day incubation period, infected individuals develop severe symptoms, including fever, malaise and headache. A maculopapular rash then develops on the face, trunk and extremities. Smallpox lesions become deep and pustular over the next 1–2 days, with scabs forming by day 10. Patient infectivity is greatest in week one, when viral shedding is at a peak, with most deaths occurring during the second week.

The discovery of vaccination – though discovery is, as we shall see, altogether too simplistic a term – is most often attributed to the work of Gloucestershire physician Edward Jenner (1749–1823). On 14 May 1796, eight-year-old James Phipps was vaccinated with bovine cowpox; days later Phipps survived deliberate infection with smallpox. Thus Jenner was, for the first time, able to induce protective immunity against the disease of smallpox. Later, in 1881, Louis Pasteur (1822–1895) adopted the word 'vaccination' – Jenner's neologism for his treatment – as a general term for immunization against any disease. In Jenner's time, vaccination had instead been known as 'cowpox inoculation' or 'vaccine inoculation'. In May 1980, the World Health Organization declared that smallpox had been totally eradicated as the result of a global programme of vaccination. No one has died of naturally occurring smallpox since. Thus vaccination, as a concept and as a practical reality, at least as used against smallpox, would seem to be an unqualified success. Yet, no idea is wholly without precedent; no concept is utterly new; no thought is without inspiration.

Ge Hong was an eminent physician, who is also credited with making important contributions to alchemy and astronomy. He became military adviser to Qi Han, author of *Nanfang caumuzhuang* (*Records of Plants and Trees in the southern region*) and one of the greatest botanists in Ancient China. Ge Hong wrote many books, including the *Baopuzi neipan* which recounts the medicinal properties of many plants and minerals. He described smallpox, and gave the first therapies for it, in the *Zhouhou Jiuzufang* (*Medical Handbook for Emergencies*), a three volume recension written to supplement the 100 volumes of *Jingui yaofang* (*Prescription in the Treasury of Medicine*), which were composed during the Jin Dynasty (266–317).

In India, smallpox was named, and its essential character described, in early Sanskrit medical treatises such as fourth century texts by Caraka and Susruta. Smallpox was called masurika, which means 'lentil' or 'pulse', since smallpox pustules resemble in shape and colour a local variety of bean. By the twelfth century, Sanskrit texts give other names for the disease, all variants of the word sitala, which means cold or cool.

The first western physician to provide an accurate description of smallpox was Ahrun (610–641), a Greek-speaking Christian Egyptian, who lived in Alexandria. In the tenth century, arguably the best early description of smallpox, and how it differed from measles, was given by one of the most outstanding physicians of the era: Abu Bakr Muhammad ibn-Zakariyya al-Razi, better known to the West as Rhazes. He was born in Rai in Persia in about AD 865. Early on he studied music, physics and alchemy, only becoming interested in medicine aged 30. Much influenced by Hippocrates and Galen, he nonetheless demonstrated independence and originality, introducing much personal experience into his texts. Of al-Razi's 36 surviving texts, the best known is his treatise on smallpox and measles. In AD 910 he described smallpox in his book *De variolis et morbillis commentaries*, noting the disease was transmitted from person to person. Al-Razi wrongly assumed that both smallpox and measles were manifestations of the disease, yet his descriptions differ only marginally from those in the famous 1892 textbook of Sir William Osler (1849–1919): *Principles and Practice of Medicine*.

## Variolation

Smallpox is a disease which cannot properly be treated but can be prevented. At some now forgotten point, a connection between infection and subsequent acquired immunity was made for smallpox: surviving the disease leads to pock marking and pockmarked individuals rarely, if ever, contracted smallpox again. A similar observation – that smallpox infection which results from a skin scratch has a greatly reduced severity – led, presumably, to the idea of variolation. It is a frustration that we do not know where or when this practice originated, whether it arose once and spread geographically through time or whether it arose independently several times and in several places.

As a prophylactic approach, variolation is something of a paradox, as it caused the disease that it was claiming to prevent. Potential benefits of variolation may have manifested themselves in two ways. Variolation, working at the level of individuals, may have caused a form of the disease much less severe than natural smallpox. At the community level, variolation might abrogate a smallpox epidemic. Moreover, by producing an augmented level of local immunity, variolation could decrease the probability that future outbreaks of smallpox might occur.

Variolation is, or was, the inoculation of uninfected individuals using dried scabs or pustular fluid obtained from smallpox lesions of recovering victims. Eighteenth century writers described the process of variolation as cutaneous inoculation with terms such as insertion, transplantation or engrafting (which has its origin in horticulture, where it refers to inserting a bud into a plant) also in common use. The term *variolation* itself was probably not used until much later: the Oxford English Dictionary, for example, says that it appeared first in 1792, although it was certainly coined earlier. The word variolation derives from the Latin *varus* for pimple, while inoculation comes from the Latin *inoculare,* meaning to graft. The term 'vaccination' has come to mean immunization by vaccine, while 'variolation' now refers only to inoculation of the normal, virulent, pathogenic agent of an infectious disease.

The technique involved first a small scratch of the person being variolated followed by the transfer of infected matter into the wound. In terms of both its underlying (and albeit poorly understood) mechanism of action and associated clinical practice, variolation is a practice quite distinct from vaccination. Postinfection fatality was much reduced for variolation (0.5–2%) when compared to naturally acquired smallpox (20–30%). Symptoms of the disease were also different, with a decreased general rash and a lessening of permanent pockmarks. Putative explanations for these differences abound. The simplest is also one of the most compelling: when variolated, a patient, who has had adequate preparation, is able to mount a full scale response and ultimately becomes immune to subsequent infection. The fact that overpreparation, and the use of strange purgative regimes, decreases the effectiveness of variolation would support this view. Likewise, another contention is that the transferred virus has been mildly attenuated. Although Pasteur-type attenuation through serial passage is generally performed many, many times, the arm-to-arm transfer seen during variolation may have afforded the opportunity for some kind of selection of less virulent virus. The variolated patient may thus receive less virulent smallpox material and incur a less severe infection compared with naturally transmitted smallpox. Another possibility posits that the physical route of infection into the body was crucial. The argument here runs thus: smallpox spreads with no little celerity through the body when introduced into the lungs; however, when introduced under the skin, as in variolation, progress is rather less rapid and the body, as manifest by the immune system, has the time to mount a proper response. Yet another hypothesis suggests that the transfer of infected material also transfers components of the innate and adaptive immune system already primed to respond to the disease. Such components may include neutralizing antibodies; or immune mediators, such as interferons, which act as natural adjuvants enhancing the immune response to the incipient infection; or Antigen Presenting Cells (APCs), such as Dendritic Cells (DCs), already presenting pathogen derived peptides. Like many complex phenomena, the relative efficacy of variolation is, in all likelihood, a result of the synergistic combination of several such mechanisms of action.

However, because the causative agent used in variolation was not wholly attenuated, or weakened, as subsequent vaccines were, the process had the significant disadvantage that variolated individuals could transmit potentially severe natural smallpox to members of the as-yet-uninfected population. Although it may have protected those wealthy families able to afford it, variolation, practiced on a sporadic basis, as it certainly was in the first half of the eighteenth century, was more a public-health hazard than it was anything else. It certainly came with many problems. Some cases were severe, and even fatal. The lancets used to transfer pustular material were seldom sterilized nor were they wielded by sterilized hands in sterile rooms. Moreover, because many inoculators preferred to take inoculum from more mature pustules, wound infections were quite common. Indeed, variolated individuals were often not isolated, and because they carried the virus yet were sufficiently well to be up and about, they were a risk to non-immunes. Indeed, the last smallpox epidemics in China in 1965, in Afghanistan in 1973, in Pakistan in 1974, and in Ethiopia in 1976 are all thought to have been caused, or at least exacerbated, by variolation. Local practitioners tried to preserve stocks of smallpox virus maintaining them by re-injecting material from consenting individuals, typically friends or family.

Moreover, there are two distinct routes of administration used in variolation: the nasal route, which is considered the more risky, and the cutaneous or skin route, which is thought to be safer. However, opinion differs on this point and it is an issue not easily resolved in the post-eradication era. The variety of variolation used in China was not the arguably safer and more effective cutaneous version, whereby crusts from smallpox pustules were inserted into cuts in the skin, which was in use elsewhere, but one enacted via the nasal route, i.e. via the inhalation, or so-called insufflation or blowing, of powdered material, obtained from dried scabs, directly onto the mucosal lining of the nose. Voltaire likened this practice to taking snuff.

## Variolation in history

It is thought that smallpox itself first entered China in the mid first century AD, co-inciding with the beginning of the Eastern Han dynasty (25–220). However, it was not until the fifteenth century, during the Tang and Song Dynasties, that progress in transportation, and concomitant increases in travel, allowed the disease to reach epidemic proportions. Among the first written reports of variolation found in Chinese records are ones that refer to the reign of Jen Tsung (1023–1063). Yu Mao Kun, in *Ke Jin Jing Fu Ji Jie* (*Special Golden Mirror and Solutions,* published in 1727), describes how, in the long Qing period of the Ming dynasty (1567–1572), variolation spread across the whole of China from the Ning Guo district of Anhui.

Many, perhaps rightly, view variolation as a great Chinese innovation, while others favour the notion that the technique had reached China, via Tibet, from India. While variolation was probably practiced in India since antiquity, there are no attested records of the procedure written before the arrival of Europeans in the fifteenth century. Subsequently, and certainly from the early eighteenth century, many settlers and merchants from Europe described the cutaneous form of variolation, which was in widespread use among the resident population. Variolation seems to have been used widely in a number of areas during the eighteenth century, including Bengal, Assam, Bihar, Orissa and Varanasi, and less commonly in parts of the Punjab, Sindh, Rajasthan and Gujarat, and occasionally in isolated regions of central India and Maharashtra. Treatments other than variolation are outlined in texts which date from the fourth century, as well as those from later commentaries, such as the eighth century Nidana of Madhava-Kara or that by Dalhana in the eleventh century, all of which belong to the Ayurvedic system. The remedies found in these works comprise both dietary changes and efforts to restore the proper balance between external forces, such as heat and cold. In India, the use of variolation was associated with worship of the goddess Sitalam, who was thought to cause smallpox. The Ayurvedic system concerning the disease and the variolation technique, with its implicit understanding of infection, formed, in thought and deed, a unified and holistic conceptualization of smallpox.

The earliest description of the practice of variolation in India is an account written in 1731 by Robert Coult. As we have said, it remains uncertain when variolation was discovered or introduced into India. Indeed, the Oriya Brahmins, who conducted indigenous variolation in northern India, were themselves unsure when the technique had been conceived or introduced into the subcontinent. In 1767, John Zephania Holwell (1711–1798), who had studied surgery at London's Guy's Hospital and saw service in Bengal from 1732 until 1760, described the Ayurvedic system of inoculation against smallpox to the Royal College of Physicians in London in a tract called *'An account of the manner of Inoculating for the Smallpox in the East Indies. With some observations on the Practice and Mode of Treating that Disease in those parts. Inscribed to the learned, the President and Members of the College of Physicians in London.'*

Arab traders were probably key disseminators of variolation. This was mirrored by the spread of smallpox itself, which occurred in the wake of the rapid territorial gains made by the burgeoning Arabic civilization that emerged in the first 150 years after the founding of Islam. This helped disseminate the disease through North Africa and Europe during the sixth, seventh and eighth centuries. Traders spread knowledge of the practice into South East Asia and, as we shall see below, probably also into Africa and Ottoman Turkey. Perhaps the most compelling evidence, however, comes from Patrick Russell (1727–1805), the noted physician and naturalist, and his brother Alexander (1715–1768). In December 1768, they published an account, in the *Philosophical Transactions of the Royal Society,* which described variolation in Arabia: it summarized the extensive observations that Alexander had made while living in Aleppo in Syria, which suggested that inoculation against smallpox was practiced extensively amongst the Bedouin tribesmen of the Middle East. It seems also to have been in common use in Persia, Georgia and Armenia, among others.

It seems certain that variolation was also widely known throughout many parts of Africa, at least from the late 1600s and, in all probability, much earlier. It is believed, for example, that variolation was introduced into Egypt by the Mameluke Turks during the thirteenth century. In 1738, Englishman Thomas Shaw wrote a discourse on his travels which said that inoculation was well known in North Africa. In 1768, the memoirs of Chais, a protestant priest from Holland, stated that an ambassador from Morocco had said publicly in 1738 that inoculation against smallpox was commonly practiced in North Africa. Also, as we shall see below from the story of Cotton Mather, cutaneous variolation was unquestionably known in West Africa from at least the seventeenth century, and was certainly practiced widely during the nineteenth century.

## Variolation comes to Britain

Despite some evidence in the Anglo-Saxon Chronicles, which may make reference to the disease, it was only in the eleventh and twelfth centuries that returning Crusader Knights, their troops, and civil entourages, coupled to the continuing expansion of trade with the Middle East, brought smallpox to Northern

Europe. The disease had become endemic in Northern Europe by the fifteenth century. By the seventeenth century smallpox had displaced bubonic plague as Europe's most terrifying and fatal disease; and it is during this century that the first accounts emerge of what can be seen as the seeds of variolation in Europe, although its origins are rooted deeply in superstition. Thomas Bartholin (1616–1680), called it 'transplantation of disease', and pronounced it 'a stupendous remedy, by means of which the ailments of this or that person are transferred to a brute animal, or to another person, or to some inanimate thing'. The practice of variolation had even reached Central Europe at this time, probably via the Balkans, where it was being used extensively in Slovakia. Indeed, in 1721, Dr Johann Reiman undertook a well-publicized inoculation against smallpox in Bohemia, now part of the Czech Republic.

By the turn of the eighteenth century, news concerning variolation had even begun to penetrate into England. Throughout much of its history, England was a small, underpopulated, geographically-remote island on the edge of a backward and fractious continent far removed from the centre of civilization. By the end of the seventeenth century this had changed, but not as much as we know it would: within a century England would have gained and lost one Empire and then gained another. The news of variolation that reached England was news in the loosest sense; what was actually circulating was a tiny handful of letters describing the practice.

In 1700, the Royal Society received several reports which described a variety of Chinese intranasal variolation: the first report on Chinese variolation is given in a 1700 account by Dr Clopton Havers (who died in 1702). The Chinese method was also described in an account (dated 5 January 1700) sent by Joseph Lister, an East Indian Company trader stationed in China. This letter, addressed to Dr Martin Lister (1638–1712), reported that:

> a method of communicating the smallpox involving opening the pustules of one who has the smallpox ripe upon them and drying the matter with a little cotton and afterwards put it up the nostrils of those they would infect.

Nothing very substantive came of either account; knowledge of the Chinese practice of *sowing the smallpox* by nasal insufflation was not to vanish: witness, for example, the book *De Various et Morbillis Uber*, written by Richard Mead (1673–1754), where it is mentioned. Moreover, the method is fully described by the Jesuit missionary d'Entrecolles in letters from Jao Tcheon (1715) and Pekin (1725), which were published in the *Lettres Edifiantes et Curieuses*.

In the following decade, reports appeared that described cutaneous variolation, as practiced in Turkey. In 1712, Dr Edward Tarry of Enfield, who had returned to England from Pera and Galata, claimed to have observed more than 4000 variolated persons. During late 1712 and early 1713, Richard Waller (1646–1715), secretary to the Royal Society from 1710 to 1714, had initiated a campaign to obtain, on behalf of the Royal Society, more and better information concerning variolation.

In December 1713, Emmanouil Timonis (1665–1741) sent an extensive eye-witness account of variolation, written in Latin from Constantinople, to the Royal Society. On 27 May 1714, this letter was called to the attention of Fellows of the Society by John Woodward (1665–1728). An English translation of the letter was later read out to Fellows of the Society on 3 June 1714, and it was formally discussed on 10 June 1714. Timonis described 'smallpox by incision': pustular material was usually only taken from healthy boys with smallpox and applied to persons of all ages, causing them only minor inconvenience. The only required preparation was to abstain from flesh for 20 days.

Despite Woodward's unpopularity with other Fellows of the Royal Society – he had formerly served on the council of the Royal Society but was expelled in 1710 for insulting Sir Hans Sloane – extracts of the note by Timonis were published in the Philosophical Transactions of the Royal Society, during May 1714, as *Timoni E. An account, or history, of the procuring of the smallpox by incision or inoculation, as it has for some time been practised at Constantinople*. Timonis was a physician, as well as an antiquarian and diplomat and, it was said, *a very learned man*. Timonis had in his youth obtained medical degrees from Padua and Oxford, and was later elected a Fellow of the Royal Society in 30 November 1703. At this time, he practiced medicine in Constantinople and served as family physician to various British Ambassadors there, including Sir Robert Sutton and, as we shall see, his successor Edward Wortley Montagu.

The report of Timonis generated some discussion and the Royal Society then commissioned an even more complete investigation, much of which occurred through already established English commercial contacts. In 8 July 1714, Richard Waller wrote to the botanist William Sherard (1659–1728), who had become a Fellow of the Royal Society in 1720, asking if he had access to more information concerning variolation. Sherard was at that time the British Consul at Smyrna (modern Izmir in Turkey), and he afterwards contacted his Venetian equivalent, a man called Iakovos Pylarinos (1659–1718), who also practiced as a physician. Pylarinos later described variolation against smallpox in a Latin pamphlet dedicated to William Sherard, printed in Venice during 1715, which was entitled *Nova et tuta Variolas excitandi per transplantationem methodus nuper inventa, in usum tracta, qua rite per acta immuniaa in posterum praesenvatur ab hujus modi contagio corpora* or 'New and safe method to excite smallpox by inoculation, just invented and put into use, performed routinely, by which the bodies acquire immunity against this infection in later years'. The pamphlet, introduced at the 24 May 1716 meeting of the Society, contained personal observations made by Pylarinos while he practiced at Smyrna and Constantinople. The pamphlet was later summarized in the *Philosophical Transactions*, appearing during 1716 as Pilarino G. *Nova et tuta variolas excitandi per transplantationem methodus, nuper inventa et in usum tracta*.

On 7 March 1716, Sherard sent his brother James Sherard (1666–1738), an apothecary and also a Fellow in the Royal Society, a letter and the printed pamphlet by Pylarinos. It seems that Pylarinos had undertaken, or at least observed, a series of three successful inoculations in or around 1701. Sherard's letter stated that two sons of Hefferman, Secretary to Sir Robert Sutton, the British Ambassador to Turkey, had been variolated in Constantinople. Pylarinos had been born on Cephalonia, and obtained degrees in law and medicine from the University of Padua and was also, amongst other things, physician to the princes of Serbia and Moldova and, for a time, chief physician to the Russian Tsar Peter the Great (1672–1725).

In 1715, Peter Kennedy, a Scottish surgeon who had visited Constantinople, also published his observations of variolation or, in his words, *engrafting the smallpox*, in a book called *An Essay on External Remedies*. The process he described involved collecting pox fluid on day 12 of the infection, keeping it warm and then introducing it to the patient through a scratch in the skin.

Knowledge of variolation was spreading, but the process of gradual dissemination, which moved with only imperceptible slowness, was haphazard and unsystematic; it came not in a rush but in an uncoordinated dribble. This drip feeding of information continued with intermittent reports of variolation percolating into England. In 1721, Jacob de Castro Sarmento (1691–1761) was able to publish a pamphlet on variolation called *Dissertatio in Novam, Tutam, ac Utilem Methodum Inoculationis seu Transplantationis Variolorum* or *A dissertation on the method of inoculating the smallpox; with critical remarks on the several authors who have treated of this disease*. His work was published first in London and then translated into German a year later. A supplement followed in 1731. His *dissertation* recommended that smallpox material taken from an inoculated individual should be used in preference to that obtained from someone in whom the disease had occurred naturally.

## Lady Mary Wortley Montagu

However, the kind of small-scale, anecdotal evidence, whether first- or second-hand, as provided by Lister, Pylarinos and Kennedy, or even that provided by Fellows of the Royal Society such as de Castro or Timonis, did little to alter the fixed and cautious opinions that prevailed amongst English surgeons and physicians. They were reluctant to adopt new and untried procedures in a cold northern climate where smallpox manifested itself as such a severe disease. In the opinion of many, these were peculiar foreign medical adventures supported by reportage little better than hearsay; they were seen as virtuoso amusements, as one-off events, as quaint oddities, similar, in many ways, to the cabinets of curiosities, which were so fashionable at the time. What was needed was a strong and persuasive advocate. This variolation received in the form of Lady Mary Wortley Montagu.

Lady Mary, born Lady Mary Pierrepont, was baptized on 26 May 1689 at Covent Garden in London. Lady Mary is, arguably, best known to history for her letters, particularly for her record of her Ottoman experiences, *Turkish Embassy Letters*, now a notable primary source for historians of the period; but in her own time she was as renowned as a poet as she was as a witty correspondent and letter writer.

Lady Mary was the eldest daughter of Evelyn Pierrepont, afterwards First Duke of Kingston. Her mother, who died while Mary was still a child, was the daughter of William Fielding, Earl of Denbigh. She was cousin to Henry Fielding, the novelist. Lady Mary conducted an animated correspondence with Edward Wortley Montagu, grandson of the first Earl of Sandwich. Lady Mary's father refused to accept Montagu as a son-in-law as he would not entail his estate on a possible heir. When, in 1712, Lady Mary's father insisted his 23-year-old daughter marry a different man, the pair decided to elope. The couple had two children, Mary and Edward. The first few years of Lady Mary's marriage were spent in parsimonious rural seclusion. Edward was elected a Whig Member of Parliament for Westminster in 1715, and shortly afterwards became a Treasury Commissioner. When Lady Mary joined him in London her beauty and her wit rapidly brought her to prominence at court.

It was Lady Mary who is now seen as being ultimately responsible for bringing smallpox variolation to Britain. While she alone was not wholly responsible for introducing the technique *per se*, she was certainly responsible for fomenting its incipient popularity, first in high circles and subsequently amongst the wider population.

Lady Mary was herself no stranger to the effects and lethality of the disease: in 1713, during the first year of her marriage, her beloved 20-year-old brother, already a husband and father, had died from smallpox, his promise yet to be fulfilled. Only 18 months after this vicarious brush with 'the speckled monster', as smallpox was rather quaintly known during the eighteenth century, Lady Mary survived a bout of smallpox; whatever its severity, the bout left her 'previously exquisite' face severely pitted and scarred, and also caused the loss of her 'very fine eyelashes'. The actual extent of her disfigurement and the relative seriousness of her attack remains, however, a point at issue: many have suggested that it was not overly severe, but the tone of her recorded poems of the period suggests otherwise.

We must remember that, for people of the time, death was everywhere: families were large, lives were short. Men, women and children, both those rich and poor, famous or obscure, all were as one before the scourge of contagious disease. Thus the perception of death and personal loss may, for them, have been very different. As Leslie Poles Hartley (1895–1972) says at the start of his most famous book *The Go-Between*: 'The past is another country. They do things differently there.' We cannot guarantee that our own sentimentalized views on personal mortality were necessarily shared by those living in past centuries.

In 1717, a few years after George I (1660–1727) had succeeded Queen Anne (1665–1714) to the British throne, Lady Mary's husband, Edward Wortley Montagu, was appointed ambassador to the Ottoman Empire in Constantinople. Tentative diplomatic relations had first been established between Britain and the Ottoman Empire in 1579 when Queen Elizabeth I (1533–1603) exchanged letters with the then Ottoman ruler Sultan Murad III (1546–1595). Earlier, in 1578, two London merchants had sent their agent William Harborne to Turkey; his mission was to obtain the right for English merchants to fly their flag in Ottoman waters, a right which had been granted previously only to the French. Later, in 1580, Harborne obtained for British merchants privileges similar to those enjoyed by the French. Subsequently, the Levant Company was established in London. For the next 200 years, Anglo-Turkish relations remained in the hands of the Levant Company: for many years it paid the salaries of English Ambassadors to Turkey; the company remained a power in the eastern Mediterranean until 1821, when it was assimilated by the British Government.

## Variolation and the sublime porte

When Montagu was appointed ambassador to the Ottoman Empire, Lady Mary accompanied him to Vienna and from there to Constantinople, via a 2 month stay in Adrianople. The Wortley Montagu's long and dangerous trans-continental journey, which was undertaken in the dead of winter, was considered something of an achievement at the time. Wortley Montagu and his retinue arrived in Adrianople (present-day Edirne) on 13 March 1717, escorted by some 500 Janissaries. They had come via Sofia and Philippopolis, and would stay for 2 months before moving on to Constantinople, where they arrived towards the end of May 1717. Adrianople had been the Ottoman capital until the fall of Constantinople in 1453 and continued to be much used by the Sultan and the Sublime Porte, as the Ottoman court was known.

Unlike so many western visitors to Turkey and the Orient, Lady Mary sought actively to engage with the upper class Ottoman world. Lady Mary learnt quickly that the Turks inoculated healthy children with a naturally attenuated, postinfection form of smallpox in order to confer immunity against the more virulent, contagious version of the disease. On April Fool's Day 1717, soon after her first arrival in Adrianople, Lady Mary wrote back to her friend in England, Mrs Sarah Chiswell of Nottingham, giving a positive yet very graphic description of the practice of variolation.

How the Ottoman Turks had learned of the practice is once again lost. One suggestion is that it came to them from India, via Arab intermediaries, in the early 1600s. Another is that the practice spread slowly from China along the Silk Road. The first extant report in the Turkish literature reports that in 1679, a man came to Constantinople from Asia Minor and variolated several children. Voltaire relates what is most probably an apocryphal tale: how, in 1670, Circassian traders, from the shores of the Black Sea north of the Caucuses Mountains, first introduced variolation to the Ottoman Court and how women from the Caucasus, who were in great demand in the royal harem because of their legendary beauty were, as children, variolated in those parts of their bodies where scars would not show. However, later travellers in the Caucuses could find nothing to corroborate such tales.

In March 1718, perhaps motivated by the family's impending return to England, and while her husband was absent, Lady Mary had her five-year-old son Edward variolated at Pera, a suburb of Constantinople. The Embassy Chaplain reportedly opposed the procedure, calling variolation an unchristian operation that could succeed only amongst infidels. Lady Mary ignored his querulous objections. Charles Maitland (1668–1748), a Scottish physician who had been retained by the Edward Wortley Montagu as surgeon to the Embassy, oversaw the process. He later wrote an account of this event:

> The Ambassador's ingenious Lady, who had been at some pains to satisfy her curiosity in this matter, and had made some useful observations on the practice, was so thoroughly convinced of the safety of it, that she resolved to submit her only son to it, a very hopeful boy of about six years of age: she first of all ordered me to find out a fit subject to take the matter from; and then sent for an old ... woman, who had practised this way a great many years: after a good deal of trouble and pains, I found a proper subject, and then the good woman went to work; but so awkwardly by the shaking of her Hand, and put the child to so much torture with her blunt and rusty needle, that I pitied his cries, who had ever been of such spirit and courage, that hardly any thing of pain could make him cry before; and therefore inoculated the other arm with my own instrument, and with so little pain to him, that he did not in the least complain of it.

The scars of this variolation later served to identify Edward Wortley Montagu when, as a boarder at Westminster School, he became notorious for absconding without sanction. Advertisements offered a £20 reward for his recovery. These notices described him as possessing 'two marks by which he is easily known; viz. in the back of each arm, about two or three inches above the wrist, a small roundish scar, less than a silver penny, like a large mark of the smallpox.' Edward grew up to be a man who almost eclipsed his mother in his eccentricity and shambolic lifestyle.

In total, the Wortley Montagus' stay in Constantinople lasted no longer than 14 months. Stanyan, Montagu's replacement, had arrived in Adrianople by May 1718, and within a few months the former Ambassador and his wife had left Constaninople, returning to England in July 1718. Within 3 years, London was again gripped by a virulent smallpox epidemic; an epidemic that was to spread to other parts of Britain during the following 2 years. Thus in April 1721 – and, we may presume, strongly motivated by this new epidemic – Lady Mary persuaded a reluctant Charles Maitland to undertake another variolation.

Maitland had by now also returned from Turkey; he had retired to the country and was living in Hertford. The variolation procedure was conducted on Lady Mary's four-year-old daughter, also called Mary. She had been born in January 1718 in Constantinople, and would, in time, become wife to the Scottish aristocrat John Stuart (1713–1792), the Third Earl of Bute; he later succeeded Pitt as Prime Minister in 1763, resigning a year later as a consequence of the Seven Years War.

The variolation of the younger Mary was to be no private event, however; indeed, and importantly, several outside physicians were present. It is unclear if these initial witnesses were there at Maitland's request or, as Lady Mary's granddaughter Lady Louisa Stuart suggests, were representatives of the government or court. Either way Maitland seemed happy to be persuaded. Lady Louisa said also that these witnesses were hostile; so hostile, in fact, that Lady Mary dared not leave her daughter alone with them, in case they should harm her and thus slander the experiment.

However, they were not all hostile. One of them, James Keith, a Scottish physician and old friend of Maitland, described below, was favourably impressed; he had himself lost two sons to smallpox, and asked Maitland to variolate his surviving son, a five-year-old, born 2 months after the death of his brothers. Fortunately, in time, this public demonstration of inoculation proved successful. Little Mary and James Keith's son both did well. Although neither variolation was widely reported, professional circles, and the rather more elevated circles in which Lady Mary moved, became well aware of these events. Shortly afterwards, the venerable Dr Walter Harris, physician to Queen Anne in her lifetime, addressed the Royal College of Physicians on 17 April 1721, subsequently adding an appendix which mentions the variolation of little Mary Wortley Montagu, and does so with a recommending tone, which was published in London in August 1721.

## The royal experiment

Eventually, and in the light of such a demonstration, word of the potential efficacy of variolation spread to members of the royal family, including an erstwhile yet like-minded acquaintance of Lady Mary: the Princess of Wales, Wilhelmina Caroline, daughter of Frederick, Margrave of Brandenburg-Anspach. Caroline was married to the heir apparent George Augustus, later George II. They had eight children, not an uncommon number in an era of high infant mortality and no contraception: Fredrick Louis (future father of George III, Frederick predeceasing George II in 1751), George William, William Augustus, Anne Princess of Orange, Amelia Sophia Eleanora, Caroline Elizabeth, Mary and Louisa. The Princess of Wales was an intelligent and strong-minded woman, with interests that included theology and philosophy; Voltaire described her, somewhat flatteringly perhaps, as a philosopher on the throne.

In order to avoid risking young royal lives, on 9 August 1721 Maitland was granted a royal license to test variolation on prisoners from Newgate Gaol. Six prisoners – three male and three female – were granted the King's favour should they survive the experiment. The variolation of these prisoners was overseen by Sir Hans Sloane and John George Steigerthal. About 25 court physicians, surgeons and apothecaries observed this exercise in experimental variolation. Most of these learned and worthy medical men were members of either, or both, the Royal Society or the College of Physicians. Also in attendance was Claude Amyand, personal surgeon to George I and, later, to George II. Fortunately, all six prisoners survived, and those challenged with smallpox proved to be immune. In the months that followed, Maitland successfully repeated the experiment on five orphaned children. These forerunners to today's clinical trials, dubiously conducted on orphans and prisoners, raised few, if any, ethical dilemmas at the time.

In the meantime, Princess Caroline consulted Sir Hans Sloane; while he would not advise her to variolate her children, neither would he advise her against it, thus fuelling her intention to act. George I gave permission for the inoculation of his granddaughters, 11-year-old Amelia and nine-year-old Caroline. His grandsons, in contrast, being more likely to succeed to the throne, had to wait for several more years. Thus, on 17 April 1722, the royal surgeon Claude Amyand variolated the two Princesses; he acted under the supervision of Sloan and Steigerthal and was directed by Charles Maitland, who also supplied the infectious material. On the same day, Amyand treated his own two children. A day later he variolated the six children of Lord Bathurst, a friend of Lady Mary. Later the same year, Caroline, Princess of Wales, was inoculated, and in 1724 the King sent Maitland to Hanover to inoculate his grandson Prince Frederick, afterwards Prince of Wales. George I was later inoculated by Amyand and Maitland.

However, on 21 April 1722, within days of these events, news came of the death of the Earl of Sunderland and his recently variolated two-year-old son, William Spencer, who had been treated by Maitland on 2 April. Moreover, one of Lord Bathurst's servants, a 19-year-old footman, who had been variolated by Maitland on 30 April 1722, after being exposed to Bathurst's variolated children on 25 or 26 April, died on 19 May; this may have resulted from natural smallpox infection as there was, after all, an epidemic of the disease underway. Several other prominent deaths followed over time, such as that in 1725 of the niece of Sir John Eyles, sub-governor of the South Sea Company.

Unfortunately for Lady Mary, many of her close friends and family were not persuaded and did not follow her lead where variolation was concerned. When Lady Mary inoculated her daughter, she also invited her sister, Lady Gower, to have her son variolated, but she declined and 2 years later he died of smallpox. Most ironical of all was, perhaps, the death, in 1726, of Sarah Chiswell, the London friend to whom Lady Mary had first written lauding Turkish variolation.

## The Boston connection

Meanwhile, on the other side of the Atlantic Ocean, the city of Boston was also being ravaged by smallpox. On 22 April 1721, HMS Seahorse, commanded by Captain Wentworth Paxon, a British ship out of Barbados, arrived in Boston. It bypassed the harbour hospital, and docked. Within a day, crewmen displayed clear signs of smallpox; soon afterwards cases appeared across Boston. Within days, about 1000 people had left the city. By mid-June, the outbreak had become an epidemic. As the disease became pervasive, panic became endemic, peaking during September to November 1721. This was to be the worst epidemic of smallpox that Boston would suffer during the eighteenth century, killing 844, of approximately 6000 infected, from a total population of about 11 000. This was the sixth epidemic to overwhelm Boston since it was founded. However, with a fatality rate of 14% of those infected with smallpox, the 1721–1722 outbreak was by far the worst.

The Reverend Cotton Mather (1663–1728) was a remarkable, and eccentric, polymath, now much derided as the archetypal Puritan clergyman: bigoted, harsh, and intransigent. He wrote in his diary on 26 May 1721: 'The grievous calamity of the smallpox has now entered the town.' Mather had also been present in Boston during the 1677–1678 and the 1702–1703 smallpox outbreaks, observing for the later epidemic that 'more than fourscore people were in this black month of December, carried from this town to their long home.' Three of Mather's children contracted the disease during the outbreak and fortunately all three survived.

Mather had thought to become a physician but abandoned this for a life as a minister. However, his interest in science persisted; his observations of various American phenomena, which were published in his *Curiosa Americana*, eventually allowed him to become, on 27 July 1713, the first native-born American to be elected a Fellow of the Royal Society.

As was mentioned above, variolation was practised widely within Africa and Mather acquired some knowledge about the practice from his African-born slave Onesimus, given to him in 1706 by some of his parishioners. Mather calls Onesimus a Garamantee or Garamante. A Garamantee is a member of a black African race (as opposed to one with a Berber or Arabic origin) from the Sahara, which is now called the Tabu; they are mostly found in northern Chad, eastern Niger, and southern Libya. However, Garamante can also be a classical reference to denizens of Libya, and Africa more generally, and so this attribution may be erroneous. Mather asked other slaves and slave traders, who corroborated the account of Onesimus. Later, Mather read the account of Timonis in the Philosophical Transactions, which described Turkish variolation, and corresponded with John Woodward on 12 July 1716; he enquired why variolation was yet to be introduced into England. Mather also told Woodward that he intended to convince Boston physicians to variolate when smallpox occurred there again.

Thus, on 6 June 1721, during the 1721 epidemic, Mather, perhaps mindful of the response which he might receive, wrote a guarded and conciliatory open letter to the physicians of Boston. The letter, which also contained brief summaries of the articles by Timonis and Pylarinos, advocated that said physicians should undertake a vigorous campaign against smallpox using the method of cutaneous variolation. All this was done quite independently, and without knowledge, of Lady Mary's activities at the British court. Only one physician responded to Mather's letter: Zabdiel Boylston. Boylston, who had himself survived smallpox in 1702, was a family friend of Mather; perhaps this personal association was sufficient encouragement in itself, either that or Boylston was too intimidated by the formidable preacher to decline.

Boylston (1679–1766) had been born in Brookline, Massachusetts. Despite receiving no formal medical training, Zabdiel Boylston, like Edward Jenner and many

others, did receive a solid grounding in practical medicine through several apprenticeships. These apprenticeships had been undertaken first with his father, Thomas
Boylston, and then as preceptor to the eminent Hiram Cutter; both men were at
the time well-known Bostonian physicians. In time, his medical knowledge and
surgical skills would gain for Boylston a not inconsiderable reputation as a man of
medicine. Nonetheless, he was subsequently alleged by his opponents to be no more
than a stone cutter. During the sixteenth and seventeenth centuries, it was common
for men to gain what medical expertise they had in this way.

Boylston may have been the first American-born surgeon to undertake a non-
trivial surgical procedure in the American colonies, although operations undertaken
in North America had previously been performed by English and Spanish surgeons.
As reported in the Boston News-Letter, on 24 June 1710, Boylston successfully undertook the surgical removal of a large bladder stone from a child named Hill. The
child recovered within the month. Boylston had already removed stones from other,
unnamed patients prior to this. In the late seventeenth and early eighteenth century,
the removal of bladder stones – being 'cut of the stone', as Samuel Pepys, another
sufferer, famously rendered it – was, like most surgery of any significance, difficult
for the surgeon and traumatic for the patient. There was, of course, no anaesthetic.
Hygiene, though often better perhaps than we are now apt to credit, was basic.
Contemporary manuals record a procedure that begins with lengthy preparation involving bleeding, purges and a series of warm baths. Alcohol was banned, and a
fixed diet involving herbal concoctions was prescribed. Patients were counselled to
have the operation in the spring when heat and cold could be avoided and there
was an abundance of natural light for the surgeon. The operation itself involved two
stages: first, passing a metal implement into the bladder via the urethra, and second,
cutting a 3 inch incision between the genitals and the anus. The bladder would then
be removed with forceps. The wound was not sealed or stitched but bound and left
to heal.

After another personal letter from Mather, dated 24 June 1721, Boylston undertook the first in a long sequence of variolations. On 26 June 1721, he wrote: 'I inoculated my son, Thomas, of about six, my Negro-Man, thirty-six, and Jackey, two
and a half Years old.' Boylston reported, in the Boston Gazette on 17 July 1721, the
successful variolation of seven more patients. Later, on 12 August, he undertook the
variolation of Cotton Mather's son Samuel. Unfortunately, Samuel Mather almost
died, and public disquiet escalated alarmingly.

Boylston was attacked in the street. Professionally, he was opposed by all his
colleagues. After a threat of hanging, Boylston was obliged to go into hiding for
2 weeks. Once, in the early hours of the morning, a small bomb was thrown through
a window in Mather's house into a room where his nephew, the Reverend Walter
from Roxbury, was recuperating from the after-effects of variolation.

By February 1722, however, Boylston had used variolation on over 247 Bostoni-
ans. Two other physicians treated another 39. The danger of death from the procedure and the strongly contagious nature of the variolated patient reduced the number
of candidates. Of the 286 individuals variolated, only six had died, and several of

these may have already been infected with naturally acquired smallpox; this equated to a mortality rate of about 2%, compared with over 840 deaths among 5889 cases for naturally occurring smallpox, or a rate of about 15% for the whole epidemic. This clear differential was no small vindication of Mather and Boylston's introduction of smallpox inoculation into North America.

Two years after the epidemic of 1721 had run its course Boylston, his reputation fully rehabilitated, was invited to London; he received honours and lectured to the Royal College of Physicians. Boylston had, perhaps, more direct first-hand knowledge of variolation than anyone in the world. As such, he was invited to write a full account of his experiences, which he duly did. Published initially in London in 1726, Boylston produced a revised, enlarged and corrected version of the book in 1730: *An historical Account of the Small-pox inoculated in New England*.

## Variolation takes hold

By the eighteenth century, with the exception of a few remote places with small populations, smallpox was endemic throughout the world; the annual death rate from smallpox across Europe had by this time reached an estimated 400 000. It killed between 12% and 20% of its victims; this equates to between 7% and 12% of deaths from all causes. Young children were particularly at risk. Smallpox might have accounted for 30% of child mortality. Thus one might imagine that inoculation, in the form of variolation, would be warmly welcomed, but not so; for there were clearly risks to being variolated. Then, as now, inoculation, whether realized by vaccination or by variolation, was regarded with great scepticism by several sections of society. Initially, variolation had some success amongst the aristocracy, yet this was only a vanishingly-small sliver of the population. The impact on variolation on other sections of society is harder to headline but the widespread use of variolation outside of the court can be seen to have begun early, if sporadically.

Shortly after the *Royal Experiment*, the effectiveness of variolation was investigated by James Jurin (1684–1750), who was both a physician and a skilled mathematician. On the basis of data collected between 1723 and 1727, he concluded that variolation protected against smallpox and that the probability of dying from variolation was much less than that of dying through natural smallpox: the death rate from natural smallpox was 2 in 17, or about 12%, while that in the 1721 epidemic had been in the region of 1 in 5 to 1 in 6, or 17–20%. The risk from variolation ranged from 1 in 60, about 2%, for data collected in Massachusetts during 1726, to 1 in 91, or just over 1%, in England. Subsequently, mortality rates for variolation dropped to around 1 in 500, as the technique was incrementally refined. Based on Jurin's sound statistical analysis, the Royal Society, together with a tranche of well-known London physicians, which included Sir Hans Sloane, John Arbuthnot, John Crawford, Samuel Brady, James Keith and Richard Mead, were happy to endorse publicly the practice of variolation.

However, the revival of variolation in Britain had already begun in the 1740s and, during the 1750s, continued to gain pace. Several factors helped foster the practice. One of the most significant factors fomenting renewed interest in variolation was the nationwide smallpox epidemic visited upon England during 1751–1753. This was, at the time, probably the most pervasive and the most lethal outbreak of the disease that England had seen. It had begun in December 1751 in London, and by the following spring the epidemic had moved out of the capital and across many other parts of England. The disease was virulent, and casualties high: during 1752, it killed over 3500 in London alone, while in Chelmsford in Essex, 95 died out of 290 infected.

Some say that this epidemic was a turning point for the practice of variolation, which went from a minor undertaking enacted on a very small scale, mainly amongst the highest echelons of society – the aristocracy and those associated with it – to a widely practiced medical treatment. Throughout the eighteenth century, much effort was expended on minimizing the inherent dangers and unwanted side effects of variolation. Unfortunately, and particularly so for the patients involved, the relatively simple technique brought to England by Maitland and others was, in time, much modified. Patients were prepared for variolation by an overwhelming succession of highly counterproductive treatments – strict and nonsensical diets, vigorous purgations and rigorous bleedings – that brought little benefit and probably did much harm. The results of this overcomplicated procedure were often disastrous: patients rapidly became exhausted and extremely weak and, as a consequence, many did not retain the strength to fight the virulent viral infection.

## The Suttonian method

The threat of death and disfigurement that came with the 1751–1753 epidemics was responsible for a significant shift in thinking concerning variolation. While opposition remained, the numbers of people who underwent the process increased appreciably. Towns and villages paid for surgeons, physicians and apothecaries to enact the procedure on their residents. The poor were variolated for the first time. Fortunately, with this renewal of interest came beneficial technical enhancements: John Ranby (1703–1773), for example, achieved remarkably low mortality rates amongst his variolated subjects. Ranby had become 'Surgeon to the Person of the King' in October 1740, and remained in post until May 1743. He succeeded Claude Amyand, who had held that curiously titled office from 1715 till 1740. The principal reason for Ranby's success was his use of the arm-to-arm technique. This approach introduced pustular matter into a superficial epidermal incision rather than into a deeper cut in the skin. Ranby, as others would do later, segregated variolated individuals and did away with much of the drastic purgings, extensive bleedings and near starvation which were typical preparations prior to variolation. These innovations were to be perfected, if perfected is not too strong a word, by several physicians, who developed enhancements to the method. However, the technique that achieved the greatest fame in England was to be the Suttonian System. Robert and Daniel Sutton improved Kirkpatrick's technique and were able to report 2514 cases without a single fatality. The resulting procedure was both less painful and more successful, with a concomitant death rate of about 1 in 2000.

The Sutton family of Suffolk physicians comprised Robert Sutton (1707–1788) and six of his sons. To a large extent, they raised the practice of variolation from a sporadic and idiosyncratic undertaking, popular amongst the aristocracy and those attending them, to the level of a lucrative medical business, which was taken up widely by all stratas of society from the gentry down to the poor. The Suttonian system included a special treatment regime before and after the variolation: abstinence from all animal food and alcohol for 2 weeks before inoculation. Afterwards he had to take exercise in the open air until such time as he developed a fever, which was then treated with cold water, warm tea and thin gruel by mouth. Once the eruption appeared the patient was persuaded to get up and walk about the garden, regular purges were given and the secret remedy was used to try and control the symptoms.

Despite several obvious drawbacks – a still appreciable death rate and the contagious nature of the newly inoculated – variolation was, following the mitigation of its worst effects, becoming better accepted by the general population, at least in Great Britain. However, religious opinions of many remained decidedly against the practice. In 1763 it was prohibited in Paris, as an official investigation showed clearly that a very virulent epidemic was kept up and increased, if not originated, by the practice. In Germany the practice, owing to the opposition of the medical profession, never made good its footing. Goethe says in his *Wahrheit und Dichtung* that 'speculative Englishmen' visited Germany and received handsome fees for the inoculation of the children of persons free from prejudice; the people as a whole, however, would have none of it. However, variolation was beginning to spread back into parts of Europe. Voltaire suggested that in order to stay alive and keep women beautiful the French should adopt the practice. Again, adoption of variolation was greatly influenced by Royal patronage. Physicians from various parts of Europe went to London to study variolation and British inoculators travelled all over the European continent. For example, William Baylies, from Bath, was invited to Berlin in 1775 by Frederick the Great to teach his method of variolation to 14 physicians from the German provinces. However, in terms of the European take up of variolation, three names figure highly: Thomas Dimsdale, Jan Igen-hausz, and Theodore Tronchin.

# Variolation in Europe

Dr Thomas Dimsdale (1712–1800), who held a medical degree from Aberdeen in Scotland, first practiced as a physician in the town of Hertford in 1734. Dimsdale championed variolation during the mid-eighteenth century, and helped to popularize it in England, publishing a book, *The Present Method of Inoculating for Smallpox,* which described variolation in 1767. His disquisition was quickly brought to the attention of Catherine II, the Great (1729–1796), Empress of Russia, at a time when a smallpox epidemic was sweeping through her country. In order to protect the Russian people, and thus set an example, she volunteered for variolation. Dr Dimsdale, accompanied by his son Nathaniel (1748–1811), was invited to Russia in October 1768 and variolated Catherine the Great and her 14-year-old son, the Grand Duke Paul, later Paul I (1754–1801). It was said that a team of horses was kept in readiness to whisk Dimsdale away should the variolation procedure fail and the Russians seek vengeance against him. Fortunately, things went well. The Empress was most generous, creating Dimsdale a Baron of the Russian Empire, a councillor of state, physician to the Empress, and showering him with gifts of furs and diamonds, together with an emolument of £10 000, £2000 in expenses, and a life-long annual stipend of £500. The Empress later bought houses in Moscow and St Petersburg, which Dimsdale was able to use as vaccination hospitals.

A family tradition holds that Thomas Dimsdale first learnt of variolation from the Suttons, although Dimsdale wrote in 1767 that he had been undertaking the procedure for over 20 years, suggesting his career had begun years before that of Robert Sutton. Initially, Dimsdale had used a method distinct from that of the Suttons: a thread was first drawn through the smallpox pustule and then placed onto an incision in the arm. In his book, *The Present Method of Inoculating for Smallpox*, Dimsdale described another method: 'a small incision is in skin for no more than an eighth of an inch and this small wound was then stretched between thumb and forefinger, so that pustular material could be smeared around its edges.'

Another prime mover, in terms of European variolation, was Jan Ingen-hausz (1730–1799), now best remembered as a pioneering plant physiologist who, together with Jean Senebier (1742–1809) of Geneva, laid the empirical foundation of what we now understand as photosynthesis. Following the death of his father, Ingen-hausz was invited to London in 1765, where he rapidly became an expert exponent of variolation. In 1768, at the suggestion of her personal physician of 23 years standing Gerard van Swieten (1700–1772), Ingen-hausz was invited to the Austrian capital Vienna by order of the Empress Maria Theresa (1717–1780), in spite of the opposition of the great clinician Anton de Haen (1704–1776). Maria Theresa had given birth to 16 children (10 of whom survived into adulthood), and has thus been called 'the mother-in-law of Europe'; an accolade – if such it was – that was also to be given, a century or so later, to Queen Victoria. She had her first child at the age of 19. Her sister, Maria-Anna, had died in childbirth. It was for this reason that van Swieten had first been called to Vienna. Maria Theresa instructed Ingen-hausz to variolate her children, including the 13-year-old Marie Antoinette. Ingen-hausz stayed on in Vienna to serve as an Austrian court physician for more than a decade, returning to England in 1779. However, as we shall see below, we are not quite finished with the story of Jan Ingen-hausz.

The great Swiss physician Theodore Tronchin was responsible for introducing variolation into a number of European countries. In 1748, in the Netherlands, Tronchin first used the practice in Amsterdam, immunizing his eldest son after his second son had barely survived a serious attack of the disease. Afterwards, in

1749, Tronchin also introduced variolation to Geneva. Samuel-Auguste A.D. Tissot (1728–1797) introduced variolation to Lausanne, Switzerland in 1754. Gerard van Swieten, also, like Tronchin, an erstwhile pupil of Boerhaave, had the practice introduced into Austria, and Sweden and Denmark took up variolation between 1754 and 1756. Van Doeveren undertook the first variolation in Groningen in 1759, and despite Boerhaave already having claimed that variolation was an effective, safe and reliable prophylactic treatment a heated debate took place resulting in a campaign against Van Doeveren.

In 1756, Tronchin was invited to Paris to treat two children of the Duc d'Orléans, the Duke de Chartres and Mlle de Montpensier, descendents of the brother of Louis XIV, and second in rank only to the King. As a result of this public demonstration and the incipient fame attached to treating royalty, a queue of fine carriages formed outside Tronchin's door: one observer likened it to the chaos seen preceding a performance by the Comédie Française. From then on, Tronchin began to introduce and popularize variolation in France, while continuing to practice it in Geneva despite popular disapproval there.

The use of variolation as a prophylactic disease countermeasure was not limited solely to smallpox however. It was also used against a variety of other diseases including scarlet fever, plague, syphilis, measles and yellow fever. Variolation was also used in animals to address a variety of infectious diseases. These included sheep-pox, cattle pleuropneumonia, rinderpest, ruminant anthrax and bovine plague, amongst others.

Sheep-pox was endemic in many countries. Since the disease had clinical signs somewhat similar to smallpox, variolation was much used to combat the disease. Cattle pleuropneumonia, a bovine lung disease, was causing havoc, decimating cattle throughout Europe. Willems, a young Belgian doctor, developed a technique for variolating at the end of the animal's tail. His method was described and discussed throughout Europe.

## The coming of vaccination

By the end of the eighteenth century, variolation was drawing to the end of its long day. Not that anyone realized at the time. Its demise would come at the hand of yet another eccentric figure; not a fire-and-brimstone Puritan minister nor yet an aristocratic poetess, but instead a quiet country doctor, living in deepest Gloucestershire: Edward Jenner. Most of us are probably well acquainted, in some form or other, with the textbook story of Edward Jenner and the discovery of vaccination: the quaint but compelling account of Sarah Nelmes, Blossom the cow, and eight-year-old James Phipps. However, rather less well known is that in the years following Jenner's work, many came to claim that they had got there first. Arguably, many had. There are many alternative claimants to being the first vaccinator: Fewster (1765), Bose (1769), Jesty (1774), Rabaut-Pommier (1780), Nash (1781), and Platt and Jensen (1791), amongst others.

Despite variolation, smallpox remained a scourge in the mid-eighteenth century. Since the 1720s, many had proselytized and lauded the benefits of inoculation amongst the aristocracy and the gentry, yet the practice remained unpopular amongst the rural and urban poor. Death tolls were high and the effects of the disease were everywhere. In the eighteenth century, for example, very few passed their whole lives without contracting either mild or severe smallpox; indeed, faces so frequently bore smallpox scarring that any woman without such marks was straightway accounted beautiful. It is thought that at this time less than 20% of the European population escaped smallpox altogether.

However, in rural areas of England, Germany, France, Italy, Holland and Mexico, there was a common folk wisdom amongst the dairy farming community: a widespread belief that cowpox conferred immunity against smallpox in humans. Cowpox, a mild, localized disease acquired traditionally when milking infected cows, manifested itself as irregular pustules on cow udders, although cattle showed no other signs of disease except for a slight decrease in milk production. Cowpox was occasionally contracted by humans, particularly dairymaids, who were well known for their flawless complexions. Indeed, the beauty of milkmaids had long been legendary. It had been extolled by the Elizabethan poets, amongst others. This was because few milkmaids exhibited the pockmarks which were so characteristic of other women. Milkmaids and others who contracted cowpox were rendered immune to natural smallpox as well the artificial, variolated version.

In 1765, Jon Fewster, an apothecary from Thornbury in Gloucestershire, sent a report '*Cowpox and Its Ability to Prevent Smallpox*' to the Medical Society of London, although subsequently unpublished it did describe how variolation provoked no response in those who had once had cowpox. Rolph, another physician from Gloucestershire, later expressed the view that no experienced physician was unaware that cowpox induced immunity to smallpox. In 1769, Jobst Böse of Göttingen reported on the protection against smallpox enjoyed by milkmaids.

Of the many who claimed precedence over Jenner as the first to perform vaccination, perhaps the best documented and most reliable case was that presented on behalf of Benjamin Jesty (1737–1816). Jesty was a successful and enlightened tenant farmer who, in 1774, dwelt in a large stone farmhouse called Upbury, situated in the village of Yetminster, near Sherborne in Hampshire. Jesty was prominent in his locality, an overseer of the poor and he attended vestry meetings. He had married Elizabeth, 2 years his junior, in 1770, and they had three children: Robert (born 1771), young Benjamin (born 1772), and young Elizabeth (born 1774). In 1797, Jesty moved his family to Downshay Manor, in Worth Matravers, a village in the Isle of Purbeck, near Swanage. Aged nearly 80, Jesty died on 16 April 1816.

Jesty had contracted cowpox, a mild disease in human beings, when he had worked alongside cattle as a young man. Convinced that cowpox could protect against smallpox, Jesty thought to substitute cowpox material for smallpox as a safer alternative to variolation. He knew, for example, that his two dairymaids – Anne Notley and Mary Reade – had both been infected with cowpox, yet neither woman had since contracted smallpox, even though they had nursed smallpox victims.

When smallpox visited his locality again, this time in 1774, Jesty resolved to protect his wife and sons. He took the family on a 2 mile walk in order to reach cowpox-infected cattle which were grazing in the vicinity of Chetnole village. Using a stocking needle, of the type used to knit the knee-length stockings worn at the time with breeches, Jesty inserted material from a cowpox lesion into the skin of his wife's arm, just below the elbow. He then repeated the insertion on his sons. The trio of vaccinated Jestys remained free of smallpox, even though they were subsequently exposed to epidemics of the disease. In 1805, Jesty was invited to the Original Vaccine Pock Institute in London, who later honoured him with a pair of gold mounted lancets, a testimonial scroll, 15 guineas expenses and had Jesty's portrait prepared by the painter Michael Sharp.

In 1781, Nash produced another reasonably accurate description of cowpox, which included discussion of how milkers' hands helped to spread cowpox through dairy herds, as well as its protective effect against smallpox. However, this account was not published until 1799, a year or so after the promulgation of Jenner's work.

In 1791 another deliberate cowpox vaccination was made, this time by Peter Plett (born in Klein Rheide in December 1766), a one-time tutor in Schonweide in Holland where he learnt of variolation. He had also learnt from milkmaids that cowpox protected them against smallpox. Later, as a tutor to another family in Hasselburg, Holstein, Plett vaccinated his employer's two daughters and another child with material taken from cows; these children were the only survivors when, 3 years later, a smallpox epidemic ravaged the area. Plett and a physician called Heinze later vaccinated over 1000 children and adults in Probstei. However, the hand of one of the children became severely inflamed and this dissuaded Plett, like Jesty before him, from undertaking further evaluation.

# Edward Jenner

Neither Jesty nor Plett ever strove to publicize their work. Thus their isolated and independent experiments did little or nothing to change medical practice. Instead, it was Edward Jenner who is now generally credited with the discovery of vaccination – perhaps rightly so, perhaps not – and the names of Jesty and Plett, and the names of others like them, have been consigned to the little-read footnotes of history. Jenner was the first to publish on vaccination with cowpox and, through his contacts, to bring it before the scientific establishment and the public.

Edward Jenner was in many ways a remarkable man; in others, he was very much a contradictory – even a paradoxical – figure. There is much in the life of Edward Jenner that his enemies and opponents could find and exploit in order to support their critical assessment of the man and his work. After a brief period of initial medical training in London, Jenner, a native of Gloucestershire, spent his entire career working as a country doctor. With the possible exception of a trip to Edinburgh, it was said that he never travelled more than 150 miles from his birthplace. Yet, one should not dismiss the man, as many have seemingly done, as no more than a parochial rural doctor. No, indeed not. He was certainly much more than that. Above all, perhaps, Jenner was well connected, making both social contacts and scientific contacts of the first water. He was part of the minor landed-gentry in the area, and he possessed that most useful thing: a modest independent income. His medical status, compounded by his many social connections, guaranteed him clients among both the local gentry and the aristocracy. Contacts made during his brief student days in London numbered many amongst the highest echelons of the British scientific and medical establishments.

Described by some as awkward, Jenner nonetheless possessed the good fortune of being able to build and maintain friendships. Indeed, he seems a fully rounded man. He was, apparently, a respected, kindly and approachable physician; indeed the kind of medical practitioner we would all like to have but seldom find, at least not in the early twenty-first century. He also played his part in the fashionable life of Cheltenham; but again, Jenner was more than well connected and convivial. His work on the cuckoo, for example, or his cataloguing of specimens from Cook's voyages, suggests that he was gifted as well as socially successful.

However, apart from his seminal contribution to vaccination, it was Jenner's ornithological observations of the cuckoo that are, perhaps, the most interesting and significant. Many naturalists dismissed his account, and it remained controversial well into the era of photography. Although in 1921 he was eventually vindicated by photographic evidence supporting his explanation, for over a century, those who opposed vaccination used supposed defects in this study to call his ideas into question. Published at the instigation of John Hunter in 1788, this work led directly to Jenner's election as a Fellow of the Royal Society in 1789.

Edward Jenner was born the fourth son of the Reverend Stephen Jenner (1702–1754), vicar of Berkeley in Gloucestershire, and his wife Sarah (1709–1754), daughter of Henry and Mary Head of Berkeley. Many biographies of Jenner exist: some are hagiographies, some are critical to the point of contumely, while yet others are more measured and analytical. We will only précis them here. Jenner's story begins in the vicarage at Berkeley where he was born. Edward Jenner's early life, of which we know relatively little, seemingly passed without note. Named after a brother who died in April 1749, he was the eighth child of nine. Only five of his eight siblings survived into adulthood. Both of his parents died when he was five years old.

Aged seven, Jenner was sent to Cirencester Grammar School. Here he encountered smallpox for the first time. During the summer of 1757, a smallpox outbreak occurred in Gloucestershire. Pupils at the school, including Edward Jenner, were variolated by a local surgeon. The concomitant trauma, it was said, stayed with him always. The variolations were undertaken by a Mr Holbrook, an apothecary from Wotten-under-Edge. Long after this event, Jenner recalled that during a 6-week preparation period, he was repeatedly purged, subjected to frequent blood lettings and kept on a diet low in vegetables. The inoculation episode itself nearly killed him. During these travails, and for many weeks after the variolation, Jenner was kept in an inoculation stables.

Jenner's schooling was completed at Reverend Dr Washbourn's school at Cirencester. Here he made a number of lifelong friends, including John Clinch and Caleb H Parry (1755–1822). Clinch was later to bring vaccination to the Americas. Jenner dedicated the first edition of his *Inquiry* to Parry. From an early age, Jenner's family decided that his education should focus on medicine. In 1763, when still only 13, Jenner, as was customary at the time, became apprenticed to Daniel Ludlow, a surgeon apothecary from Chipping Sodbury, near Bristol. Later, in August 1764, Jenner became apprenticed to country surgeon George Hardwicke, also of Chipping Sodbury.

Between 1770 and 1772, Edward Jenner received invaluable medical training as a private pupil of the great John Hunter (1728–1793) at St George's Hospital, London. Moving into Hunter's house on Jermyn Street, Jenner paid him £100 per annum, which included both board and lodging, and hospital fees. Hunter was one of the foremost surgeons of his age, a skilled comparative anatomist, and a physician who insisted that medicine be based upon evidence and sound scientific method rather than unsubstantiated theory persisting from remote antiquity. Hunter was to profoundly influence the life and career of Edward Jenner. Hunter taught Jenner to value observation over received authority. He initiated and fomented many important friendships which Jenner developed during his brief sojourn in London. Amongst the friends and acquaintances that Jenner was to make were such future luminaries as Joseph Banks, later president of the Royal Society, and Henry Cline and Everard Home. Both lodged with Hunter and both later become president of the Royal College of Surgeons.

Even after his return to Berkeley, Hunter continued to mentor Jenner, encouraging his interest in natural history. On his recommendation, Jenner involved himself in cataloguing the varied and various botanical specimens which Joseph Banks had brought back to England from the first expedition made by Captain James Cook to the South Pacific. Jenner discharged his duties with sedulousness and flair, and was even prevailed upon to join Cook's second expedition. He demurred, however, deciding instead to establish a rural practice back in Berkeley.

On 6 March 1788, Jenner married elegant and accomplished Catherine Kingscote (1760–1815) of Kingscote near Berkeley. She was niece to the Countess of Suffolk and possessed a rich father. However, she had contracted tuberculosis and spent most of her life as a valetudinarian, eventually becoming virtually a permanent invalid. Despite this, Edward and Catherine had three children: Edward (1789–1810), Catherine (1794–1833), and Robert Fitzharding (1797–1854). While recovering from typhus in 1794, Jenner established a second medical practice in fashionable Cheltenham.

## Cowpox

Ideas relating to the powerful putative prophylactic powers of cowpox may have come initially to Jenner in 1770 while he was still an apprentice. A dairymaid, treated by Ludlow for a pustular skin infection, was confident that her infection could not be smallpox as she had previously had cowpox. Another pleasing, if probably apocryphal, story relates to a supposed encounter in 1778 when Jenner heard a Bristol milkmaid boast: 'I will never have smallpox for I have had cowpox. I shall never have an ugly pockmarked face.' Certainly, in *The Origin of the Vaccine Inoculation*, Jenner says many of his patients who had contracted cowpox through milking resisted variolation. This was apparently well known among local farmers; as was discussed above, it is certainly true that this relationship was well known in the eighteenth century – witness Jesty, Plett and all the rest. Jenner probably did know of the connection well before he went to London. Certainly, he had begun to explore a link between smallpox and cowpox early in his career.

By the late 1770s Jenner, already an experienced variolator in his own right, was actively gathering data with which he hoped to validate the link between smallpox and cowpox. These data were mostly cases reported retrospectively but also, from 1782, new examples as well. Information accumulated steadily, most deriving from routine variolations done after 1792 by Jenner and his nephew, and assistant, Henry. They collected 28 cases, each representing instances where cowpox had been previously acquired directly from a cow or horse, and where immunity was subsequently measured through variolation or natural exposure to smallpox. These observations seemed consistent with the hypothesis that cowpox lesions were protective against subsequent smallpox infection.

Jenner eventually sought to test these ideas formally. He reasoned that cowpox inoculation should and would be safer than variolation, since cowpox in humans seemed benign. Thus on 14 May 1796, Jenner extracted fluid from the cowpox pustule on the hand of Sarah Nelmes, a dairymaid, and inoculated this fluid, through two half-inch incisions, into the arm of an eight-year-old child. The child, a boy named James Phipps, developed local vesicles and a mild fever from which he soon recovered. About 6 weeks later, on 1 July 1796, Jenner variolated two sites on Phipps's arm; the boy was unaffected and did not develop any of the symptoms of smallpox. Jenner repeated the variolation exercise a few months later; again without effect.

Jenner wanted to publish immediately, but was dissuaded by the Royal Society, who felt more data were needed. How things change. They warned him ' . . . not [to] promulgate such a wild idea if he valued his reputation'. So, instead, he collected more case histories, and undertook a further sequence of vaccinations during March and April 1798. Jenner's work remained controversial. So, based on these 12 vaccinations, together with the 16 additional case histories he had collected between the 1770s and 1790s, Jenner published privately a book of 75 pages in 1798. This book – *An Inquiry into the Causes and Effects of the*

*Variolae Vaccinae, a Disease, discovered in some of the Western Counties of England, particularly Gloucestershire, and known by the name of Cow Pox* – was to become a classic text. Over the next few years, Jenner wrote several more books which sought to develop and expand these ideas, as well as detailing extra experiments and more supporting evidence. The books were: *Further Observations on the Variolae Vaccinae* (1799), *A Continuation of Facts and Observations Relative to Variolae Vaccinae or Cowpox* (1800) and *The Origin of the Vaccine Inoculation* (1801).

Jenner presented evidence that cowpox material could be transferred through four generations and could provide protection against challenge by variolation; 'These experiments afforded me much satisfaction, they proved that the matter in passing from one human subject to another, through five gradations, lost none of its original properties.' His assertion 'that the cow-pox protects the human constitution from the infection of smallpox' laid the foundation for modern vaccinology.

The *Inquiry* was divided into three sections. The first section explored Jenner's belief that cowpox was originally a disease of the horse. The second section concerned how cowpox infection protected against smallpox. It contained the key observations and case histories supportive of this view. The third section was a lengthy polemic concerning how Jenner's results related to smallpox.

In the book, Jenner drew some important conclusions: that inoculation with cowpox conferred lifelong protection against smallpox; that this protection could be propagated, via arm-to-arm inoculations, from person to person; and that inoculated cowpox (unlike inoculated smallpox) never induced fatalities, producing only local lesions (not generalized pustular eruptions) and was not itself infectious. However, vaccinations resisted challenge by smallpox, though this was only assessed after a matter of a few weeks. Notwithstanding this final and important caveat, Jenner felt that vaccination was better and safer than variolation.

Parliament gave Jenner grants of £10 000.00 in 1802 and £20 000.00 in 1807. The first figure equates to over £660 000.00 in 2005 money and the second figure to more than £1 173 000.00. In part, these grants were meant to reward and honour the great man, and partly, it has been suggested, it was intended to compensate him for making his findings freely available. These are not insubstantial sums yet Parliament, dominated then, as now, by politicians as ignorant of science and medicine as they are of the dark side of the moon, remained decidedly ambivalent towards Jenner and vaccination. Despite the grants given to Jenner – and the fact that they abolished the practice of variolation by act of Parliament in 1840 in favour of vaccination – when, in 1858, a statue of Jenner (sculpted by noted nineteenth century artist, Calder Marshall) was erected in London's Trafalgar Square, Parliament took grave exception: 'Cowpox was a very good thing in its proper place, but it has no place among the naval and military heroes of the country,' The statue was taken down as a result and relocated to Kensington Gardens.

## Vaccination vindicated

However, as we know, time was to prove Parliament wrong; vaccination owing to Jenner has raised him, in fact if not in public estimation, far above a Marlborough or a Nelson or a Wellington – indeed far above any other national hero, military or otherwise. Nonetheless Jenner was, in his own time, and despite the views of certain parliamentarians, praised and fêted by gentry and aristocracy alike. He became something of a celebrity in Cheltenham, and a celebrated figure across Europe. Inoculation using the Jennerian method became the cornerstone of burgeoning national health programmes. Governments seized upon mass vaccination as a means to trumpet their desire for healthy citizens and demonstrate their forward-thinking attitudes to science and medicine.

In his later years, Jenner, beset by physical ill health and depression, withdrew slowly from public life, spending his final days back in Berkeley. The mounting sorrows of his life had long oppressed him. In 1810, aged 21, Edward, his eldest son, died of tuberculosis. His sister Mary died the same year; his sister Anne 2 years later. In 1815, his wife also died from tuberculosis. In 1820, Jenner suffered a stroke. He survived and continued his medical practice, albeit intermittently. On January 24, 1823, he visited his last patient, a dying friend. The next morning, Jenner did not appear at breakfast; he had died as the result of a massive stroke – or apoplexy, to use the equivalent terminology of the time. Without regaining consciousness, Jenner died on Sunday, January 26, 1823. Jenner was interred on 3 February in Berkeley parish church beside his wife, son and his parents. An epitaph to Jenner reads: 'His glory shines in every fresh and healthy face . . . his monument is not in one cathedral but in every home.'

Much of the remaining history of vaccination in the nineteenth century – at least until the time of Pasteur and his successors – was to be characterized by the polarization between opposing views: enthusiastic vaccinators on the one hand and passionate antivaccinators on the other. This mirrors a similar dichotomy between variolators and antivariolators seen in the eighteenth century. The potential loss of a highly remunerative monopoly engendered trenchant opposition from practitioners of variolation. Jan Ingen-hausz, himself a noted variolator, wrote in October 1798 refuting Jenner's theory that naturally acquired cowpox protected against smallpox.

Within 2 years of the publication of Jenner's main pamphlets, 100 000 people had been vaccinated across Europe, and vaccination had begun in the United States, spearheaded by Harvard professor Benjamin Waterhouse and President Thomas Jefferson. In 1803, King Charles IV sent the Balmis Expedition to the Americas to begin vaccination in Spain's colonies. Before disembarking on the so-called Royal Expedition of the Vaccine, Francisco Xavier de Balmis rounded up five orphans from Madrid; they acted as an arm-to-arm transfer chain keeping fresh the vaccine until the expedition reached the Americas. Napoleon Bonaparte had the highest regard for Jenner and vaccination. When Jenner wrote to request the release of an imprisoned British officer, Napoleon's response was: 'Anything Jenner wants shall be granted. He has been my most faithful servant in the European campaigns.'

Napoleon had all his troops vaccinated in 1805 and all French civilians a year later. By 1810, cowpox vaccine was widely used throughout Europe, the Middle East, the Americas, India, China and Australia.

# Louis Pasteur

The development of vaccinology stalled somewhat after the ground breaking efforts of Jenner and his forebears. Indeed it was almost another century before the development of the next acknowledged vaccine. However, if we relax the constraining eye of hindsight, this interregnum seems hardly surprising. While in the two centuries that intervene between Jenner and ourselves, a potent and appealing dogma has arisen – what Plotkin is want to call 'the doctrine of *for each disease, a vaccine*' – yet to the minds of late eighteenth century scientists such a persuasive and compelling idea was by no means a foregone conclusion. Jenner's achievement, and the achievement of those who preceded him, helped, or partly pre-empted him, is all the more remarkable because it was achieved without any knowledge of the underlying immunological basis of disease. This was to change significantly, however, as the intervening years unfolded. A prime force in the mediating of this change was the work of Louis Pasteur and Robert Koch.

Louis Pasteur, a legendary polymath amongst legendary polymaths, was without doubt one of the greatest, and certainly among the most celebrated, scientists of the nineteenth century or, indeed, of any other century. He was born on 27 December 1822, the son of a tanner. Pasteur studied chemistry in Paris at the École Normale Supérieure and received his Doctorate in Crystallographic studies in 1847. He was appointed to the post of Professor at Strasbourg in 1849. In 1854, he became Professor of Chemistry at Lille and was simultaneously elected a member of the French Academy of Medicine. In 1857, Pasteur returned to Paris as Director of Scientific Studies at the École Normale before moving to become Professor of Chemistry at the Sorbonne in 1867. Later, in 1874, he moved back to the École Normale as Director of Physiological Chemistry. Despite suffering a stroke aged 46, which partially paralysed his left side, he continued his research. Pasteur's last years, from 1888 until his death, were spent as Director of the newly founded Institute Pasteur. In 1887, he suffered a second stroke, which affected his speech significantly. He died on 28 September 1895 at Garches, Seine-et-Oise.

In 1856, while living and working in Lille, Pasteur was asked by brewers and wine manufacturers from Northern France to look at ways to extend the lifetime of their products. Thus he began work on the properties of fermentation; this would ultimately lead Pasteur to make major advances in our understanding of what would later become known as germ theory. During the latter half of the nineteenth century, many physicians and scientists were becoming interested in how diseases of humans and animals might be related to micro-organisms. However, it is clearly wrong to attribute all of the major initial steps in microbiology to the triumvirate of Koch, Pasteur and Lister. Nonetheless these three, together with innumerable if unenumerated colleagues and coworkers, made large and abiding contributions to the fomentation of the discipline, building it into a major science, opening the way to the acceptance of the germ theory and thus to vaccine development, antisepsis and surgical asepsis.

Pasteur's work on how sugars were fermented by yeast into alcohol indicated that this process was mediated by micro-organisms. Since fermentation displayed several similarities to the observed putrefaction seen in wounds, Pasteur came to believe that other specific ferments, or 'germs', were responsible for specific diseases. He conjectured that these invisible 'germs' travelled about in the air and through physical contact, an idea much deprecated and disparaged by his critics. Pasteur's proof that diseases were caused by air-born 'germs' proved to be an epoch-making discovery.

## Vaccination becomes a science

Perhaps the greatest, and for us the most relevant, of Pasteur's many achievements was his pioneering work in vaccinology. He made vaccinology – if not quite into a science in its own right – into something which at least used scientific methods; this is analogous, perhaps, to the way in which linguistics and archaeology, while not quite sciences in themselves, nonetheless make use of scientific techniques to do the things they do. Pasteur thus made vaccinology into something rather more general, complete and useful than it had been previously. He discovered that one could artificially modify, through various means, the intrinsic virulence of an infectious micro-organism. The process produced attenuated or 'weakened' microbes which were capable of inducing subsequent protection against disease. Chickens, for example, treated with attenuated bacteria survived infection by the virulent form, or sheep, vaccinated with attenuated anthrax bacteria, showed protection versus the virulent strain and hence the disease.

Following on from his work on fermentation, and the ideas of germ theory that they engendered, Pasteur began work on disease in general, and human infections in particular, in or around 1877. His initial studies included some on cholera in chickens. In 1880, a piece of stupendous serendipity came his way. An oversight by a technician had resulted in a stock of cholera bacteria being locked away in a cupboard for several weeks during hot summer weather. This culture had not been exposed to light or air during this period. Emile Roux (1853–1933), one of Pasteur's closest confidants, chanced on this sample and was intrigued by the qualities of this aged culture. He had it injected into healthy chickens, which subsequently developed only mild symptoms which passed away quickly. As a control, he then had a new stock of cholera bacteria prepared, which he again had injected in the same tranche of chickens, who survived this second insult unscathed. Fresh, untreated chickens obtained from a local market succumbed rapidly to the virulent cholera bacteria. Roux and Pasteur reached the conclusion that the attenuated culture offered chickens viable protection against cholera.

At this time, the attention of Pasteur and his colleagues was also directed towards anthrax, a zoonotic disease caused by *Bacillus anthracis*, a spore-forming bacterium. Anthrax affects many animal hosts including sheep, cows and humans. It occurs frequently in grazing herbivores, which become infected either by inhaling or ingesting spores from soil. Humans are infected by contact with anthrax-infected animals or animal products. Hence 'wool sorters disease', a common epithet for anthrax.

Pasteur and their colleagues competed hard with Toussaint, a Professor in the Toulouse veterinary school, to be the first to vaccinate against anthrax. Eventually, Toussaint won, being the first to produce a vaccine. However, it proved near to impossible to industrialize. Meanwhile, Louis Pasteur and his team had developed a live attenuated anthrax vaccine for animals. They found that the virulence of anthrax-infected blood was contingent upon oxygen and temperature. Following Koch's work on anthrax spores, Pasteur's group showed that cultures grown at elevated temperatures had lower virulence. These cultures only induced mild symptoms in sheep. Pasteur's anti-anthrax vaccine was demonstrated successfully in a well-publicized experiment conducted at Pouilly-le-Fort on 5 May 1881. Healthy sheep were protected against anthrax by inoculating them with attenuated bacteria. The egregious level of publicity which this demonstration garnered both nationally and internationally helped open up new possibilities in the immunization against infectious diseases.

Pasteur, and his young colleague Thuillier, were asked to help find a method of protection against swine erysipelas, then a problem in southern France. In March 1882, Thuillier discovered the microbe responsible for the disease: the bacterium *Erysipelothrix rhusiopathiae*. It had been discovered, quite independently, by Detmers in Chicago. Pasteur and Thuillier attempted to reduce the virulence of the erysipelas bacterium by passage through pigeons. These experiments actually increased virulence when tested in pigs and pigeons. However, when they passed the bacteria through rabbits, which were marginally susceptible to the disease, they saw increased virulence in rabbits but a decreased virulence in pigs. The resulting vaccine was the first experimental use of repeated passages through weakly or nonsusceptible species to reduce pathogen virulence in its target species.

## Meister, Pasteur, and rabies

Pasteur's most impressive success, and arguably his best known, was his development of antirabies vaccination. What Pasteur actually created was a rabies antitoxin; it worked as an antidote post-infection primarily because the rabies virus possesses such a long incubation period. However, whatever the vaccine actually was, Pasteur and his colleagues were able to attack a well-known and much feared disease – rabies. The significance of the achievement in itself was matched and reflected in the lead it gave to others. Ideas – and scientific ideas especially – naturally permeate and propagate themselves.

Working with Chamberland, Roux and Thuillier, Pasteur became interested in finding a rabies vaccine. Initially, Pasteur had tried to decrease the virulence of the street rabid virus by serial passages through monkeys. This did not work, and Pasteur was obliged to find another approach. He rejected saliva, the commonest medium for transmitting rabies, as it proved wholly inappropriate and inadequate as a source of virus since it was heavily contaminated with infectious bacteria. Instead, Pasteur and his colleagues decided to use nervous tissues originating in the brain or spinal cord of a rabbit. Material was injected into the brain of other rabbits directly after trepanning under ether anaesthesia. In this way, it proved possible to retain a convenient and uncontaminated supply of virus. Several serial passages later, they generated a strain of rabies that had increased virulence in rabbits: death in 8 days rather than 15 in all vaccinated animals.

Pasteur and his group then changed their choice of experimental animals from rabbits to dogs. They also passed the virus from dog to monkey and then from monkey to monkey and found that the resulting virulence was attenuated at each transmission. If the attenuated virus was inoculated back into dogs, rabbits or guinea pigs, it remained attenuated. However, virulence increased at each passage from rabbit to rabbit or guinea pig to guinea pig.

The precise details of the next stage of this process are hazy, but resulted in the attenuation of rabies virus. Pasteur, Roux and colleagues suspended the spines of rabbits killed by the same laboratory strain of rabies in dry air until they obtained material which lacked all virulence. The greater the duration of the drying process the less virulent the resulting virus. After 14 days of air drying, spinal cord material no longer transmitted rabies to other rabbits. They inoculated the dogs with fragments of infected spinal cord, which had been dried for between 1 and 14 days. Each day of drying decreased virulence: on day 1 the virus was fully virulent but by day 14 it had lost all virulence. The result of all this was the ability to fine-tune the virulence or degree of attenuation. Thus, Pasteur and his coworkers had managed to generate an attenuated rabies vaccine, and with it they successfully immunized 50 dogs. At the end of the treatment, the animals were totally resistant to rabid bites or the inoculation of virulent rabies virus, even intracranially.

On Monday 6 July 1885, a shepherd boy from Alsace called Joseph Meister, then aged nine, was brought to see Pasteur. The child had been badly bitten by a rabid dog 2 days earlier. With some reluctance, Pasteur was persuaded by two experienced physicians Drs Vulpian and Grancher of the Académie de Médecine – to vaccinate the child with emulsion from rabies-infected rabbit spinal cord which had been dried in the air for 2 weeks. The child received another 13 inoculations over 10 days. Each inoculation was with progressively more virulent extracts. After 3 months and 3 days, they could announce that the child was in excellent health.

Meister had become the first person publicly to receive the rabies vaccine. On 20 October, Pasteur successfully treated another patient bitten 6 days earlier by a rabid dog. Fortunately, this second case also ended successfully. By 1886, Pasteur and his colleagues had treated 350 patients from Europe, Russia and America. After these events, and the ensuing publicity, Pasteur's approach to treating rabid animal bites was widely and rapidly adopted. Thousands of vaccinations were made and few of these inoculated individuals died of rabies. Success indeed and, ultimately, the kind of success everyone is interested in.

Many thus view his work on rabies as Pasteur's most significant and remarkable success. With hindsight, it is easy to agree with such arguments. However, it has subsequently emerged that Pasteur's published account of these events – the one we described above – had been subject to significant redrafting. This obscured the fact that Pasteur had violated prevailing ethical standards for human experimentation; these had been established, in part, by Pasteur himself. Despite the polemics, a skill in which Pasteur was to become well versed, the treatment had not been thoroughly tested on animals before being administered to Meister. Pasteur suggested his vaccine had been tested on a 'large number' of dogs. Pasteur's notebooks indicate something else entirely. They show that Meister had been treated using what was, essentially, a newly devised approach previously untested on animals. The dog was very probably rabid but not certainly. Had the veracity of Pasteur's account been greater, or the experiment ultimately less successful, Pasteur would have been embarrassed, perhaps even disgraced. Instead, his heroic status simply grew.

Moreover, in light of the want of ethics that Pasteur hid from the world, not least his patient, there is a rather melancholy postscript to these events. Later in life, Meister served for many years as commissionaire of the Pasteur Institute. During the dark days of the Second World War, 55 years after his first vaccination, the Germans then occupying Paris ordered Meister to open Pasteur's crypt. Rather than acquiesce, Meister is said to have taken his own life.

## A Vaccine for every disease

In the years after Pasteur, scientists continued to work assiduously in pursuit of new or improve vaccines against a plethora of contagious diseases: plague, typhus and yellow fever, cholera, and tuberculosis being prominent among them. Others worked with equal diligence to address diseases of cattle, such as foot-and-mouth disease and bovine pleuropneumonia.

The methods they employed were largely of two kinds. The first set of approaches derived from Pasteur. Pasteur's vaccines were developed in the absence of any proper understanding of the immune system or how it works. Moreover, in the case of rabies, he had no direct evidence – other than that provided by its contagious nature – that a micro-organism was actually involved in mediating the disease. Nonetheless, the use of an attenuated micro-organism was the cornerstone of Pasteur's approach to vaccination. He developed four methods which gave rise to attenuated microbes: ageing in the presence of oxygen, which he used to develop a vaccine for chicken cholera in or about 1880; prolonged cultivation at higher than normal temperatures, used for anthrax in 1881; passage through different host species, used for swine erysipelas (1883); and lastly drying, used for rabies in 1885.

The second set of methods was based on a wholly different concept. In 1886, Smith and Salmon published their work on a dead hog cholera virus vaccine. At that time, virus meant a pathogen agent rather than a microbe based around infective DNA. The experimental model they used was salmonella killed by heat which, when injected into pigeons, protected these animals against an attack from the same virulent bacteria. The idea implicit in this work did not require the use of a weakened but still living – and thus potentially pathogenic – microbial organism. No, it was based on using some nonliving version or component derived from the original pathogenic organism by some kind of fractionation or chemical inactivation. A paper of Roux and Chamberland, in 1887, described the same phenomenon. Pasteur and the growing clique of vaccinologists were greatly interested by these observations, which had opened the door to a new kind of vaccine that might prove easier to produce and also to quantify. Pasteur was to argue that these observations were first obtained in the Pasteur Institute, which was palpably untrue, as the initial publication had come from North America. These nonliving or 'dead' vaccines were chosen on the basis that they still possessed the capacity to be recognized by the immune system and gave rise to protection against the disease mediated by the pathogen in question. Thus these vaccines might comprise immune-active dead pathogens, or their products, or their denatured toxins. Killed bacteria were the first to be explored as tools for potential vaccination.

For either approach, several problems presented themselves. The first was to identify the specific pathogen or set of pathogens which gave rise to the disease in question. A clear limitation to vaccine development in the period following Pasteur was the effective and efficient production of microbial pathogens or their components. To an extent this remains true today. While bacteria were easily grown, viruses needed to be produced either in live animals or in eggs. Moreover, certain viruses could not be grown *in vitro*, while protozoan parasites often had intractably complex life cycles involving one or more host organisms.

## In the time of cholera

In the days before bacteriology, diseases spread by contaminated water supplies – cholera, typhoid and paratyphoid fevers and dysentery – were often confused. However, when microbiology had identified their causative agents, science could begin to identify vaccines effective against them. The first palpable success was cholera. Cholera is an acute disease caused by the bacterium *Vibrio cholerae*. Cholera is often mild and without symptoms, yet in severe cases, particularly during epidemics, symptoms include major disturbances of the gastrointestinal tract, including profuse watery diarrhoea. Other symptoms include vomiting, terrible muscle cramps and rapid loss of body fluids which, in turn, leads to dehydration and shock. Without treatment, death can occur in hours.

Cholera was another of the great infectious diseases of the nineteenth century: four pandemics swept outward across the world from cholera's endemic centre in northern India. The disease had been endemic along India's Coromandel Coast since at least the 1770s, and probably long before. The Ganges basin was the likely initial reservoir. Progressing by land and sea, the disease propagated itself along trade routes into Russia, then into western Europe, and from Europe it crossed the ocean to North America. The exact dates of these several pandemics remain points at issue, although each was clearly distinct from the other. The first major outbreak of cholera in western records is the Indian epidemic of 1781–1783. Five thousand British soldiers travelling through the Ganjam District were struck by the disease; 1143 were hospitalized, several hundred succumbed.

The first of the four major cholera pandemics lasted from 1817 to 1823. It began in the town of Jessore near Calcutta in Bengal and spread with rapidity across India, entering Sri Lanka in December 1818. Eventually, the pandemic reached as far as China in the east and the Caspian Sea in the west, before receding. The second pandemic lasted from around 1829 till about 1851. It reached Europe during 1832. In London, it was the worst outbreak in the city's history, claiming 14 137 lives. In Paris, 20 000 died from a total population of 650 000; 100 000 died in the whole of France. Cholera first reached North America by sea in 1832. It first entered the United States at New York and entered Canada at Quebec. The New York outbreak lasted for 6 weeks with 3000 fatalities. Health records for April through June 1832 were destroyed to hide the fact that Irish immigrants had brought cholera with them. By June, 300–400 cases per day were being reported in Quebec and Montreal, with a mortality rate running at about 50%. Cholera struck New Orleans in late October; the disease propagated itself through the city with staggering celerity. The outbreak lasted less than a month, yet 5000 died.

The third pandemic (1852–1860) affected Russia most severely, causing a million deaths. An outbreak in Chicago during 1854 killed about 5.5% of its population. The fourth pandemic of 1863–1875 mostly affected Europe and Africa. It arrived in North America in 1866, but was much less severe; a final, and rather limited, cholera outbreak occurred in 1873. Because of rapid advances in public health subsequent pandemics had little affect on Europe, North America and other parts of the developed world. However, Russia was still badly compromised by cholera.

Working in London, John Snow demonstrated the waterborne transmission of cholera in 1854. A cholera epidemic had struck the city then claimed 10 738 lives. Snow made a detailed epidemiologic study of the disease and showed that 73 deaths occurred close to the Broad Street pump. He conjectured that sewage was leaking into the well. A quaint, and probably apocryphal, story has since grown up concerning his removal of the handle from the well pump, thus stopping the epidemic. In fact, reality was slightly different and the epidemic decreased slowly in the face of many other factors.

# Haffkine and cholera

Waldemar Mordecai Wolff Haffkine (1860–1930) was born Vladimir Aronovich Chavkin in Odessa, Russia. He was the third of six children born to Aaron and Rosalie Chavkin, part of a family of Jewish merchants. His mother died before his seventh birthday. In 1872, Haffkine entered the *Gymnasium* at Berdyansk before studying Natural Sciences at Novorossiysk University from 1879 to 1883. In 1886, the Odessa Society of Physicians commissioned him to learn about antirabies vaccination in Pasteur's laboratory. When he returned to Russia Haffkine began the first antirabies clinic outside of France. He also studied cholera, anthrax and pneumonia. A sequence of pogroms induced Haffkine to leave for Geneva. In 1889, he joined Mechnikov at the Institut Pasteur, working as assistant librarian. He enrolled in a course on microbiologic technique run by Emile Roux (1853–1933); in 1890 Haffkine became his assistant when Alexandre Yersin sailed away to Indochina as a ship's physician.

In 1891, Prince Damrouy, the King of Thailand's brother, asked Pasteur to find a cure for cholera. Pasteur turned to Haffkine. During the 3 year period from 1889 to 1892, Haffkine approached the problem systematically and was able to protect various laboratory animals against the disease. At that time, it was thought that live vaccines generated greater immunity than killed ones. Thus, Haffkine used two different live vaccines: an attenuated strain grown at 39°C with aeration, and a passaged strain with augmented pathogenicity. He published a brief paper on this in 1892.

Haffkine vaccinated himself and three politically-likeminded fellow émigrés: Georgi Yaveyn, Georgi Tomamshev and Ivan Vilbouchevich. Haffkine experienced malaise, elevated temperature and pain at the site of injection, but had no intestinal problems. Subsequently, all three volunteers were also vaccinated with both vaccines, and had similarly mild reactions. Haffkine reported his minitrial on 30 July 1892. This brought immediate interest, since France was experiencing a cholera epidemic with a death toll of 4542.

News of Haffkine's work on cholera spread rapidly. Lord Dufferin, a former viceroy of India, who was then British ambassador at Paris, wrote to the secretary of state for India asking that Haffkine be allowed to work in what many saw as the 'home' of the disease. Thus, Haffkine arrived in Calcutta in March 1893. Haffkine carried with him a supply of killed vaccine, as this did not require refrigeration or transfer to fresh culture medium. Haffkine began his vaccination campaign in April. After injecting himself and four Indian doctors, he induced some villagers from the Bengal cholera belt to volunteer for vaccination. His plan was to inoculate where cholera was endemic and then analyse vaccinated populations. The British authorities required all vaccinations to be voluntary, ruling out a comparison between protected and unprotected groups. Buoyed by his early successes, Haffkine travelled through northern India. Thus, from 1893 to 1896, Haffkine's vaccines were tested on a large scale through a substantial part of the subcontinent.

The efficacy of Haffkine's vaccine was far from complete, and its success in mass vaccination trials in India was limited. Modern statistical analysis indicates that only some of his trials were properly efficacious. In Calcutta, during 1894–1896, protection was only seen from day 5 to day 416 post-vaccination. Nor was vaccination an effective treatment of those already infected. Haffkine's vaccine was protective but not therapeutic. Cholera vaccines available today still only provide short-term protection. Cholera is treated by replacing lost fluids and electrolytes, and by administering antibiotics.

Haffkine suffering the debilitating effects of both overwork and malaria contracted while in India. In September 1895, Haffkine returned to recuperate back in France. He arrived back in India in February 1896, and resumed anticholera vaccination. By this time, Haffkine had concluded that his first attenuated vaccine was not necessary. Again, he tested this conjecture on himself, vaccinated with three times the typical dose of virulent vaccine. Since it was 2 years since his last anticholera vaccination, he reasoned that any residual immunity against the disease had long since lapsed. From the summer of 1896, only Haffkine's second vaccine was used on humans. However, in August of the same year, Haffkine was obliged to begin investigating a virulent outbreak of plague. The cholera vaccination programme was now to be managed by the Indian Medical Service.

Cholera is now no longer a significant issue in the developed world. Sanitation has always been vital to the control of cholera. This resulted from the treatment – filtration and chlorination – of the water supply, and an improved understanding of the etiology and transmission of the disease. As with many diseases, such as tuberculosis, there is mounting evidence that cholera is becoming resistant to many antibiotics.

# Bubonic plague

During 1894, Haffkine moved to work on a virulent outbreak of plague which was then affecting India. Bubonic plague is a systemic invasive disease, caused by the gram-negative bacterium *Yersinia pestis*. The plague-causing bacterium has a complex life cycle and is transmitted to humans by flea bite, the fleas living in the coats of animals. Indeed, in excess of 200 different species of mammal have been reported to be naturally infected with *Yersina pestis*. However, of all potential animal reservoirs of the disease, rodents are by far the most important. Indeed other carriers are of little importance in the long-term survival of *Yersina pestis*, other than as agents spreading plague between different rodent populations.

The plague pandemic probably began in the Chinese province of Yunnan in around 1855. Moving with war traffic spread the disease to the southern Chinese coast, reaching Hong Kong in 1894 and Bombay in 1898. By 1900 the disease had swept across the globe, reaching every inhabited continent. By 1903, the plague was killing a million Indians year; over 12 million inhabitants of the Indian subcontinent may have died of it from 1898 until the end of the First World War. Improvements to public health, coupled to the introduction of antibiotics and vaccines, greatly mitigated the potential effects of bubonic plague in the nineteenth and twentieth centuries.

At the height of the Hong Kong plague outbreak, during June 1894, Alexandre Yersin and Shibasaburo Kitasato announced, more or less simultaneously, separate isolations of the microbial source of bubonic plague: *Yersinia pestis.* Haffkine was asked to investigate the plague epidemic which swept across India during the summer of 1896. He set up a plague laboratory at Grant Medical College, Bombay, and there he worked on an antiplague vaccine utilizing principles he had used successfully for his successful cholera vaccine. Haffkine quickly realized that protective immunity could be generated using killed rather than attenuated bacteria. By December 1896 a vaccine was ready. Haffkine's successfully immunized rats against plague, publishing his results in 1897. By January 1897 Haffkine felt able to test his vaccine on himself. In the following few months around 60 people – prison inmates and Indian volunteers – were vaccinated successfully. The vaccine gave substantial, though incomplete, protection, and there seemed to be no major side effects. Haffkine now tested his vaccine on a larger scale: over 42 000 were immunized. His results were valuable, yet the protection afforded by Haffkine's vaccine was short-lived – at most lasting a few months. Sceptics questioned the vaccine's utility and plague vaccination in general. Was it feasible, they asked, to vaccinate the whole of India in time to slow the disease?

Indian hostility to plague vaccination deepened considerably after November 1902 when a tragedy struck the Punjab village of Malkowal, where a cohort of 19 (out of 107 vaccinated) developed tetanus post-vaccination and later died. An Indian Government commission reported that the vaccine had been contaminated before reaching Malkowal. The reaction of many was to blame Haffkine and the staff of his laboratory. This incident left Haffkine something of a broken figure. He left India in 1904 under a cloud of suspicion. Subsequently, no firm evidence against Haffkine or his laboratory could be found, and in 1907 he was asked back. Although he did return, he was a most unhappy figure. Haffkine retired in 1914. He returned to Paris, where he lived until 2 years before his death in 1930.

During the 1910–1911 Manchurian outbreak, Wu recognized that the epidemic was the pneumonic form of plague and instituted the use of protective measures against aerosol spread of the disease. The works of Meyer and associates advanced our understanding of vaccine and antibiotic efficacy, animal models and the pathology of the disease. The studies of M. Baltazard provided early descriptions of the role of resistant or silent enzootic reservoirs in the maintenance and epidemic outbreaks of plague.

Bubonic plague, as opposed to the rather rarer pneumonic and septicemic plagues, is the principal form of the disease. The disease is spread by flea bite or exposure of open wounds. Symptoms of the disease include fever, headache, chills and, within 2 to 6 days post-infection, nausea, vomiting and diarrhoea are also common. However, the single most characteristic symptom is the presence of very tender, swollen and discoloured lymph nodes – the so-called buboes from which the disease is named. *Yersinia pestis* is now beginning to show worrying signs of multiple drug resistance. Both antibiotics and vaccines have been used to prevent *Y. pestis* infections. Two types of plague vaccine are in current use. The live vaccine derives from an attenuated strain; and the killed vaccine comes from a formalin-fixed virulent strain. Another killed vaccine was developed in the early 1940s to immunize American military personnel.

The current vaccine is manufactured from *Yersinia pestis* 195/P and is injected into muscles as a sequence of three prime doses. Two booster shots are given at 6-month intervals, followed by an additional boost every 1 to 2 years. Antibody-mediated protection wanes quickly, necessitating subsequent immunizations. Vaccines are only administered to those at very high risk. Quoted vaccine effectiveness is based on small numbers of confirmed plague cases in individuals vaccinated during the Second World War and the war in Vietnam. The current vaccine shows adverse reactions in many; these are usually mild, but are occasionally severe.

## The changing face of disease

By the end of the nineteenth century, there were five human vaccines that had been developed: three killed bacterial vaccines (cholera, plague and typhoid) and two live attenuated vaccines (smallpox and rabies). We have traced their story above, but as the story of vaccinology enters the twentieth century, it ceases to be a single tale; it is no longer a continuous, unbroken narrative that can be easily followed as if it were a simple, single plotline. Instead, it begins to split into many concurrent stories moving in parallel through succeeding decades.

Though she may not thank me for saying so, my maternal grandmother was born during the First World War. As we all know, in the 90 years or so since that war, an unprecedented series of technical advances has all but remade the world. The cumulative impact of all these individual changes, each with its own dramatic impact on some particular aspect of our daily existence, has been to engender an unmatched paradigm-shift in the way we live. During those same 90 years, the nature of prevalent disease has also changed dramatically. In 1900, the primary causes of human mortality included influenza, enteritis, diarrhoea and pneumonia, which together accounted for over 30% of deaths. Yet cancer and heart disease were only responsible for 12% of deaths. Compare that with the final quarter of the seventeenth century, when average life expectancy was less than 40 years. The principal cause of death was also then infectious disease: smallpox, tuberculosis, malaria, yellow fever and dysentery, which affected adult and children alike. Plagues and pestilence, epidemics and pandemics, ravaged the population contributing greatly to both morbidity and mortality. Disease struck swiftly, without warning, and seemingly at random. Seemingly little had changed in the intervening 150 years. Today, the picture is radically different, with infectious disease accounting for less than

2% of deaths, and chronic disease now accounting for more than 60% of deaths in developed countries.

Patterns of disease have changed over the past 100 years and will change again in the next 100 years. Some of these changes will be predictable, others not. Nonetheless, many diseases, at least in the western world, have been beaten (or seemingly beaten) or at least subdued and kept in check. This is due to many factors which have militated against the severity and spread of disease; these include improvements to the way that life is lived – precautionary hygiene, nutrition, water quality, reduced overcrowding and improved living conditions – as well as more significant, interventionary measures, such as quarantining, antibiotic therapy and, of course, vaccines.

Looking back from the early years of the twentyfirst century we can see how the methodological advances in microbiology, biochemistry and immunology, amongst others, have opened the door to a proliferation of disease-targeting vaccines (see Table 1.1). We will now look at five further diseases: typhoid, tuberculosis, polio, diphtheria and whooping cough. Several vaccines were developed before the Second World War, including tuberculosis and the first trials of a whooping cough vaccine in the 1920s. Yellow fever, for example, was isolated initially in 1927, leading to a vaccine against the French strain of the disease in 1932. A vaccine with fewer side effects, which acted against the 17D strain, soon followed. Two killed vaccines against influenza were developed by 1936. A live and longer-lasting vaccine against the disease followed in 1937. Vaccines against typhus and Q fever appeared in 1937, and were heavily used during the Second World War.

## Almroth wright and typhoid

Enteric fevers, or fevers of the intestines, include typhoid and paratyphoid. Typhoid, or typhoid fever, is a serious acute infection which is transmitted through contamination of water or food by urine and faeces; the causative agent is the bacterium *Salmonella typhi*. Typhoid is a disease characterized by prolonged fever, a bright red rash and intestinal inflammation with ulceration. Paratyphoid is a milder form of enteric fever caused by species of Salmonella other than *S. typhi*. Typhoid should not be confused with typhus, or typhus fever, which is another serious infection of high mortality caused by *Rickettsia prowazeki* derived from flea bite. During the nineteenth century, typhoid infection proved to be a public health problem of significant proportions in England and elsewhere.

Soon after the agents which caused both typhoid and paratyphoid were discovered by German bacteriologists, a vaccine against typhoid was developed independently, yet almost simultaneously, by Almroth Wright (1861–1947) and by the German researchers Richard Pfeiffer and Wilhelm Kolle in 1896. In 1867 William Budd had reasoned, by analogy to smallpox, that typhoid (which is characterized by a lesion on the lining of the intestine) must be contagious, and that infective material must be present in the lesion and hence excreted with the

**Table 1.1**  Introduction of major vaccines*

| Live attenuated | Killed whole organism | Subunit, toxoid or engineered | Carbohydrate or conjugate | Combination |
|---|---|---|---|---|
| **Eighteenth century** | | | | |
| Smallpox (1798) | | | | |
| **Nineteenth century** | | | | |
| Rabies (1885) | Typhoid (1896) | Tetanus (1890) | | |
| | Cholera (1896) | | | |
| | Plague (1897) | | | |
| **Twentieth century** | | | | |
| Tuberculosis (BCG) (1927) | Pertussis (1926) | Diphtheria (1923) | Pneumococcus (1977) | DTPw (1957) |
| Yellow fever (1932) | Influenza (1936) | Tetanus (1927) | Meningococcal (1980) | DTIPV (1961) |
| Adenovirus (1957) | Typhus (1938) | Staphylococcus Aureus (1976) | H. influenzae b (1988) | DTPIPV (1966) |
| Polio (OPV) (1958) | European encephalitis (1939) | Hepatitis B (1981) | Meningitis C (1999) | MMR (1971) |
| Measles (1963) | Japanese encephalitis (1954) | Pertussis toxin (1981) | | DTPwIPVHib (1993) |
| Mumps (1967) | Polio (IPV) (1955) | Tick-borne encephalitis (1982) | | DTPa (1994) |
| Rubella (1969) | Hattaan B (1989) | Lyme Disease (1998) | | DTPwHB (1996) |
| Variceila (1984) | Hepatitis A (1991) | | | DTPaHib (1997) |
| Zoster (1994) | E coli (1995) | | | DTPaIPVHib (1997) |
| Junin Virus (1996) | | | | |
| Rotavirus (1998) | | | | |
| Anthrax (1998) | | | | |
| **Twentyfirst century** | | | | |
| | | Pertussis (2005) | Pneumococcus (2001) | DTPaHBIPV (2000) |
| | | Human papilloma virus (2006) | | DTPaHBIPVHib (2000) |
| | | | | DTPaIPV (2004) |
| | | | | Td/IPV (2004) |

List, with dates, of the introduction of major vaccines. Dates of primary introduction vary by country. Those stated equate to the USA or UK.
*Partial list, after Plotkin (1999).

intestinal discharge. This speculation led him to demonstrate the waterborne-nature of typhoid.

A prominent figure in Edwardian medicine, Sir Almroth Edward Wright was known for a variety of achievements of varying provenance: his 1911 work on pneumonia in South Africa; for developing vaccines against enteric tuberculosis; for advancing a therapy based on vaccines prepared from bacteria drawn from the patient's own body; and for his advocacy of scientifically-based medicine. Indeed, he sought yet failed to transform the medical establishment so that diagnosis and prognosis were based not on a physician's whims and fancies but on scientifically-sound, scientifically-based laboratory medicine. As medical opinion turned its figurative back on Wright's vaccine therapy, so it also turned away from his vision of what medicine should be.

Wright was convinced that vaccination against typhoid would save thousands of lives, and determined to fight for its adoption. Wright considered that using a live bacterial vaccine against the disease was unsafe and so instead developed one based on using heat-killed *Salmonella typhi*. He was, in a way, fortunate to be working with a vaccine against typhoid fever. Humans are the only reservoir for the typhoid bacteria; it causes no disease in animals and so there was, practically speaking, little real need for animal testing. Nor were animals needed for production. Wright was not so fortunate when testing his vaccine on humans. Initially, he tried it out on himself and several volunteers. In February 1897, he published a short account of his work in the *British Medical Journal*. Wright now sought an extended trial. After a few months a serious typhoid epidemic in Maidstone in Kent provided him with his chance. There was an outbreak among staff at the Kent County Asylum and Wright was called in. He vaccinated 84 of the 200 staff; none caught typhoid, while four of the unvaccinated cohort did succumb.

During the Boer war in South Africa, Wright took the opportunity to trial his vaccine. Two factors conspired against him. First, his inability (and the inability of those around him) to keep adequate records and, secondly, serious problems in maintaining the viability of stored vaccine. Thereafter the army suspended vaccinations against typhoid. Yet, during the Boer War, Wright's typhoid vaccine was used widely with a mortality of over 16% in nonvaccinated individuals versus 8% in the vaccinated cohort. By the outbreak of the First World War, however, typhoid vaccination had been rehabilitated and the practice was adopted widely in the army and among certain civilian populations. Wright persuaded the British army to prepare 10 million doses of vaccine. At the beginning of the First World War, this made Britain the only country to have soldiers with immunity to typhoid and this proved to be the first war where more British soldiers died in combat than from disease.

Within a decade of its discovery there were several different variants of typhoid vaccine in production. The French and the Germans both developed their own. In Britain, Wright's vaccine was the first to receive extensive testing. Pfeiffer and Kolle also showed that one could vaccinate with dead salmonella. The priority of the discovery was a subject of dispute for a long time.

# Tuberculosis, Koch, and Calmette

At the turn of the last century, among the greatest of all killers was tuberculosis. Tuberculosis (or TB from *Tubercle bacillus*) was, and is, a prevalent bacterial infection caused by *Mycobacterium tuberculosis*. The disease can affect many regions of the body, but is found most often (80% of cases) in the lungs, where it is known as 'pulmonary tuberculosis'; the TB sufferer develops a persistent 'dry' cough, weakness and chest pains. TB also affects the central nervous system, as well as the bones, joints and the circulatory, lymphatic and urogenital systems. Like the 300 or so varieties of the common cold, TB is spread between individuals through droplet infection: sneezing, coughing and spitting.

Without doubt TB was, during recent centuries, amongst the most significant global causes of death and disease. As a disease endemic among the urban poor, TB was a major public health issue during the nineteenth and early twentieth centuries. Considering the prevalence, infection rate and fatalities from the disease, such concern was well founded. Twelve years after his identification of the bacterium that gave rise to anthrax, on 24 March 1882, the great Robert Koch (1843–1910) was able to show that the causative agent of TB was a bacterium: *Mycobacterium tuberculosis*; proving unequivocally that tuberculosis was indeed an infectious disease. He showed that *M. tuberculosis* bacteria were present in tubercular lesions of both human and animals. Using bacteria grown using coagulated bovine or ovine serum, Koch was able to inoculate otherwise healthy animals with live TB bacteria and produce typical tuberculosis. Classical staining did not initially reveal the bacteria, however. Success was later achieved using a serendipitous preparation of methylene blue containing added alkali. When treated with Bismarck brown, only the TB colonies stayed blue: the rest of the slide turning brown. Koch received the 1905 Nobel Prize for Medicine for this and, in the process, became arguably the best remembered bacteriologist of them all.

In 1890, Robert Koch announced a glycerine extract of *M. tuberculosis* culture medium – which he later named *tuberculin* – which he thought might act as a vaccine against TB. It is now known that tuberculin actually produces a cell-mediated delayed-hypersensitivity reaction and, indeed, tuberculin proved ineffective. However, subsequently tuberculin became the basis for a useful skin test for the detection of active presymptomatic tuberculosis. In 1891, Albert Calmette (1863–1933), a former pupil of Louis Pasteur, was appointed to be the founding director of the newly-opened Pasteur Institute in Saigon. As part of his work there, Calmette studied Koch's tuberculin treatment for tuberculosis and soon found it to be ineffective against TB, although he would subsequently investigate its effectiveness against leprosy, but again without positive result.

In 1893, Calmette was forced by a severe bout of dysentery to return to Paris and the Pasteur Institute. The city of Lille established its own Pasteur Institute 2 years later and Calmette was, at Pasteur's suggestion, offered the post of director. Among other things, Calmette recognized that endemic TB posed perhaps the greatest risk to Lille's corporate well-being, since the death rate from TB infection was in the region of 300 per 100 000. Calmette decided that his new institute should, at least in part, focus its endeavours on TB. Over a 30-year period, Calmette's quest to treat TB properly became a veritable obsession. He opened an antiTB dispensary in 1901, the first such clinic in continental Europe, and later founded the first public TB hospital in France during 1905.

## Vaccine BCG

As part of his efforts to address the pressing issue of TB, Calmette returned to the search for a vaccine. He realized that he needed to understand the disease better and, in particular, the route of infection. Prompted by the work of the pioneering German bacteriologist Emil von Behring (1854–1917), Calmette investigated whether pulmonary TB could be acquired through intestinal absorption. He was helped in this, and later work, by the veterinarian and vaccine researcher Camille Guérin. Together, they demonstrated that ingestion of virulent *M. bovis* by goats led to serious lymph node infection followed by secondary infection in the lungs. Moreover, they also found that young cattle, after intestinal absorption of the less virulent human *M. tuberculosis*, developed immunity to a subsequent administration of virulent bovine bacteria. This is how, as smallpox variolation so amply demonstrates, the prophylactic power of virulent agents is invariably compromised on safety grounds. Calmette speculated at the time that heat-modified bacteria might be effective for oral vaccination of neonates. Although, in time, this proved a fruitless avenue of investigation, nonetheless he and his coworkers continued their sedulous search for a live antigenic strain of mycobacteria for use as a vaccine against TB.

   Calmette's quest was ultimately to bear fruit in the form of the vaccine BCG (Bacille Calmette-Guérin), which consists of a live attenuated strain of *Mycobacterium bovis*. Today BCG is amongst the most widely used vaccines throughout the world. The vaccine was initially used mainly on the continent of Europe, and it was not until 1956, following much work, that its prophylactic effect was accepted and the vaccine became commonly used elsewhere. During its 80 year history, BCG has been given to more than 3 billion people. Even I have had it. BCG is effective for both animals and humans because bovine and human TB bacteria are sufficiently close genetically that they are cross-protective, to use some immunological jargon. BCG is safe because the live bacteria it contains are poorly virulent. It is still not clear why it works, despite rigorous comparisons of the genome sequence of BCG and virulent *M. Bovis*. Or why it works in some parts of the world and not others. Currently, BCG is produced by over 40 separate manufacturers around the world. However, resistance to BCG use is strong in North America, and it is little used there. Despite its limited use there, it can be beneficial in certain high-risk groups and in those communities where the tuberculosis infection rate is high.

In Calmette's time, bacteria were routinely cultured using glycerinated potato. Using this medium, *M. bovis* became tightly clumped and stubbornly difficult to suspend. However, Calmette and Guérin found that the addition of sterile beef bile greatly improved its ability to form a fine suspension. It may have been the Norwegian physician Kristian Feyer Andvord (1855–1934) who suggested that Calmette might be able to produce successively less virulent tuberculosis bacteria on a medium with added ox bile. After a sustained cultivation on media with ox bile, the bacteria had lost the ability to induce disease in cows. Later, an optimal growth medium was formulated. This consisted of potato slides treated with 5% glycerinated beef bile, a highly alkaline medium rich in lipids. Replanted every 21 days, the culture began to change morphology. Although apparent virulence increased in year 1, subsequent years saw it decrease regularly. Calmette and Guérin began a long and exhaustive series of experiments, involving both continuing passage of the bacterial cultures and animal tests, mostly conducted on cattle, of the attenuated protovaccine. Over a period of 13 years, from 1908 to 1921, Guérin and Calmette produced increasingly avirulent subcultures by repeatedly cultivating *M. tuberculosis*.

During the First World War, Lille was occupied by German forces, and this difficult period, which involved Calmette being suspected of spying and his wife being held hostage by the Germans, rather interrupted ongoing efforts to develop a vaccine. After the eventual cessation of hostilities, Calmette became Sub-Director of the Pasteur Institute, yet he stayed in Lille for several months reforming his teams. After returning to Paris, he and Guérin were joined by L. Neagre and A. Boquet. After 231 serial passages, made between 1908 and 1924, the vaccine finally offered the desired protection in animal models. Calmette and his team believed that they had created an attenuated yet immunogenic variant of *M. bovis*. In 1924, the successful vaccination of infants using BCG began.

The original BCG strain was maintained at the Pasteur Institute in Paris by repeated passage. Before this original BCG strain was lost, however, samples were sent to laboratories in dozens of countries around the world, each of which made its own BCG vaccine, which again they maintained by serial passage. Clinical use of BCG vaccines started during the 1920s. Norwegian tuberculosis experts were anxious to test the vaccine. Its use was supported by 1926 trials conducted by Heimbeck among nursing students at Ulleval in Norway. This demonstrated 80% protection in those vaccinated with BCG when compared with those who did not receive the vaccine. By the 1940s several other clinical studies had confirmed the evidence of protection of BCG vaccines, and it took until then for BCG to received widespread acceptance in other countries.

After the Second World War, tuberculosis rates increased leading many international health organizations to support BCG vaccination. In the 1960s, the WHO developed recommended routine BCG vaccination. BCG was incorporated into the Expanded Programme on Immunizations infant vaccination programme in 1974 and mass vaccination was undertaken in various countries, including Japan, Russia, China, England, France, Canada and several other countries.

## Poliomyelitis

Another great success for vaccination and public health controls has been the near eradication of polio. The words polio, meaning grey, and myelon, meaning marrow and indicating the spinal cord, are of Greek derivation. It is the effect that poliomyelitis virus has on the spinal cord that generates the classic paralysis characteristic of polio. In the past, many odd ideas had flourished concerning the possible cause of the disease. These included bad smells from sewage, flour which had gone mouldy, poisonous caterpillars, infected milk bottles and, of all things, gooseberries. In 1908, however, the polio virus was finally identified by the Austrian immunologist Karl Landsteiner (1868–1943). He produced a primate model of the disease and showed that observed spinal cord lesions matched those seen in human poliomyelitis. He was later awarded a Nobel Prize, but not for his work on poliomyelitis; he received the 1930 Nobel Prize for Medicine for his contribution to the discovery of human blood groups. By 1912, it had become clear that polio was indeed an infectious viral disease with the capacity to give rise to epidemics. After this, polio became a reportable disease. A major advance, for which they were awarded the 1954 Nobel Prize for Medicine, had come when John Enders (1897–1985), Thomas Weller (1915-) and Frederick Robbins (1916–2003) cultured three polio serotypes in non-neural human tissues.

Two vaccines appeared during the 1930s. Both were highly touted yet at best both proved decidedly ineffective. During 1935, Maurice Brodie and William H. Park of the New York Health Department tried to inactivate poliovirus by treating it with formaldehyde. Using this formalin inactivated vaccine 20 primates were treated; this regime was then extended to include 3000 children. However, results did not prove satisfactory and Brodie's vaccine was never deployed again. John Kolmer of Temple University in Philadelphia later attempted to use live attenuated virus, yet this also proved inefficacious. Indeed, it would later be derided as a 'veritable witches' brew', and was suggested to have induced polio many times.

Before 1900, outbreaks of polio had been rare and sporadic. The first European outbreaks occurred in the early nineteenth century and the first in the United States in 1843. For the next 100 years, polio epidemics of increasing severity were reported from the Northern Hemisphere during the summer and autumn. Before the eighteenth century, polioviruses probably circulated widely. Initial infections occurred in early infancy, when acquired maternal immunity was high. Exposure during life probably provided recurrent immunity, while paralytic infections were probably rare. The disease altered in the late nineteenth century from a mild and endemic form to a variety that was new and virulent. The age of patients with primary infection increased along with disease severity and the number of polio deaths. The size and severity of polio epidemics grew continuously through the first half of the twentieth century.

Polio affected advanced, affluent, hygienic countries disproportionately, and during the early to mid-twentieth century the United States suffered significantly. The first significant polio outbreak in the United States occurred during 1916, when around 7000 people died and 27 000 were paralysed. In all, it affected 26 states, primarily those in the north west of the country. New York was hit especially hard: 2448 died out of about 9000 reported cases, which equates to an incidence of 28.5 cases per 100 000 people. The average, non-epidemic rate was about a quarter of this figure. Almost all cases were in individuals under the age of 16. The 1916 epidemic began in midsummer and continued until late October, when cooler autumnal weather arrived. The American poliomyelitis epidemic of 1931, which was again centred on the north west, killed a total of 4138 out of around 33 918 reported cases. Later, an extended polio epidemic, which lasted from 1943 to 1953, was also visited upon the United States. It proved to be arguably the most severe epidemic of its kind, eventually peaking during 1952 when over 57 000 cases were reported.

Franklin Delano Roosevelt (1882–1945), when aged 39, was paralysed in both legs following an attack of poliomyelitis on 10 August 1921. In 1938, after Roosevelt had become President, he instigated the formation of the National Foundation for Infantile Paralysis (NFIP) under the directorship of Basil O'Connor. O'Connor was a long-term friend and former law partner of the President. The mission of NFIP was to find a cure for polio, and its aims were to support professional education, patient care and polio prevention, and to foment research into the disease. It acted as a fundraising body, with a tenth of its funds being directed at research. In NFIPs heyday, from 1941 to 1955, the foundation was widely seen as a public institution, and it drew its funding mainly from the middle class. It was said that during the early 1950s, NFIP, which was run solely on donations, spent ten times more fighting polio than did the US National Institutes of Health. It was a grass-roots organization, with 3000 local chapters staffed by 90 000 volunteers, supervised by five regional directors. Another 2 million volunteers collected money during the annual January fund drive. NFIP raised $1.8 million during its first year; this figure rose to almost $20 million by 1945; by 1954, NFIP was garnering close to $68 million. During the period 1938 to 1962, NFIP had received a total of $630 million in donations. Only the American Red Cross raised more. NFIP spent about half its income caring for polio patients and about $55 million on research into polio. Eventually, of course, with progress in the development of effective polio vaccines, the work of the foundation was rendered obsolete, and during the 1960s it changed its focus to look at birth defects.

## Salk and Sabin

Following the Second World War, during the late 1940s, the incipient World Health Organization created an Expert Committee on polio, which undertook to adumbrate the main areas needed for research into poliovirus and the disease it caused. Attempts to develop a polio vaccine continued. In 1955, Jonas Salk (1914–1995) developed an inactivated poliovirus vaccine and widespread immunization began. Later, in 1960, a live attenuated oral vaccine was developed by Albert Sabin

(1906–1993). Salk and Sabin have been described as scientists both brilliant and ambitious.

Jonas Salk was born a New Yorker and was an outstanding student. He studied at New York University (NYU) Medical School. Salk's mentor at NYU was bacteriologist Thomas Francis, whom he followed later to the University of Michigan. There, Salk spent a year helping to develop inactivated influenza virus vaccines; experience he would use in developing polio vaccine. Later, Salk set up an NFIP-funded laboratory for poliovirus typing in Pittsburgh in 1948.

Albert Bruce Sabin was born to a Jewish family at Bialystok in what is now Poland. Fleeing racial persecution, his family moved in 1921 to Paterson, New Jersey, in the United States. After graduating in 1928, Sabin spent a year furthering his training in London. In 1935, he joined Rockefeller University before moving to the Cincinnati Children's Hospital in 1939, where he worked on viruses, including polio. Sabin worked for the US army during the Second World War, isolating the virus which caused sandfly fever, studying Japanese encephalitis viruses and helping develop a dengue fever vaccine. After the war, he returned to Cincinnati. Sabin showed that poliovirus first invaded the digestive tract and then the nervous system. He was also among those who identified the three types of poliovirus.

Salk and Sabin took divergent paths towards the ultimate development of safe and effective human polio vaccines, and throughout their separate careers, each kept to his own approach to the development of a vaccine. Salk opted for an approach based on using killed virus, akin to the one he had seen used to combat influenza. Persuaded by the apparent efficacy of vaccines for vaccinia and yellow fever, Sabin had become certain that the best hope for an effective vaccine lay in attenuated live viruses, believing they had a greater chance of being both immunogenic and protective. Thus, he began attempts to attenuate the three polio serotypes.

As we have said, America suffered its worst polio epidemic during 1952. Although both Salk and Sabin had received considerable funding from NFIP, the director, Basil O'Connor, concluded that in light of the pressing need for a vaccine Salk's would likely be available sooner. As a consequence, the NFIP backed Salk's work. When the Salk vaccine became available for field trials, having been first studied in small groups of children, Basil O'Connor recruited Thomas Francis to organize and direct it. By 1954, this vaccine had demonstrated its effectiveness against the three poliovirus serotypes.

During the 1954 trials, in excess of 1.8 million children were randomly assigned to vaccinated or nonvaccinated groups. Vaccination decreased the incidence of polio to below 50%, and when a vaccinated child did contract the disease, it was usually nonparalytic. Results of this extraordinary trial were disclosed with much fanfare during a press conference held on 12 April, 1955, 10 years to the day after the death of President Roosevelt. Salk, perhaps rightly, became an overnight global hero, since the trial had demonstrated rates of protection of about 80% with three doses of vaccine. He further endeared himself to the public at large by refusing to patent or to profit directly from his vaccine.

Salk's inactivated poliovirus vaccine (IPV) was licensed immediately and was used widely until the early 1960s. Soon over 4 million children had received IPV. However, as the general acceptance of Salk's vaccine made it almost impossible for Sabin to conduct large trials in the United States, he chose to collaborate with Soviet investigators and vaccinate children in Eastern Europe with oral poliovirus vaccine (OPV). Later, the WHO sent a group to analyse his studies, which brought back a positive report. The effectiveness was demonstrated in field trials (1958 and 1959).

Eventually, it became clear that Sabin's live attenuated oral vaccine was superior in many respects: it was cheaper and more cost-effective; as an oral vaccine it did not require injection and could be delivered by non-expert personnel in both sporadic and mass vaccination contexts; it provided immunity over a much longer time; the list goes on and on. Arguably, however, the most important factor in its favour, at least in terms of the eradication of polio from the developing world, was that it generated mucosal immunity via the intestine, reducing the spread of wild polio.

In 1961, type 1 and 2 monovalent oral poliovirus vaccine (MOPV) became available in the United States followed, in 1962, by type 3 MOPV. In 1963, trivalent OPV began to displace IPV, becoming the prime polio vaccine against polio in the developed world. Polio vaccination had dramatic effects: reported cases fell from 28 000 in 1955 to 15 000 in 1956. In North America, the prevalence of polio dropped by over 90% in the 5 years of IPV, a decline continued by OPV. In 1960, there were 2525 paralytic cases – by 1965, only 61. The last case of paralytic poliomyelitis caused by endemic wild virus was in 1979, due to an outbreak among Midwest Amish communities. An enhanced-potency IPV was licensed in late 1987, becoming available in 1988. During the 1980s and the 1990s, 144 cases of vaccine-associated paralytic polio caused by live OPV were reported. Since 2000, OPV has been replaced in North America by IPV; OPV is no longer available. No case of polio has been reported since 1999.

# Diphtheria

Let us turn to two other pediatric diseases: diphtheria and whooping cough. Diphtheria is an acute, toxin-mediated infection caused by the bacterium *Corynebacterium diphtheriae*. The disease was named by French physician Pierre Bretonneau in 1826 and derives from the Greek word diphthera, meaning leather hide. Diphtheria was once a major paediatric disease. During the 1920s, 100 000 to 200 000 cases were recorded in the United States, with 13 000 to 15 000 deaths. During the 1930s, in England and Wales, diphtheria was among the top three causes of death for children under 15.

An early yet effective treatment was discovered in the 1880s by physician Joseph O'Dwyer (1841–1898); his tubes could be inserted into the infected throat preventing suffocation. In 1888, Roux and Yersin, working in Paris, purified a heat-labile exotoxin in bacterial filtrate. In the 1890s, Emil von Behring developed a neutralizing antitoxin which, although not killing the bacteria, did mitigate the disease and its effects. Beginning in 1890, von Behring and Kitasato showed that the resistance of animals immunized against diphtheria toxin could be transferred to other animals. This was used immediately to protect against diphtheria in human patients. Von Behring successfully treated the first patient in 1891 in Berlin. However, the first results were not clear-cut because of the quality and quantity of antisera produced in small animals. For this, and his development of a tetanus antitoxin, von Behring was awarded the first ever Nobel Prize in Medicine in 1901.

Beginning in the early 1900s, prophylaxis was attempted using mixtures of toxin and antitoxin. Glenny and Hopkins prepared diphtheria toxins, using them to vaccinate horses and obtain antidiphtheria serum. They found that keeping toxin in a container sterilized by formalin reduced its toxicity but not its immunogenicity. They called the product 'toxoid'. At the same time, Ramon found that the combined action of heat and formalin reproducibly produced antitoxin. These vaccines were much safer but generated a much reduced immune response.

Toxoid, although developed around 1923, did not come into widespread use until the 1930s; combined with tetanus toxoid and pertussis vaccine it became used routinely during the 1940s. However, antibiotics effective against diphtheria were not developed until after the Second World War. In any case, cases of diphtheria had dwindled in number over time, as a result of improving public health measures, reaching around 19 000 cases in 1945. A more rapid decrease began with the widespread use of toxoid in the late 1940s. From 1970 to 1979, 196 cases per year were, on average, reported in the United States. Diphtheria was frequently seen in lower socioeconomic populations including Native Americans. From 1980 to 2000, 53 cases of diphtheria were recorded in North America and only five cases since 2000.

# Whooping cough

Let us now look at another distressing childhood disease. Pertussis, better known as whooping cough, is an acute infection caused by the bacterium *Bordetella pertussis*. Pertussis epidemics were first recorded in the sixteenth century. In the twentieth century, the disease became one of the great childhood scourges causing the death of many children in developed countries. Before the 1940s, over 200 000 cases were reported each year. From 1940 to 1945, over 1 million cases of pertussis were recorded, averaging 175 000 cases annually. After whooping cough vaccine was introduced in the 1940s, incidence of the disease in the United States dropped gradually, reaching 15 000 cases in 1960. By 1970, there were less than 5000 cases, and during the 1980s there were only 2900 cases per year.

Whole-cell pertussis vaccine is a suspension of *Bordella pertussis* cells inactivated by formalin. Developed in the 1930s, it was in widespread use by the 1940s. Efforts to develop an inactivated pertussis vaccine began soon after the causative bacterium was first cultured in 1906. In 1925, Danish physician Thorvald Madsen tested a whole-cell vaccine, controlling an epidemic raging in the Faroe Islands. In 1942, Pearl Kendrick combined pertussis vaccine with antitoxin 'toxoids' against tetanus and diphtheria to create the first combined DTP vaccine. Controlled trials of the 1940s indicated that four doses of whole-cell DTP vaccine were between 70% and 90% effective against whooping cough. Protection dropped with time so that protection disappeared 5 to 10 years after the final dose.

The widespread use of pertussis vaccine has decreased incidence of the disease by over 80%; yet during the 1970s and 1980s, whooping cough vaccination proved controversial. In Great Britain, for example, many feared that whole-cell pertussis vaccine induced brain damage, resulting in levels falling below 30%. This was repeated in Japan and Sweden. Reactions to the vaccine include redness, swelling, pain at the injection site, fever and other mild systemic events. More severe reactions, such as convulsions and hypotonic hyporesponsivity, were uncommon; acute encephalopathy was rare.

It was known that the pertussis component of DTP was responsible for most side effects. Experts disagreed as to whether the vaccine caused brain damage, but did agree that if it did so, it did so very rarely. As a consequence of herd immunity, a dramatic rise in the incidence of whooping cough followed drops in the overall population vaccination level. Two outbreaks of whooping cough in the United Kingdom caused more than 30 deaths, and many of the infected children suffered brain injury. Several published studies have shown no causal link between vaccine and brain damage. However, emotive, highly publicized anecdotal evidence of vaccine-induced disability and death engendered an antiDTP movement, similar to the more recent MMR controversy. In the United States, many manufacturers worried by the economics of litigation stopped producing DTP vaccine during the 1980s. The cost of vaccine escalated dramatically leading to a shortage. Only one American manufacturer remained by the end of 1985.

Safety concerns led to purified acellular pertussis vaccines with a lower incidence of side effects. Yugi Sato developed an acellular pertussis vaccine consisting of pertussis toxin and filamentous haemagglutinin, which were secreted into the culture medium by *Bordetella pertussis*. Sato's vaccine was used in Japan from 1981, and was licensed in the United States in 1992, as part of DTaP. However, whooping cough remains a significant health problem for children of the Third World; an estimated 285 000 deaths resulted from the disease in 2001. Although the whole-cell DTP vaccine is not much used in developed countries, the WHO still purchase and distribute it as it is currently cheaper than the acellular alternative.

## Many diseases, many vaccines

As our story moves through the twentieth century it looses, or starts to loose, the romantic veneer which distance in time affords. Now, instead, it takes on the meaner, fragmented, more disagreeable air of the recent past or present. The apparent medical heroism of Jenner and Pasteur gives way to the anonymous activities of the corporation and the government laboratory. Apart from Sabin, Salk and Hilleman, few vaccine discoverers active in the second half of the twentieth century have gained any prominence or fame. There is no one now to champion and mythologize the modern day vaccinologist. As it progresses towards the present day, the history of vaccinology and vaccination becomes ever more splintered and concurrent. If we are to deal with it, we must quicken our pace. Table 1.1 is, in effect, an overview of the history of vaccine discovery. A number of technical breakthroughs have driven and directed the course of vaccine development since the Second World War. During the 1940s, tissue culture techniques had a huge impact on vaccine development and production. As we have seen, it led directly to the development of polio vaccines. During the 1960s, vaccines against mumps, measles and Japanese encephalitis appeared followed, in the 1970s, by the appearance of those which acted against German measles and chickenpox.

The RA 27/3 vaccine against German measles or rubella is based on a live attenuated virus. The virus was first isolated in 1965 at the Wistar Institute from infected fetal material. The virus was later attenuated by 25 to 30 passages through human diploid fibroblasts. Chickenpox is an acute infection caused by the *Varicella zoster* virus. In the early 1970s, Takahasi first isolated the virus upon which the initial antichickenpox vaccine was based. Subsequent work led to a live attenuated vaccine in Japan. Chickenpox vaccine was licensed for general use in Japan and South Korea in 1988, and introduced for paediatric and adult use in the United States in 1995.

In the 1980s, Merck and GlaxoSmithKline both developed recombinant vaccines for hepatitis B. The first such vaccine was licensed in the United States in 1986, and was the first produced by recombinant DNA technology. A second, similar vaccine was licensed in 1989. Earlier, a hepatitis B vaccine had been licensed in the United States in 1981 but later removed in 1992. It had been produced from HBsAg particles which had been purified from human plasma. Australia antigen, later known as hepatitis B surface antigen (HBsAg), was first described in 1965 and was, in time, expressed in large amounts, forming the immunogen in several effective vaccines. Although the vaccine was safe and effective it was not taken up.

A polysaccharide-based vaccine against *Haemophilus influenzae* Type b was licensed in 1985, but was not effective in the very young. HbPV was used until 1988, but is no longer licensed in the United States. Hepatitis A vaccines were licensed in 1995 and 1996 and provide long-term protection against the disease. Pediatric pertussis subunit vaccines were licensed in 1991 and 1996.

The first efforts to find pneumococcal vaccines began in 1911, but it was only in the late 1960s, that progress was made to develop a polyvalent vaccine. The first such vaccine was licensed in the United States in 1977; it was composed of capsular polysaccharide antigen from 14 different pneumococcal bacteria. In 1983, a 23-valent polysaccharide vaccine (PPV23) was licensed and replaced the 14-valent vaccine, which is no longer produced. PPV23 consists of polysaccharide antigen from 23 pneumococcal bacteria, which cause 88% of human pneumococcal disease. The first conjugate vaccine appeared in 2000.

The first meningococcal polysaccharide vaccine was licensed in America during 1974. The first monovalent (group C) polysaccharide vaccine was licensed in 1974 and the current quadrivalent polysaccharide vaccine in 1978. Meningococcal conjugate vaccine has been licensed in the United Kingdom since 1999 and has been extremely successful in ameliorating type C meningitis. Menactra, a meningococcal conjugate vaccine from Sanofi Pasteur, was licensed in the United States during 2005; while the first pneumococcal conjugate vaccine was licensed in the United States in 2000, and a quadrivalent conjugate vaccine was first licensed in the United States in 2005.

## Smallpox: Endgame

Let us return briefly to where we began: smallpox. Let us remind ourselves through the perusal of a few statistics what a horror smallpox was. At its height, smallpox killed 10% of Swedish children within their first year. In London, more than 3000 died in a single smallpox epidemic in 1746, and during the period of 1760 to 1770, the city lost another 4% of its population to the disease. By the end of the Second World War, smallpox had receded to the point where it had all but disappeared from the developed world. It remained, however, a very significant problem of the Third World. Even as recently as the late 1960s, there were 10–12 million cases in 31 countries, with 2 million deaths annually. Yet, as we know, the disease is, apart from a few hopefully well-guarded stockpiles, a thing of the past. There have been no cases in the last 25 years. It is the only disease to have been eradicated through the use of vaccination. It was realized in the decades after the Second World War that global eradication of the disease was theoretically possible, though many felt it to be an unattainable goal. Nonetheless, in 1958 the World Health Organization (WHO) made smallpox eradication a key objective. At that time, a programme to eradicate malaria was eating up much of the WHOs time and resources; initially, funds committed to work on smallpox was, by comparison, nugatory. In 1967, however, the WHO committed itself wholeheartedly to eliminating smallpox within a decade. A 10 year effort, costing over $300 million, eventually succeeded in completely eradicating smallpox. The campaign succeeded, in part, by means of a strategy of containment involving surveillance, isolation and vaccination of contacts. The WHO was eventually able to declare smallpox officially eradicated in 1979.

Smallpox is gone – eradicated. To many, eradication – the reduction of incidence to zero followed by the total elimination of the causative pathogen – has become the ideal; a means to greatly reduce, if not eliminate, the economic and human health costs of disease itself. Indeed, the eventual eradication of disease is a tenet consciously or unconsciously implicit within much of vaccinology. However, there may also be both significant short- and long-term consequences of eradication. As we have seen, this has been achieved for only one disease – smallpox; though the eradication of polio remains tantalizingly close. Time – in the form of 25 long years since the eradication of smallpox – has greatly dulled our collective recollection of this dread disease. It is now only in the pages of textbooks that we can see terrible images of human suffering brought about by this scourge. The aim of many is to see this repeated for scores of diseases across the world and, in many ways, we are now better placed to see this happen than ever before.

As we shall see in Chapter 2, the current landscape within commercial vaccine development is one characterized by optimism rather than pessimism. While the development pipelines of new small molecule drugs of many pharmaceutical companies both large and small are fast running dry, the vaccine arena is rather more buoyant. Moreover, widespread technical breakthroughs in both pure and applied bioscience and medicine make the prospects of developing a whole tranche of new vaccines seem very positive indeed. Many strands – many techniques of great promise – combine to affect this sea change, not the least of which is immunoinformatics and *in silico* vaccinology.

## Further reading

What the story of vaccinology cries out for is a comprehensive yet accessible text able to draw out all the fascination and excitement implicit in the subject. There are no recently published and wholly satisfying examples, yet all the required hallmarks of popularity are are to be found there: drama and danger, eccentricity and character, excitement, importance and controversy. In fact, everything you need to sell books. However, many, many books have been written on the subject of smallpox, none better than that by Hopkins (ISBN 0226351688). Lady Mary Wortley-Montagu is a fascinating topic and several biographies have appeared in the last decade. My recommendation is *Lady Mary Wortley Montagu: Comet of the Enlightenment* by Isobel Grundy (ISBN 0198187653). Pead discourses over much of relevance in his book *Vaccination Rediscovered* (ISBN 0955156106). There are few recent, decent biographies of Pasteur and Haffkine, though Almroth Wright is well served by Dunnill's book *The Plato of Praed Street* (ISBN 9781853154775). *Polio: An American Story* by David Oshinsky covers Salk and Sabine in depth.

# 2
# Vaccines:
# Need and Opportunity

*Inventions reached their limit a long time ago, and I see no hope for further development.*

—Julius Sextus Frontius (40–103)

## Eradication and reservoirs

The reader who worked their way through Chapter 1 will now be familiar, albeit superficially, with the context and history of vaccines, vaccination, and vaccinology. More than 80 infectious agents are known to be regularly pathogenic in humans; of these there are now more than 30 licensed individual vaccines targeting 26 infectious diseases, most of which are either viral or bacterial in nature. About half of these 30 vaccines are in common use and are, in the main, employed to prevent childhood infections. The lasting effects of vaccination work to greatly reduce the morbidity and mortality of disease, often conferring lifetime protection.

Smallpox elimination was a remarkable and – regrettably – a unique phenomenon necessitating an unprecedented, and seldom repeated, level of international cooperation. The campaign was effective because of three factors which, when combined with effective multinational surveillance and public education, made eradication feasible. First, an effective vaccine was made readily available on a large scale, and technical problems with transport and storage were solved. Second, since variola virus produces an acute illness, disease is relatively easy to identify and to differentiate from other infections. Moreover, there is no chronic carrier stage. Thirdly, the only reservoir for smallpox is a human one; there are no known equivalent reservoirs

---

*Bioinformatics for Vaccinology*   Darren R Flower
© 2008 John Wiley & Sons, Ltd

in animals. Although animals have been infected with the variola virus, this has only been undertaken in the laboratory. Thus, humans are the sole natural host.

As we have seen, it may be justly argued that the eradication of smallpox was the greatest single achievement of twentieth century medicine; however, attempts to finally put an end to other infectious diseases have not met with the same success. Currently, the only other disease for which elimination is, within a short time frame, a viable objective is polio. Humans are again the only reservoir for poliovirus, there is no asymptomatic carrier state and disease transmission is mediated by those already infected. Polio has also been the subject of a coordinated worldwide campaign which aimed to have eradicated the disease by the turn of the twentyfirst century. A polio eradication programme conducted by the Pan American Health Organization led to the elimination of polio in the Western Hemisphere in 1991. The Global Polio Eradication Programme has dramatically reduced poliovirus transmission throughout the world. In 2003, only 784 confirmed cases of polio were reported globally and polio was endemic in six countries. Yet today, polio remains endemic in Nigeria, Afghanistan, Pakistan and India.

A number of other serious diseases are also restricted solely to human reservoirs. These include meningitis (approximately 10% of adolescents and adults are asymptomatic transient carriers of *N. meningitidis*, and a majority of strains are not pathogenic), diphtheria (most carriers are also usually asymptomatic – in outbreaks, most children are transient carriers), Hib (again asymptomatic carriers are the only reservoir; Hib cannot survive in the environment), measles (no known asymptomatic carriers have been documented), *S. pneumoniae* (its reservoir is the nasopharynx of asymptomatic human carriers), rubella (although infants may shed rubella for long periods, a true carrier state is yet to be described), and even influenza types B and C, although obviously influenza A also infects animals. Although other primates have been infected in the laboratory, HBV only affects humans.

Measles is an acute disease mediated by viral infection. The first measles vaccines were licensed in 1963, when both an inactivated and a live attenuated vaccine (Edmonston B strain) were introduced. The inactivated type of vaccine was withdrawn in 1967 as it offered inadequate protection. Recipients of this vaccine often developed atypical measles, if subsequently infected with the wild measles virus. Edmonston B was withdrawn in 1975 since vaccinated individuals often developed fever and rash. Another attenuated vaccine (Schwarz strain) was introduced in 1965, but later withdrawn. Yet another attenuated vaccine (Edmonston–Enders strain), introduced in 1968, caused fewer reactions than the original. Before the first introduction of the vaccine, infection was almost universal during childhood: over 90% of the population were immune by 15. However, measles remains a common and potentially fatal disease in the Third World. The WHO estimates there were 30–40 million cases and 745 000 deaths from the disease during 2001.

Rubella is another disease which has been greatly suppressed if not actually eradicated. The name derives from Latin, meaning 'little red'. Rubella was first described as a separate disease in the German medical literature in 1814, hence

'German measles'. Three rubella vaccines were licensed in North America in 1969: HPV-77:DE-5, HPV-77:DK-12 and GMK-3:RK53 Cendevax strains. HPV-77:DK-12 was later removed. In January 1979, the RA 27/3 strain was licensed and all other strains were discontinued.

Given appropriate vaccine tools, and the political will, the diseases listed above are, on this basis at least, all suitable candidates for eradication. Other diseases, such as insect-borne malaria, are not. Diseases with multiple hosts and complex life cycles are much harder nuts to crack. Tetanus, for example, is found in soil and the intestinal tracts of animals, as well as humans. The main reservoirs for anthrax are again soil and infected animals. Moreover, anthrax spores are extremely resistant to physical and chemical assault; they can persist in the environment, remaining dormant in certain kinds of soil for many decades.

## The ongoing burden of disease

So, if we have had such success, and so many diseases have been dealt with, why is the development of new approaches in vaccinology still regarded as something of importance? Surely, the key work was done long ago? Surely, nothing of any value remains to be done? Surely, there are no more threats for vaccinology to face? Obviously, we know that the answer to most, if not all, of these questions is a resounding no. Threats abound in nature: potential new or re-emergent or as-yet-unconquered diseases or new ways of contracting infections. The rise of chronic noncommunicable diseases, the application of vaccination to allergies and so-called lifestyle vaccines give rise to new opportunities for vaccinology. Our response to new and continuing threats is equally important. The reduction of childhood mortality and morbidity through vaccination is the greatest public health success that history has witnessed. However, there remain many uncontrolled targets for vaccination: new and improved vaccines must continue to emerge to meet the challenges of today and the challenges of tomorrow. History will judge us both by how well we grasp our opportunities and by how well we deal with threats.

## Lifespans

To a first approximation life expectancy has, on average, escalated consistently throughout the last few thousand years. Obviously, a few great epidemic diseases – principally the Black Death – have, on occasion, made not insignificant dents in this inexorable upward progression. Citizens of the Roman Empire enjoyed a mean life expectancy at birth of about 22 years. By the Middle Ages, life spans had, in Europe at least, risen to about 33 years. Even the rich and powerful were prone to the terrible and ineluctable predations of disease. By the middle of the nineteenth century general life expectancy had risen to roughly 43 years. In the early 1900s, mean lifespans in more developed countries ranged from 35 to 55 years.

Life expectancy has accelerated over the last hundred years or so and today over 40 countries have an average life expectancy exceeding 70 years. The average lifespan across the whole human population is somewhat lower, however, estimated at 64.8 years: 63.2 years for men and 66.47 years for women. Iceland heads the most recent 2003 league table with a mean life expectancy of 78.7 years, next is Japan (78.4 years), followed by Sweden (77.9 years), then Australia (77.7 years). Next are Israel and Switzerland jointly with 77.6 years, Canada (77.4 years), then Italy (76.9 years), New Zealand and Norway jointly (76.8 years) and then Singapore with a mean life expectancy of 76.7 years. The United Arab Emirates is in 10th place with 76.4 years, followed by Cyprus (76.1 years), and in joint 12th place Austria and the United Kingdom (76.0 years). Perversely, perhaps, the richest and most economically successful country on Earth, the United States of America, only manages 20th place (74.6 years); while the newly emergent tiger economies of China (69.9 years, 41st place) and India (61.8; 77th place), which threaten to dominate the economic and fiscal landscapes of the coming century, come even lower on the list.

The population in many developed countries is now said to be ageing which puts burgeoning pressure on social welfare systems. However, this so-called ageing is only comparative, and comparative to the past. In fact, around 27% of the global population are aged 14 or under; of this, 0.91 billion are male and 0.87 billion are female. The majority of this age range is of school age. An estimated 100 million children do attend school; a relatively small yet still significant proportion of the total 1.8 billion. The gender imbalance also varies across the world. In Hennan province, the most populous region of China, the balance is skewed 118:100 in favour of boys, probably due to elective abortion; the average in industrialized nations of the First World is 103–108:100. The global average is 104:100. 65.2% of the world's population are between the ages of 15 and 64, with a ratio of 2.15 billion men to 2.10 billion women. Globally, only 7.4% of people are actually 65 and over, with a male to female ratio of about 0.21 billion to 0.27 billion. However, the number of people aged 60 and above will rise from about 600 million today to around 1.9 billion by 2050.

When compared to centuries past, however, this shift is remarkable. One might call it a lurch, it has been so rapid. One way in which this shift manifests itself is in the vastly increased longevity of the individual, as well as an increasing proportion of the population reaching old age. This phenomenon is partly a by-product of the First World's more comfortable and more urbanized post-industrial environment. Coupled to decades of better nutrition, medical advances in both new medicines and treatment regimes have allowed an ever-larger section of the population to exploit their individual genetic predisposition to long life. Demographic estimates in the United States suggest that by 2050 those living beyond the age 100 would be well in excess of 100 000. Buoyed by such statistics, many have predicted a future where the average span of human life will be routinely stretched to 120. However, while reaching 100 is now so commonplace as to lose all newsworthiness, the total global population of so-called supercentenarians – those living beyond 110 – is roughly 80; and, as is often quoted, only one in 2 billion will live beyond 116.

## The evolving nature of disease

With this growth in life expectancy, has come a concomitant growth in the diseases of old age. It presents the world with unprecedented epidemics of noncommunicable chronic diseases. These include hitherto rare, or poorly understood, neurodegenerative diseases, such as Parkinson's or Alzheimer's disease, which proportionally affect the old more, cardiovascular diseases and stroke, the prevalence of which is also increasing: around 60 000 people die as the result of a stroke annually in England and Wales and about 100 000 suffer a nonfatal first stroke. The WHO estimates that chronic disease accounts for about 60% of the 57 million annual deaths and roughly half the world's disease burden. By 2020, the burden resulting from chronic disease will increase to over 60%.

One may perceive a bias here; an unfair concentration on the West. However, in the increasingly globalized economy of the twentyfirst century, developing countries, principally India and China, aspire to the egregious economic growth and prosperity that the United States and, to a lesser degree, other countries of the First World have enjoyed for the last 50 years. Apart from the unsustainable burden placed on the Earth's strained capacity for survival, with this growth will come the plethora of chronic diseases that characterize overfed, under-exercised, addictive western societies. As globalization, and the mad gallop of developing countries to emulate the economic growth and prosperity enjoyed by the First World, takes hold, chronic diseases suffered in the West today will increasingly become a problem shared, at least in part, by the whole world. So we must look to the world's gross consumer America, and its affluent allies, for the future trends we shall be seeing throughout the world.

At the other end of the spectrum, life expectancy in what used to be called underdeveloped countries has climbed rather more gradually. There are many countries for which reliable data are simply not available. However, of those countries which we do know about, the last 10 places are filled by Swaziland with a mean life expectancy of 32.1 years, followed by Lesotho (34.6 years), Botswana (35.9 years), Zimbabwe (37.3), Zambia (37.9), Central African Republic (38.4), Angola (39.3), Sierra Leone (39.4), Malawi (39.8), Mozambique (41.1), and Rwanda (42.1). It is no surprise that all these countries are African, since Africa, in particular, is imperilled by a potent combination of disease and starvation, exacerbated by war, corruption and economic decline. A heady mixture of diseases ravage the continent: principally AIDS in many of these nations, but also TB, diarrhoea, pneumonia, malaria and measles, among others. These ills are made manifest in burgeoning rates of infant mortality: misery is weighted out to those least able to resist it. Each year sees almost 6 million children die from hunger or malnutrition.

## Economics, climate, and disease

Hunger and disease have dire and far-reaching economic effects; they prevent poor nations from helping themselves. An estimated 852 million people were under-nourished during 2000–2002. In sub-Saharan Africa, the number of malnourished people has grown from 170.4 million to 203.5 million during the last 10 years. The share of the global disease burden borne by developing countries is disproportion-ate. The WHOs big three infectious diseases – malaria, HIV/AIDS, tuberculosis – are the most visible part of a complex, minatory background. Potential zoonotic pandemics pose a threat to rich and poor alike. Economic growth, when it does come, will be patchy at best. It will bring with it chronic noncommunicable dis-eases which will increase suffering in the developing world.

Infectious diseases are to blame for around 25% of global mortality, particularly in children under five. Expressed as millions of deaths per year, the leading causes of death are 2.9 millions of deaths per year for tuberculosis, 2.5 million for diar-rhoea and related diseases, especially rotaviruses, a rapidly escalating 2.3 million for HIV/AIDS and 1.08 millions of deaths for malaria. Many infections caused by viruses have proved stubborn and recalcitrant threats to human health and well-being. 350 million people carry hepatitis B (HBV). 170 million carry hepatitis C (HCV), and 40 million carry human immunodeficiency virus type 1 (HIV-1). Each year, 5–15% of the world's population become infected by a new variant of the in-fluenza virus, causing 250 000–500 000 deaths. Latent bacterial infection can be even higher: there are, for example, over 2 billion people infected with TB.

Nascent changes to our climate induced by run away carbon emission or the damming of rivers and lakes or other thoughtless human interventions have brought with them potentially dramatic changes to the geographical spread of diseases for-merly thought confined to limited regions of the topics. In a similar way, millennia-old cultures and ways of living are altering at an unprecedented rate, sweeping away the accumulated behaviour of centuries. Mechanisms as diverse as the consumption of bush meat or the close proximity of humans and domesticated or semidomesti-cated animals have opened us up to new threats from zoonotic disease. As a highly interdependent global society, we are also threatened in a more direct way by dis-ease used as weapons of ideology. Bioterrorism, though often exaggerated in its capabilities, is nonetheless a real and potent threat.

## Three threats

We face three separate and rapidly burgeoning threats from emerging infectious disease. First, the geographical spread of endemic diseases previously restricted to parts of the Third World. The world continues to warm, and with weather patterns altering and becoming less and less predictable, the geographical spread of many tropical infectious diseases changes also, expanding to include many regions pre-viously too temperate to sustain them. Notable among these threats are West Nile

Fever, Dengue Fever and Dengue Haemorrhagic Fever, all caused by flaviviruses. As global warming and other abuses of the planet take an ever tighter and tighter hold, the problems of the Third World today will increasingly become the First World's problem tomorrow. The coming of a warmer and wetter world will bring new illness and disease inexorably in its wake.

Secondly, we are faced by the resurgence of long-standing and long-established diseases (previously susceptible to antibiotics), such as tuberculosis. The threat from infectious disease which, in the First World at least, has been mostly in abeyance for the last 50 years, is poised to return, bringing with it the need to develop powerful new approaches to the process of antimicrobial drug discovery. Antibiotics were one of the great discoveries of the twentieth century. Drugs like penicillin, which are able to destroy pathogenic bacteria without harming their human host, or at least to mitigate their effects while they were cleared by the body, have saved countless lives. Yet microbial organisms are prone to rapid genetic change and resistant bacteria have evolved quickly to fill the niche created by the profligate use of antibiotics by prescription-happy medics and pharmacists. We are now threatened by, amongst others, antibiotic-resistant TB and so-called 'superbugs', such as MRSA and *Clostridum difficile*.

Finally, the third threat, that of recently emergent diseases, such as HIV/AIDS, SARS or avian influenza. These dangerous, poorly understood and unpredictable diseases form part of the dauntingly complex jigsaw comprising the global disease burden. The world at the beginning of the twentyfirst century is thus threatened by a plethora of diseases that range greatly in lethality. However, arguably, the most serious long-term threats are represented by the three infectious diseases branded in 1997 by the WHO as global emergencies: tuberculosis, AIDS and malaria. To those we may add the more acute potential threat represented by influenza and other zoonotic diseases.

# Tuberculosis in the 21st century

TB is a chronic bacterial infection of the first magnitude: it probably causes more deaths around the world than any other disease. It was once thought to be consigned to the ash heap of history, yet its return has been unequivocal, killing one victim every 15 seconds. Around 1.7 billion people, between a quarter and a third of the world's population, are infected with latent tuberculosis. In 2004 there were 8.9 million new cases of TB; approximately 140 cases per hundred thousand. Although most infected individuals never develop active TB, over 14.6 million have developed it and are living with the disease, as the epidemiological euphemism has it. Again in 2004, 1.69 million died of TB, a case rate of 27 per hundred thousand. Hopes that TB might, like smallpox and polio, be largely eliminated have been more or less dashed as a consequence of the rise of antibiotic-resistant *M. tuberculosis* during the 1980s. Tuberculosis cases in Britain, for example, have risen significantly from a figure of 5500 in 1987 to around 7000 in 2000. New York has had to deal with over 20 000 unnecessary TB patients infected with resistant strains. On-going poverty and homelessness, tourist travel, and economic migration have increased TB exposure in developed countries.

The need to thwart once more many diseases thought formerly to pose no threat has become a key imperative in an era of burgeoning antibiotic resistance. The infection rates of formerly curable bacterial diseases are now rising again. For example, there has been a sharp rise in the number of nosocomial infections; up to 60% of these in the developed world are now caused by drug-resistant and often opportunistic pathogens like *Pseudomonas aeruginosa* and *Staphylococcus aureus*. Through the rise of antibiotic resistant bacteria – such as TB and MRSA – the era of conventional antibiotics seems to be drawing to a close. Several factors have contributed to this rise in resistance. In the five decades since penicillin became commercially available, misdiagnosed illness by health workers, patients failing to adhere to treatment, the widespread misuse of antibiotics with animals and the wrong prescription given for a particular disease, have all contributed to the problem. Within a competitive environment, resistance is able to spread quickly through the resident bacterial population. While antibiotics kill most susceptible cells, the residual resistant bacteria quickly colonize the empty niche, and pathogenic species can obtain a significant amount of their genetic diversity this way. Horizontal or 'lateral' gene transfer between distinctly related species adds to the problem; resistance and/or virulence factors can be exchanged between a virulent donor and a recipient avirulent strain to produce new pathogenic varieties.

## HIV and AIDS

Much has been written on the topic of HIV and AIDS; it seems more than pointless to even try to reiterate it here. About 40 million men, women and children are currently infected with the virus, two-thirds of whom live in sub-Saharan Africa. More women than men are now HIV-positive; more than 10 million children in Africa have been orphaned by AIDS. In 2005, there were about 4 million new infections with HIV and 2.9 million AIDS-related deaths. This equates to a daily increase of 14 000 new HIV infections and 8000 extra deaths from AIDS. Worldwide, AIDS results in, perhaps, one in every 18 deaths.

Hitherto, most vaccines have induced long-term antibody-mediated responses that neutralize a high proportion of invading pathogens, such that any persisting agent can be dealt with by normal immune responses. Unfortunately, such vaccines have not proved successful in protecting against an ever-increasing list of diseases, particularly ones exhibiting significant antigenic variation, such as HIV. Up to 30% of residues in the gp120 envelope antigen can vary. Many scientists wrongly blame all of the recalcitrance of HIV vaccine discovery on this prodigious variability. Nonetheless, after over 20 years of intense and continuous effort, there are still few high titre monoclonal neutralizing antibody preparations against antigenically different HIV isolates. One of these (IgG1b12) interferes with viral binding to the CD4 co-receptor. As a vaccine against AIDS is urgently needed, HIV-1 has become a model to see if a vaccine evoking a very strong CTL response will clear, or control, subsequent infection. If so, then a vaccinated person who subsequently becomes infected might survive much longer and be less infectious.

AIDS has, perhaps, now become the most studied disease in history. For a complex variety of contradictory, and even conflicting, reasons, governments have poured money into research addressing AIDS and HIV. The NIH in America invests around half a billion dollars a year in studying the disease, for example. This has been directed at two main objectives: first, an enhanced understanding of the disease and the host's immune response to it; second, the search for an as-yet-unrealized AIDS vaccine. Over 50 different vaccines have entered clinical trials in the last 20 years. It does not need me to reiterate that despite the vast sums of money and goodwill expended on this search, we are not much closer to a viable AIDS vaccine. Nor is there any real chance that there will be any significant breakthroughs in the foreseeable future. Witness Merck's STEP vaccine.

## Malaria: then and now

Malaria is the third disease of the WHO's big three. Malaria is a palpable threat across much of the developing world. Previously extremely widespread, the disease is now confined to certain tropical and subtropical regions, including parts of Asia, Latin America, and principally sub-Saharan Africa, where 85–90% of malaria fatalities occur. In 2002, the last year for which we have a reliable estimate, malaria deaths totalled around 1.27 million. Malaria is also a chronic condition and it has infected over 408 million people around the world. Children and pregnant women are particularly vulnerable. According to the World Bank, malaria costs Africa an estimated $100 billion in lost economic opportunity. The WHO has said that malaria slows African economic growth by 1.3% annually.

Malaria is caused by protozoan parasites, principally *Plasmodium falciparum* and *Plasmodium vivax*, although certain other species, such as *P. ovale* and *P. malariae,* are also infective. Malaria parasites are transmitted by female anopheles mosquitoes. The parasites reproduce in erythrocytes, inducing fever, chills and various flu-like symptoms, as well as anaemia, followed in certain cases by coma and death. Despite enormous efforts, no effective malaria vaccine yet exists.

In passing it is worth noting the synergy operating amongst these three diseases. Infection with HIV clearly weakens the relative strength of the immune system, increasing the probability that people will contract other diseases. The rapid spread of AIDS, especially in developing countries, has contributed to the sudden increase in TB cases in recent years. In fact, one third of the world's HIV positive population is now coinfected with tuberculosis. HIV and malaria also synergize, causing them both to spread faster. Individuals with AIDS, when they contract malaria, experience a tenfold increase in their HIV viral-load, making them more capable of transmitting infection to others. It has been estimated that perhaps 5% of total HIV infections and 10% of malaria infections can be blamed on co-infection.

## Influenza

There are, however, many other important diseases beyond the WHOs big three. The most topical is, of course, that most contagious of viral infections, influenza. The first known worldwide influenza pandemic occurred in 1580; while at least three influenza pandemics occurred in the nineteenth century (1830–1831, 1836–1837 and 1889–1891), and three in the twentieth century (1918–1920, 1957–1958 and 1968–1969). The greatest of these was the 1918–1919 pandemic. So-called Spanish influenza resulted in a huge death toll, which is variously placed between 22 and 50 million deaths across the world. This is probably larger than the combined toll from the First World War (estimated at 8.5 million) and the Second World War (estimated at 20 million), yet visions of the trenches, Gallipoli, the Blitz, and the Normandy Landings have all but effaced thoughts of this pandemic from the world's collective memory.

Antigenic shifts are significant changes in either or both influenza H or N surface antigens probably resulting from genetic recombination between viruses. Influenza viruses, unlike many of the more easily eradicable diseases, have animal hosts (notably birds), as well as humans. Efficient person-to-person transmission is a prerequisite for a particular influenza virus to become a pandemic. The last pandemic in 1968 occurred when a significant antigenic shift caused H3N2, or Hong Kong, influenza to replace completely the previously prevalent strain: H2N2, or Asian, influenza. Influenza pandemics typically start from some focal point and propagate along routes used for trade and travel. The extreme celerity and thus popularity of inexpensive air travel has greatly compounded the problem. The influenza A virus was isolated from ferrets in 1933; influenza B in 1936, the same year that the virus was found to grow in chicken eggs. This led to the eventual development of inactivated vaccines, whose protective efficacy was determined in the 1950s. Several influenza vaccines are now available.

Trivalent inactivated influenza vaccine, or TIV, has been available since the 1940s. It is delivered intramuscularly and is available in adult and paediatric formulations. TIV has been manufactured in the United States by three companies: Fluzone made by Sanofi Pasteur; Fluvirin, manufactured by Chiron; and Fluarix from GlaxoSmithKline. Because influenza varies considerably, at least in terms of its major surface antigens, vaccines against it are in something of a state of flux, needing to keep pace with genetic change in the virus. TIV currently comprises three inactivated viruses: type A (H1N1), type A (H3N2) and type B.

Current annual production of TIV is close to 290 million doses, or a global coverage less than 5%. Even in the United States demand often exceeds supply, although TIV stocks exceed 100 million doses. In 2003, live attenuated influenza vaccine, or

LAIV, was licensed in the United States. It is delivered intranasally and contains the three TIV viruses. LAIV is temperature-sensitive and does not replicate at body temperature, but it does replicate effectively in nasal mucosa.

Many experts on influenza are concerned by the increasingly wide geographic distribution of the highly pathogenic avian virus (H5N1). Newspaper scare stories and media hyperbole aside, there is genuine concern this could exacerbate the probablility of another antigenic shift, resulting in an easily transmitted influenza virus lethal to humans. There are 15 types of avian influenza. The most infectious strains, which are usually fatal in birds, are H5 and H7. There are nine different forms of the H5 strain; some are pathogenic, while others cause no harm. Avian flu virus was first identified in China during 1996; it killed six people in Hong Kong in 1997. The H5N1 strain found in Asia has proved to be fatal in humans, infecting 270 people and killing 164 worldwide – most in South East Asia – since 2003. Cross infection to humans is relatively rare, occurring where people live in close contact with infected birds. Although H5N1 can infect humans who are in direct and prolonged contact with infected poultry, the virus is not transmitted efficiently between human hosts.

The spread of a lethal strain of avian flu during the past few years has led many to anticipate a new pandemic: H5N1 transferred by birds migrating to Europe and Africa or the close proximity of human and bird resulting from present farming methods might accelerate the spread. Others argue that H5N1 has existed for so long that it probably does not have the capacity to mutate into a form capable of staging a pandemic. Experience from the past indicates 25–35% of the human population worldwide may be infected. The estimated death toll may be anywhere between 2.0 and 7.4 million. However, this reasoning is based on the 1957 flu pandemic, which was much less virulent than that causing the epidemic of 1918–1919.

## Bioterrorism

Finally, in this brief discussion of present and future threats, we come to bioterrorism. Bioterrorism is an aspect of biological warfare. The utility of biological weapons has been clear to military commanders from time immemorial, since disease often kills more men than does the enemy. Biological warfare originated in ancient times and has evolved through the centuries. Over time, biological warfare has grown from the crude, indiscriminate and serendipitous use of pre-existing infectious material as weapons to the wilful development and deployment of designed biological weapons.

Before and during the World Wars the more developed nations explored, and even used, a variety of biological weapons. During the First World War, the Germans were alleged to have tried to spread cholera in Italy, plague in St Petersburg, and to have dropped biological bombs from Zeppelins over Britain. Between the wars, the Japanese used biological warfare against China. In active military campaigns during the Second World War, an estimated several hundred thousand people, primarily Chinese civilians, fell victim to biological attacks by the Japanese. Allied scientists also experimented with biological agents. For example, in 1941, the British government experimented with open-air anthrax weapons on Gruinard Island in Scotland; subsequent entry to the island was prohibited for the next 48 years.

After the Second World War, biological warfare was practiced primarily at the state-sponsored level. The United States Army, for example, undertook research into biological agents, developing Camp Dietrick (now Ft Dietrick) in Maryland, while the British developed facilities for research into biological and chemical weapons at Porton Down in Wiltshire. At the end of 1969, possibly prompted by Vietnam War protests, President Richard Nixon ended the United States offensive biological warfare programme and ordered all stockpiled weapons to be destroyed. From that point, the United States, and its NATO allies, changed to research into biological defence countermeasures, including the development of vaccines.

Today we face threats from biological warfare originating from several sources. Viewed from the perspective of a developed western nation, such as Britain or the United States, threats come from three rather broad categories. First, the rather anomalously-named 'rogue states'; this also includes former or future superpowers – Russia or China in other words. Many have, for example, suspected the Russian government of using biological weapons in their interminable war in Chechnya. Secondly, threats from so-called *failed states*. Many of these cluster together in the Middle East: Iraq, Iran or the Yemen are principal examples. North Korea is another. Indeed, the Koreans have been suspected of stockpiling FMDV for use against livestock and accumulating stocks of influenza virus for use against the human population. Thirdly, threats originating from terrorist organizations. Al-Quieda is a clear and obvious example. This final category also includes the single fanatic working alone, as well as large scale, well organized, well funded groups. The characteristics of each type of threat are different, but all pose a potential risk of no little significance.

The West has feared the Soviet capacity for germ warfare for decades. Today the West is perhaps concerned more by the possibility of old stocks falling into the hands of criminals and terrorists. In this context, the disease which has most exercised the imagination is smallpox. Smallpox eradication has left much of the world's population susceptible to zoonotic orthopoxviruses. This makes smallpox a potent biological weapon. In this sense, the world is as vulnerable to smallpox now as the New World was in the days of Columbus. Since the disease was eradicated at the end of the 1970s, the only known stocks of the smallpox virus are held at CDC in Atlanta and at the State Research Centre of Virology and Biotechnology in Koltsovo, Russia. As the Soviet Union's biological weapons programmes crumbled in the early 1990s, and their scientists became disillusioned, it was thought possible that expert virologists and bacteriologists might have been lured to rogue states such as Iraq. By the end of the first Gulf War, Iraq was believed to have made weapons of anthrax, botulism toxin and aflatoxin. In the face of Iraqi denials, UN weapon inspectors spent long years looking to confirm this programme. Certainly, Iraq unleashed chemical weapons during the Iran–Iraq War and against rebel Kurds in the north of the country. Yet we have no unequivocal evidence that the Iraqi state has ever successfully engaged in biological warfare.

Nonetheless, it is really only state-sponsored research – be that conducted by a superpower (future or former) or by a rogue state – into biological warfare that has the capacity to engage the full power of modern molecular biology to develop new bioweapons, and to develop the necessary technological capacity to deliver them properly. Only they have the means, the knowledge, the experience and the equipment needed to develop novel biological weapons. In the 1970s, the public was worried about men with suspiciously heavy suitcases bringing to major cities the threat of home-made nuclear devastation. While much plutonium has gone missing over the years, there is no publicly available evidence to suggest that this was ever a realizable danger.

Attention has now turned to biological weapons as tools for terrorists and isolated fanatics. Examples of terrorist organizations dabbling in biological warfare are diverse to say the least. For example, during the Vietnam War, the Viet Cong used spear traps contaminated by human solid waste. Other groups famously involved in bioterrorism have included the Japanese Aum Shinrikyo cult; the Minnesota Patriots Council, an extreme right-wing militia group from America; Rajneeshee religious cultists; the Red Army Faction; the Weathermen, a left-wing group opposed to the Vietnam War; and the right-wing 'Order of the Rising Sun', amongst others. There has been some debate, from the media through to the secret services and the heart of government, about the possibility that terrorists will use the vast amount of data now publicly available over the internet to create new engineered weapons of mass destruction. While such a possibility cannot be wholly discounted, such people would find it better to direct their attention to the bewildering array of existing virulent infections and zoonotic diseases sitting waiting to be used as bioweapons.

## Vaccines as medicines

In the context of the various threats enumerated above, unmet medical need is a constant stimulus to the discovery of new medicines, be they small molecule drugs, therapeutic antibodies or vaccines. This unmet need arises from infectious, genetic or autoimmune disease, as well as other conditions that impinge deleteriously upon the quality of life. As we have said, patterns of disease have altered significantly over the past 100 years and will doubtless change again in the next 100. We can hope to predict some of these changes, but not all. Medical need is ever changing and is always at least one step ahead of us. Thus the challenge to medicine has never been greater.

Fortunately, the power of research technology deployed in pharmaceutical companies and academia has never been greater, nor based on a sounder understanding of the problem and its potential solutions. Vaccinology is slowly evolving into immunovaccinology, a discipline that uses the rapid advances in immunological understanding extant with the last few decades to affect a paradigm shift in thinking. Reverse immunology approaches offer the tantalizing prospect of short cutting the process of vaccine discovery and also producing safer and more effective vaccines.

Vaccination has, until relatively recently, been a highly empirical science, relying on poorly understood, nonmechanistic approaches to the development of new vaccines. As a consequence of this, relatively few effective vaccines have been developed and deployed during most of the two centuries that have elapsed since Jenner's work. Yet today, literally dozens of vaccine candidates have passed through phase II clinical trials. During the last decade, the number of new vaccines in active development has more than tripled to about 150.

In particular, issues of funding have been central to the steady development and distribution of vaccines, as have concerns with contamination and safety. Furthermore, public reactions to vaccines are usually quite strong, and have varied from awe to scepticism and outright hostility. Beyond the far-reaching microbiological and immunological discoveries that have transformed vaccinology over the past century, vaccinology has been shaped increasingly by regulations governing research ethics and the enforcement of health and safety standards.

Traditionally, drivers in the First World have been paediatric vaccines – a tranche of vaccines which long-ago defeated an array of childhood diseases – and travel vaccines which protect those visiting regions where tropical disease still reigns. A few years into the new millennium, we find that the commercial world inhabited by vaccines has been transformed from that which existed during the early to mid-1990s. This has been prompted by a diverse range of motivating factors, including worries over the emergence of antibiotic resistance, the threat of pandemics such as avian influenza, and bioterrorism. The vaccine market, once almost moribund, has grown tenfold over the last decade or so. In 2000, the annual sales of vaccines stood at approximately $5 billion; the global vaccine marketplace was valued at $10.8 billion in 2006. Of course, such a figure needs to be set against the total size of the pharmaceutical market. In 2000, the total sales for all human therapies (small molecules, vaccines, therapeutic antibodies, etc.) were about $350 billion. By 2004, global sales had reached $550 billion. This represented a 7% increase on 2003 sales, which in turn was a 9% rise compared with 2002. At the same time, the farm livestock health market was worth around $18 billion and the companion animal health market was valued at about $3 billion.

## Vaccines and the pharmaceutical industry

Established pharmaceutical companies are, in general, all suffering from an inconvenient coincidence: developing product droughts (caused, in the main, by weak or dwindling internal pipelines) coupled to severe earnings pressures which result from the expiry of highly remunerative patents on major flagship products. The industry's revenue growth for 2003 to 2004 was roughly 7% compared with a mean for all industry of 10.3%. Over this period pharmaceuticals did not register a growth in profit. Using Forbes figures for 2005, we see Pfizer ranked first (sales of $51 billion); followed by GlaxoSmithKline ($37 billion); Sanofi Aventis ($32 billion), which is ranked first in Europe; then Novartis ($30 billion), Roche ($26 billion), Merck & Co more or less equal with Abbott Laboratories and AstraZeneca (all at or about $22 billion), then Wyeth ($18 billion). Unlike, say, the retail sector, there is no runaway winner amid pharmaceutical companies. No one totally dominates the marketplace, since these top companies each control less than 10% of the world drug market.

However, after a long and relaxed period of sustained yet unsustainable profitability, the pharmaceutical industry is now facing a pressing need to increase efficiency. Competition increases all the time, as do regulatory controls; in the past 10 years this has seen a cyclic pattern of mergers, acquisitions and divestments. The emphasis is now on reducing time-to-market. However, at the same time tightening by regulatory bodies has increased and companies have uniformly failed to exploit new drug and vaccine targets. The time it takes to approve each new NCE: 19 months in 2001 was up from only 13.5 months in 1998. Attrition is the loss of compounds at various stages of the development process. This can occur for various reasons: insufficient *in vitro* potency during the research phase or insufficient efficacy in humans at a late stage; poor pharmacodynamic properties or unexpected side effects – the list is long and grows longer every day. Estimates of the rate of attrition within the pharmaceutical industry vary. Depending on how the calculation was performed, and on what basis, the rate lies somewhere between 0.25 and 0.001. Only about one in 12 compounds entering the development phase will eventually reach market. Even getting to market can be a mixed blessing. If we put aside so-called blockbusters, i.e. drugs grossing over $1 billion annually, then the 'average' drug will struggle to recoup its development costs. Moreover, two out of three marketed drugs fail to yield a positive return on investment.

Currently, then, vaccines form only a very small part of the wider marketplace for medicines and pharmaceutical therapy. Compared with glamour drugs designed to battle cholesterol, high blood pressure and depression, vaccines have long been the poor relations of the pharmaceutical industry, and it is still true that vaccines remain a neglected corner of the global drug industry. Indeed, at $10.8 billion, vaccines make less than the $13 billion generated by Lipitor, currently the world's top seller. Likewise, we see a similar phenomenon if we compare vaccines to the protein therapeutics market, which was valued at $57 billion in 2005. The market for therapeutic antibodies was worth an estimated $13.6 billion, accounting for more than 24% of the total biotech market. However, sales of vaccines have been growing at or about 10–12%, compared to a more modest annual figure of 5–6% for small-molecule drugs. Annual growth in the vaccine sector is expected to approach 20% during the next 5 years.

## Making vaccines

Viewed commercially, vaccines have many attractive characteristics; compared with small-molecule drugs vaccines are more likely to escape the development pipeline and reach market, with 70% of programmes gaining regulatory approval. Vaccines also enjoy long product half-lives. About 90% of all vaccines are sold directly to governments and public health authorities, and so they have much smaller marketing costs. However, until relatively recently, vaccines were not considered to be an attractive business, with very tight profit margins.

During the 1980s, the vaccine manufacturing landscape seemed highly fractured, with over 20 vaccine manufacturers. Today there are only five main players: France's Sanofi-Aventis, Merck and Wyeth in the United States, Britain's GlaxoSmithKline and now Novartis. In 1989, there were less than 10 active research-based biotech vaccine companies, now there are nearly 200. 2005 saw something of a sea change for the vaccine sector. Frantic commercial activity included significant corporate consolidation, manifest through a series of acquisitions: ID Biomedical was purchased by GlaxoSmithKline, Chiron was snapped up by Novartis and Bruna was acquired by Crucell. Pfizer are now getting into the act, acquiring Powderject as well as creating in-house expertise.

This partial renaissance has, in part, been fuelled by remarkable growth in the market for influenza vaccines: double-figure growth has expanded the marketplace to about $1.6 billion in 2005. Of the 18 manufacturers of influenza vaccine in nine countries, the 14 largest make up 90% of the total global supply. Sanofi-Aventis is the leading player, with revenues of $835 million in 2005 and a 58% market share in 2005. Novartis is now the second-largest flu-vaccine producer, with 11% of the market. Several big players have been galvanized into action, significantly expanding their manufacturing capacities.

## The coming of the vaccine industry

Another economic driver of growth in the vaccine sector is the rise of the so-called life-style vaccines. These target, for example, addiction to nicotine or cocaine, the control of hypertension and blood cholesterol levels, and obesity, as well as more familiar diseases such as psoriasis or Alzheimer's disease. As the population ages, these will become ever more important contributors to the vaccine marketplace. Currently, obesity devours 5% of American health expenditure. Even in other countries, it accounts for 2–3.5% of medical expenditure. Projections see this figure rocketing by the middle of this century.

Commercially, prospects within the vaccine market have improved out of all recognition. The threats and opportunities alluded to in this chapter, coupled to continuing scientific advance, altered regulatory policy, and changes in governmental and pan-governmental health care strategy have enormously improved the economics of the vaccine business. Although economic (profit and cost) and clinical (safety and efficacy) criteria remain priorities, legal reforms have nonetheless reduced the liability of pharmaceutical companies to acceptable levels, helping to make the discovery of vaccines more economic.

Yet competing concerns still require reconciliation and this will hopefully emerge from the interaction of all interested parties: the government and the governed; the pharmaceutical industry and academia; and the companies, charities and governmental and nongovernmental organizations that administer and fund vaccine discovery, development and delivery. Charities, typified by the Bill and Melinda Gates Foundation, have become increasingly important players in the world of vaccines. As well as the five big players – GlaxoSmithKline, Wyeth, Sanofi Pasteur, Merck and Novartis – there has also been renewed interest from many smaller companies; yet it is the big five that still drive the economics, if not necessarily the innovation, of commercial vaccine discovery. In terms of delivering future drugs from current pipelines, conventional small molecule drug discovery has been seen to stall, making vaccines an enticing alternative market and a vital new revenue stream.

# 3
# Vaccines: How They Work

*That which does not kill us makes us strong.*

—Friedrich Nietzsche (1844–1890)

## Challenging the immune system

One of the most widely cited quotations from the works of Friedrich Nietzsche originates in his 1878 book, *Thus Spake Zarathusra*: 'That which does not kill us makes us strong.' Whatever inference the author may have intended, he is unlikely to have had in mind an explicit reference to vaccinology. However, this nonetheless fits well the notion that we can battle with the threat from infectious disease, and other dangers, by challenging our immune systems. These challenges may be artificial, such as vaccines, or they may be naturally endemic or environmental in nature. As we have seen, the term vaccine can be applied to all agents, either of a molecular or supramolecular nature, used to stimulate specific, protective immunity against pathogenic microbes and the diseases they cause. Vaccines work to militate against the effects of subsequent infection as well as blocking the ability of a pathogen to kill its host.

Vaccination, of course, pre-dates Nietzsche; it began in the closing years of the eighteenth century. The words 'vaccination' and 'immunization' are sometimes used interchangeably, especially in nonmedical parlance; the latter is a more inclusive term because it implies that the administration of an immunologic agent actually results in the development of adequate immunity. As the definitions of 'vaccine', 'vaccination' and 'immunization' have changed over time, becoming more scientifically precise, many of the basic patterns and problems of vaccinology have remained constant. Infectious disease, of course, predates vaccination, having stalked humanity since the first emergence of the human species. Indeed,

*Bioinformatics for Vaccinology*   Darren R Flower
© 2008 John Wiley & Sons, Ltd

infection is likely to have been a feature of life since at least the first appearance of multicellular organisms, and possibly before.

## The threat from bacteria: Robust, diverse, and endemic

Infection is the natural enemy of medicine and medicine is the natural enemy of infection. Infection is mediated by obligate and opportunistic pathogens: protozoan parasites, fungi, viruses and bacteria. The bacterial genome is perhaps the most directly amenable to immunoinformatic analysis; as such, it has generated the greatest interest amongst immunoinformaticians. The wealth of legacy data that has accumulated within the literature during the last 150 years or so provides a remarkable resource upon which to draw when developing predictive methodologies. More than that, the bacterial cell can seem – in some respects at least – like a simplified version of the eukaryotic cell. It has a conveniently small number of distinct membrane-bound compartments – cytoplasm, periplasm and extracellular space, and membranes separating them – where proteins can be localized, and it uses many of the same mechanisms for transport and secretion. These features can be utilized to our advantage when attempting to predict antigens. Viruses, on the other hand, seem recondite and mysterious things by comparison, whose close integration with the host cell can be confounding. Protozoa and fungi are likewise more complicated both structurally and functionally.

One of the reasons that bacteria remain a potent threat is their innate adaptability. Bacteria have adapted to every potential environment – every climate, every habitat, every exotic ecological niche – that the earth has to offer. Something in the region of $10^9$ bacterial species and over $10^{10}$ bacterial genes are spread throughout the diverse consortium of ecological systems comprising the global biosphere. These numbers may be underestimates. Bacteria live everywhere we live, and many places besides. Deep underground, in the cold of the upper atmosphere, deep beneath the sea – bacteria are everywhere. In the past few decades it has become clear that microbial life has colonized, evolved and thrived in various deep subterranean ecosystems. Recently, a thermophilic anaerobic bacterium from the genus *Bacillus* was found at a depth of 2700 m below the ground. Bacteria found living near hydrothermal vents on the sea floor show unexpected similarities to human pathogens, such as *Helicobactor pylori* (which cause ulcers) and *campylobacter* (which gives rise to food poisoning).

Bacteria – and other microbial life – can survive extremes of ionizing radiation, heat, pressure, salinity, ionic strength and pH. Such extremophiles take many forms. Thermophiles can live at temperatures up to 350K, while hyperthermophiles thrive at temperatures of 393K, such as are found in deep-sea thermal vents. Halophiles need salt concentrations over 2M to survive. Endoliths are microbes that perpetuate themselves within microscopic voids in rock – the spaces between aggregate grains or groundwater-filled fissures or within fissures and aquifers deep underground. Lithoautotrophs, such as *Nitrosomonas europaea*, are bacteria that use exergonic inorganic oxidation to fix carbon from carbon dioxide. These bacteria affect geochemical cycling and the weathering of bedrock into soil. Piezophile bacteria live at high hydrostatic pressure, as is found far underground or deep in the ocean. Xerophiles thrive in highly desiccating areas, such as deserts. Cryophiles grow at or below 15 °C, temperatures common in permafrost and snow, polar ice and in the cold oceans. Radioresistant bacteria, as typified by *Deinococcus radiodurans* the most radioresistant organism known, can tolerate high levels of ionizing radiation, such as ultraviolet radiation, or resist natural or artificial nuclear radiation.

For the past $10^9$ years – give or take the odd decade or millennia – bacteria have exerted a significant selective pressure shaping the evolution of eukaryotic organisms, not least through the frantic quatrain characteristic of host-pathogen interactions. Bacteria themselves adapt more rapidly to new selective pressures than many eukaryotic organisms because bacteria have relatively small genomes and relatively short generation times. Moreover, their genomes are fluid, which enables them to transfer en masse whole biochemical pathways and thus gain novel biological functionality at a stroke. Horizontal gene transfer allows bacteria to acquire new mechanisms of virulence or survival, while others lose whole pathways to reduce virulence and become parasitic, and yet others are able to become fully symbiotic.

## Microbes, diversity, and metagenomics

In trying to address diseases mediated by single microbial species we must not lose sight of the rich complexity of microbial ecology. The key player here is the newly emergent discipline of environmental or meta-genomics, which seeks to use genomics, proteomics and bioinformatics to measure microbial diversity. Metagenomics avoids the need to culture the unculturable by recovering genes directly from microbial populations.

Microorganisms embody the largest single component of global biodiversity. The air we breath, the water we drink, the surfaces we touch, and the ground we walk on are all home to a bewilderingly vast community of interrelated, interacting microbial life. Consider the oceans, home to vast numbers of different microorganisms. The bacterium *Pelagibacter ubique*, which has a tiny genome, accounts for one in four marine organisms: there are perhaps 20 billion billion billion *Pelagibacter* scattered through the oceans of the world. Marine viruses are mostly bacteriophages. They kill marine bacteria and archaea, which dominate the oceans, keeping the concentration of marine microbes down to approximately $5 \times 10^5$ cells per ml of sea water. Phages affect microbial evolution by killing specific microbes. Theory predicts that as one microorganism becomes dominant, a phage kills it, opening up a niche that a phage-resistant variant can use. This may explain the enormous microdiversity seen in microbial communities. Phages also directly affect microbial evolution by transferring genes between hosts.

A recent viral metagenomic analysis of 184 viral assemblages collected over a decade and representing 68 sites in four oceanic regions (the Arctic, the coast of British Columbia, the Gulf of Mexico and the Sargasso Sea) indicates that most of the viral sequences were not similar to those in current databases. It also shows that viruses are widely dispersed and that viral communities vary with geographic regions. Global viral diversity is in the region of 200 000 viral species, but regional diversity is also very significant. Certain viral species are endemic and others are ubiquitous, with most being widespread and common to several marine environments. Most of the differences between sites are explained by the altered occurrence of the commonest viruses and not by the absence of particular viral groups.

However, the biggest metagenomic data-set currently available, also oceanic in origin, focuses on bacteria: J. Craig Venter's *Sorcerer II* expedition to the Sargasso Sea and his more recent global ocean sampling (GOS) expedition. Initially, Venter identified over 1.2 million genes and inferred the existence of more than 1800 distinct bacterial species. Combining this with subsequent work, Venter identified a combined data-set comprising 6.3 billion base pairs, roughly two times that of the human genome.

## The intrinsic complexity of the bacterial threat

Our corporate perceptions of the nature of bacterial interactions have also changed dramatically in recent years; most significant for me at least is the concept of bacterial multicellularity. Dismissed or ignored for decade after decade, multicellularity is now a clear and well-established phenomenon shared not by a handful of obscure species but by most if not all bacteria. Under appropriate conditions, the most standard of bacteria will exhibit coordinated multicellularity displaying pattern formation and regulated colony growth. When a colony is formed, different cells will become specialized and adopt distinct functions.

The word biofilm has become a catch-all watchword for microbial communities. Other than marine microbes, which live unicellular lives in the open ocean, most bacteria exist as part of biofilms: highly organized, cooperative microbial communities, often encased by a matrix, exhibiting significant three-dimensional structure and morphology. Biofilms can also play an important role in disease transmission. Toxic *Vibrio cholera* exists within the aquatic environment in a primarily dormant and unculturable state. During the interregnum between seasonal epidemics, biofilms provide cholera with an additional reservoir of robust and long-term viability.

Many bacteriologists now view bacteria as predominantly social and cooperative, only existing as single cells in, say, batch culture where exhibiting multicellularity is not needed for survival. Key to cooperativity is quorum sensing, a widespread mechanism linking the environmental state experienced by a microbe to gene expression and function. Quorum sensing is mediated by small messenger molecules, such as peptides and lactones, and has been implicated in regulating biofilm formation and swarming motility. Signalling molecules may have evolved as metabolic by-products and then evolved gradually into a means of communication. Bacterial functions affected by quorum sensing include bioluminescence, genetic competence and sporulation. This mechanism is found in hundreds of bacterial species and operates both within and between species. Quorum sensing is also a key mediator of infectivity in many pathogenic bacteria – for example *Vibrio cholera* – where virulence factor production is often orchestrated through this mechanism.

Symbioses, which have coevolved between multicellular organisms and bacteria, are a major aspect of life on earth. The nature of symbiotic relationships differs. Differences can include how transmission occurs between generations, i.e. via the female parent or via environmental colonization, or the physical relationship between host and symbiotic partner – is it extracellular or intracellular, for example? Most interestingly of all is whether the symbiotic association is between a host and a single microbe or between a host and a collection of different microbial species. Single cooperative association (or binary symbiosis) is typical in invertebrates. Consortial symbiosis – cooperative association between a host and numerous microbial species – is common in vertebrates and is of particular importance in humans and other large animals, particularly livestock.

## Microbes and humankind

Human symbiosis with our own resident microbes is of the greatest interest and the most pertinent to the present discussion. Throughout life we happily coexist with our indigenous microbial populations of bacteria and also fungi, protozoans and viruses. It is the view of many that human and microbial cells are best thought of as a single whole: a composite superorganism known as the 'microbiome'. Adherents to this paradigm contend that the balanced relationship between the body and its normal flora is crucial to the maintenance of health and proper function. The microbiome undertakes a variety of function roles: control of pathogen growth, they aid the breakdown of food, produce vitamins, confer cross-reactive immunity and aid tissue development. Such an important and exquisite relationship is contingent upon a complexity of interactions which occur both within and between the host, its resident microbial population and the environment. The role of the microbiome in supplementing host defence is most pertinent here. Stable populations of indigenous microbes provide critical protection against environmental disease-causing pathogens. Since every niche is filled, pathogens cannot out-compete the resident microbes.

The total number of bacteria residing in or on the human body exceeds 100 trillion; equating to 10 per human somatic or germ cell. The total number of different microbial genes in the human body is thought to outnumber human genes by up to 1000 to one. The human microbial population is composed of an ever escalating number of species, which now number well in excess of 1000 different species. The reason humans do not resemble biofilms is the enormous difference in size between prokaryotic and eukaryotic cells. A large virus will be about 1000 Å or 100 nm across, while megaviruses range between 400 and 800 nm. Unicellular protozoa, such as amoeba, have a size range between 90 and 80 μm. Archaeal cell sizes range from that of *Thermodiscus* (with a diameter of 0.2 μm and a disk thickness of 0.1–0.2 μm) to the very thermophilic *Staphylothermus marinus*, whose cell size can reach 15 μm in culture. Bacteria exhibit an even greater range: small bacteria, such as mycobacteria, are only 150–250 nm across, and are roughly the size of the lysosomes they infect; *E. coli* are 2 μm; mitochondria, which are of probable endosymbiotic origin, are 3μm, and chloroplasts 5 μm in length. However, there are many bacteria which greatly exceed such values.

Several extremely large bacteria have been identified in the last 20 years: *Epulopiscium fishelsoni*, *Beggiatoa sp.* and *Thiomargarita namibiensis. Fishelsoni*, a rod-shaped heterotrophic bacterium found in the gut of fishes, reaches 80 μm in diameter by 600 μm in length. *Namibiensis* is a chain-forming, spherical sulphur bacterium discovered on the Nambian sea floor. It can reach 750 μm in diameter. Indeed, *Namibiensis* is visible to the naked eye, forming chains that shine white like pearls on the black mud of the ocean floor. As a comparison, about four *namibiensis* are needed to cover an average tea leaf.

At the other extreme are so-called nanobacteria. Controversy rages as to the nature of these entities – some dismissing them as artifacts, others championing their status as a new form of life. Accepting for a moment that they exist, they are minute with sizes ranging from 20–500 nm. The smallest nanobacteria can be filtered by membranes with 100 nm pores. They are observable by electron microscopy, appearing as rods or spheres.

Eukaryotic cells, as typified by human tissue, range from 1 μm (the diameter of a neuronal axon) to 9 μm for an erythrocyte to 100 μm for a human egg cell. A megakaryocyte is up to 160 μm. Most animal cells range between 10 and 30 μm and most plant cells range between 10 and 100 μm. A eukaryotic cell may have 10 times the cell volume of an average bacterium. However, cells in other animals can be much larger: the squid giant nerve cell is 1 mm in diameter, while an ostrich egg may reach 120 mm, although certain dinosaurs may have had much larger eggs.

## The nature of vaccines

Vaccinology is an empirical science and it can be argued, at least in a utilitarian sense, that vaccinology is the foremost amongst all empirical sciences. Until recently, vaccinology has lacked a consistent understanding of the molecular phenomena of immunology which underpin it. It was more a complex set of tried and tested practices than a cohesive and intellectually unified scientific discipline. Things were done because people had seen that they worked rather than because they fully and completely understood why. Until recently, vaccinology has been based not on fundamental paradigms about immunology and host–pathogen interactions but on working hypotheses and time-honoured, atavistic ways of working.

Nonetheless, vaccination and vaccinology are intimately involved with matters of life and death and their success has been almost unmatched in their benefit to society.

This chapter will cover vaccinology from a slightly more rigorous biological perspective. The purpose of this chapter is twofold. First, it will place later discussion in context by outlining a rudimentary view of the general science of vaccinology. Secondly, it will attempt to provide rather more detailed information about specific aspects of molecular immunology, cell biology and biophysics which will serve as background for later chapters. As scientists, even computational ones, we should strive hard to understand the basis of vaccinology that resides in the workings of immunological mechanisms and the machinations of microbial systems interacting with host biology. This is what we set out to do in this chapter. Strictures of space, combined with my own partial and inadequate grasp of the subject, will necessarily limit our success. It is in such knowledge, however, that we shall see how attempts to integrate computational approaches can be based.

What we are not trying to do is reproduce the full context of any of the many excellent immunology textbooks that you can find littering the shelves of academic and university bookshops, since a truly detailed discussion of immunology is both beyond the scope of this current text and is also probably unnecessary, and most certainly unedifying, in the present context. Instead, we will address some pertinent basic issues and those which are often underexplored by immunological encyclopaedists. That is not to say that reading the great immunology textbooks of our time is in any way a bad idea; on the contrary, anyone with the time and self-discipline to do so will find that this complements, and indeed supersedes, the current work.

Nonetheless, when all is said and done, some basic understanding of immune function is a fundamental requirement if we are to understand how vaccines work and how informatics can help in their discovery. Thus a card-carrying immunologist would doubtless snort in derision at the facile simplicity of the description that follows. Vaccines exploit host immune responses to disease. To vaccinate against diseases such as smallpox, diphtheria or polio, physicians give patients a small amount of a modified disease agent or a key active ingredient to which the body will respond. The disease agent in the vaccine is killed or weakened so that it is unlikely to induce disease. Fragments of pathogens also work well in vaccines. The reactive components of vaccines trick the immune system into acting as if it had been exposed to a *bona fide* disease-causing agent.

Vaccines can be either prophylactic or therapeutic in their mode of operation. Prophylactic vaccines act by preventing or mitigating the effects of a future infection by pathogenic organism. Therapeutic vaccines are a treatment functioning post-infection or against, say, cancer. Vaccination is the use of a vaccine, in whatever form, to produce prophylactic active immunity in a host organism. A vaccine is a molecular or supramolecular agent which can elicit specific protective immunity and ultimately mitigate the effect of subsequent infection. Immunity is an outcome of the proper functioning of the immune system and represents the ability of an organism to tolerate endogenous substances (such as proteins, lipids, carbohydrates, etc.) intrinsic to the host and to clear exogenous or foreign matter. This discrimination can provide defence against infectious disease, since most microbes can be readily identified as foreign by the immune system. By potentiating immune memory, protective immunity is an enhanced adaptive immune response to re-infection by pathogenic microbes. Protection manifests itself through the survival of the host, the destruction of pathogens and by mitigating the effects of re-infection. Immunity can be passive or active. Passive immunity is protection through the transfer, from organism to organism, of biological products. Passive immunity often generates effective short-term protection, but this can reduce over time, usually over a span of weeks. Active immunity is, typically, permanent protection generated by a host's own immune system.

As well as protecting individuals, vaccines can be effective also in protecting communities and populations. This is known as 'herd immunity'. As disease passes from one individual to another, it needs both infected groups and susceptible groups for transmission to occur. Herd immunity reduces the susceptibility of a group. When the number of susceptible individuals drops low enough, the disease will effectively vanish as there are no longer enough individuals to carry on the infection cycle. The greater the proportion of vaccinated members of the community, the more rapidly a disease will ebb away. This is why captive populations – school children, operational military contingents – are often systematically vaccinated *en masse*. Childhood vaccination has resulted in the marked decrease of many once-common diseases including whooping cough, polio, and others. An efficacious vaccine strategy should induce strong responses in the host organism that are both long-lasting and of sufficient broadness to forestall the effects of escape mechanisms within the pathogen and also to protect against other pathogens.

## Types of vaccine

A live, virulent micro-organism would now be considered a poor vaccine since it would likely induce the very disease it was intended to prevent. This was one of the principal disadvantages of variolation as a preventative measure for smallpox. Vaccines have, until recently, been exclusively attenuated whole pathogen vaccines such as BCG (for TB) or Sabin's vaccine against polio. More recently, issues of safety have lead to the development of other strategies for vaccine development. The most successful alternative has focused on the antigen – or subunit – vaccine, such as recombinant hepatitis B vaccine.

The first step in creating a vaccine is thus to tease apart those aspects of an infective organism which cause disease from those which merely evoke a safe, manageable, non-life threatening immune response. We need to distinguish or discriminate virulence from immunogenicity or antigenicity. In practice, this will require the isolation or creation of an organism, or a part thereof, which is simultaneously unable to induce a dangerous disease state, yet retains those antigens which give rise to an immune response.

Vaccines may be living, weakened strains of viruses or bacteria that intentionally give rise to infections which are either very mild or undetectable. Vaccines may also be killed or inactivated organisms or purified products derived from them. There are several kinds of traditional vaccine. The first is the live attenuated vaccine, first developed by Louis Pasteur. Examples include vaccines against measles, rubella, yellow fever, mumps and tuberculosis. This way of making a vaccine does so by 'attenuating' or 'weakening' a pathogen; that is to say it reduces the inherent or intrinsic virulence exhibited by a virulent micro-organism through, say, altering its growth conditions in some way. These vaccines are thus live micro-organisms, bacteria or viruses, which have been cultured under conditions which reduce their capacity to cause disease while leaving their immunogenic properties untouched.

Attenuation involves selecting mutated microbes that grow at reduced rates or have lost virulence factors that attack the host, yet have retained sufficient immunogenicity to generate an immune response. Live attenuated vaccines are thought to induce robust, longer lasting immune responses. They are often very successful vaccines, as they multiply within the host invoking large systemic responses. As they can mutate back to a virulent form, inducing rather than protecting against disease, live attenuated vaccines are intrinsically risky. In healthy patients, immunity induced by attenuated vaccines can be lifelong and they will not require booster shots. However, attenuated vaccines are not recommended for immuno-compromised patients.

Another, now seldom used, way of creating vaccines is to do what Jenner did: take an organism similar to but distinct from a virulent organism which does not cause disease. BCG is an example of this, protecting against mycobacterium tuberculosis. However, BCG was also attenuated; it is part way between a vaccine as Jenner might have defined it and a vaccine as understood by Pasteur. Current BCG is a strain of TB-related *Mycobacterium bovis* weakened by serial passage.

Historically, the second kind of vaccine was a previously virulent micro-organism that has been killed by treating it with chemicals, such as formalin, or heat; they are known as 'inactivated' or 'killed' vaccines. Examples of killed vaccines used today include those against poliomyelitis, typhoid, influenza, cholera, bubonic plague and hepatitis A. Such vaccines typically induce incomplete or short-duration immune responses, necessitating booster shots.

Subunit vaccines constitute a third way to make vaccines; they comprise individual pathogenic proteins, often being called 'acellular vaccines'. Examples include vaccines against HBV, human papillomavirus and *Haemophilus influenzae* B. Subunit vaccines, which comprise highly immunogenic protein or carbohydrate, such as cell wall components, can stimulate measurable if typically weak immune responses, necessitating booster shots to sustain protection long-term, yet are deemed safe for immunocompromised patients.

Since they are based on single proteins, vaccines based on toxoids – a toxoid is a treated or inactivated toxin – share similarities with subunit vaccines and as such need adjuvant to induce adequate immune responses. Diphtheria and tetanus vaccines are toxoid-based and are usually combined with the pertussis vaccine as adjuvant. Toxoid vaccines require booster shots every decade.

## Carbohydrate vaccines

Not all vaccines are protein-based. A key type of vaccine is instead based on polysaccharides. Carbohydrate vaccines have a long history stretching back, at least, to the observations of Heidelberger and Avery in 1923. However, despite a flurry of early work, culminating in the identification of long-lasting immunity generated by pneumoccocal capsular polysaccharide vaccines, the subsequent development of small molecule drugs, specifically antibiotics, reduced interest in carbohydrate vaccines. Several factors, such as nascent antibiotic resistance, have combined to renew interest.

Immunity to carbohydrate vaccines is generally mediated by antibodies, although certain carbohydrate vaccines can activate T cells via major histocompatibility complexes (MHCs). As with all vaccines, problems remain: tolerance and the lack of significant immunogenicity necessitating the use of adjuvants. One means of addressing this is to couple carbohydrate moieties directly to an innately immunogenic adjuvant protein. Such vaccination using artificial glycoproteins offers lasting protection to both paediatric and adult populations. Mixtures of oligosaccharides derived from degraded bacterial cell surface capsular carbohydrates can act as vaccines. Several successful vaccines are based on carbohydrates: targeted bacteria include *Streptococcus pneumoniae*, *Neisseria meningitides*, *Haemophilus influenzae*, *Salmonella typhi*, *Shigella dysenteriae*, *Group B Streptococcus* and *Klebsiella pneumoniae*. Presently, several injections are needed to administer carbohydrate and conjugate vaccines to infants; this is increasingly being overcome by combining together several vaccines, such as DTaP.

## Epitopic vaccines

Carbohydrate vaccines rely on identifying polysaccharide epitopes. In principle, vaccines can also be based on other types of peptide epitope. Vaccines can be based either on epitopes or on sets of epitope: the epitope is the minimal structure necessary to invoke an immune response. In some senses, it is the immunological quantum that lies at the heart of immunity. Epitopes must come from proteins accessible to immune surveillance and to be specific for a particular pathogen or tumour. Targeting amino acid sequences as epitopes, as recognized by neutralizing antibodies or which bind MHCs, rather than whole protein antigens has the advantage that many sequences able to induce autoimmunity are eliminated. Likewise, these vaccines are potentially much safer: they contain no viable self-replicating microorganisms and cannot cause microbial disease.

Amongst others, epitope-based vaccines for rheumatic fever and malaria are undergoing clinical trials, yet single epitope delivered as peptides have not thus far proved successful as vaccines, although poly-epitope constructs or epitope-cocktails seem more hopeful. Any peptide-based vaccine will need adjuvant to enhance immunogenicity. Whole organisms contain not one or even a handful of epitopes, but vast numbers of all kinds, as well as abounding with adjuvant-like natural products and danger signals. Thus it is little surprise that single epitopes are not as immunogenic as, say, live attenuated vaccines. The ability to tailor epitopes in light of our understanding of MHC restriction suggests that epitope-based vaccines will play an important role, particularly in cancer vaccines. More-over, they afford the opportunity to bring computational methods to bear on the problem.

## Vaccine delivery

Molecular vaccines are very much less immunogenic and require adjuvants. They have properties similar to those of protein therapeutics. They can be delivered into the host in many ways: as naked DNA vaccines, using live viral or bacterial vectors, and via antigen-loaded antigen-presenting cells (APCs).

A relatively recent development, generating much interest, involves vaccinating a host directly with DNA encoding antigenic material (subunit or epitope vaccines) rather than some complex cocktail of microbial products or recombinant proteins. The approach is sometimes called 'naked DNA', in part to distinguish it from vector based approaches. The DNA is inserted into a plasmid behind an appropriate pro-moter, and injected into muscle, where it becomes incorporated into host cells and expressed as protein, which ultimately triggers an immune response. The expressed product is recognized as non-self by local dendritic cells (DCs). The immune system will hopefully recognize the protein and then respond to it and the cells expressing it. DNA vaccines are easy to produce and to store, and immune responses to them are typically strong and persistent. DNA vaccination does not seem to be harmful, nor does it lead to permanent integration into the host genome.

Despite the success evinced by naked DNA, the goal of many vaccinologists remains live viral and bacterial vectors capable of expressing antigen in vaccinated hosts. A recombinant vector, adroitly combining the physiology of one microbe with DNA coding for arbitrary antigens from another, is indeed appealing. Up to 10% of the vaccinia genome can be replaced by DNA coding for antigens from other pathogens. The resulting vector generates strong antibody and T cell responses, and is protective.

Viruses commonly used as vectors include poxviruses, varicella, polio and influenza. Bacterial vectors include both *Mycobacterium bovis* and *Salmonella*. Adding extra DNA coding for large molecule adjuvants greatly exacerbates anti-body or T cell responses. However, creating vectors with such desirable proper-ties is difficult and their effectiveness may be compromised by their capacity to down-regulate other immune responses. The efficient and rational design of effective vaccine vectors is an area where informatic techniques could play a large role.

Antigen-pulsed APCs, in particular DCs, which can ingest and process antigens presenting them as peptide-MHC complexes to T cells, have also been utilized as vectors for delivering vaccines. They can induce robust immune responses which vaccination with antigens alone will not achieve. It is over a decade since the first report on DC-based vaccines. Monocyte-derived DCs can be prepared *ex vivo* and then re-administered to the patient. Such bespoke, personalized vaccination is both costly and labour intensive, and thus unsuitable for large-scale immunization.

Many issues remain for APC-based vaccines. What is the ideal source and preparation of APCs? What is the role of DC maturation? What are the optimal vaccination route and the optimal dose? New areas being explored include the discovery of novel ways to load APCs, specifically loading antigens *in vivo*, requiring delivery of antigen via specific cell surface receptors.

## Emerging immunovaccinology

Because of its many successes, the lack of a sound theoretical basis for much that vaccinology is, or does, has never been perceived as a major problem. However, over time, it has become increasingly of concern. In its place, people had begun to evince immunovaccinology – vaccinology based on our understanding of the immune system – as necessarily succeeding it. Thus modern vaccinology is, or believes itself to be, routed firmly in such an understanding. It is an understanding that we must attempt to share if computational approaches are to deliver their inevitable dividend quickly and efficiently.

With the exception of BCG, which is mediated primarily through cellular mechanisms, essentially all licensed vaccines induce the production of specific neutralizing antibodies, which typically act early in infection. This statement can lead to two competing arguments. One is essentially pessimistic and cynical. It states that future vaccines will be hard to find, as all facile vaccines have been found, since vaccines based on T cell epitopes are so difficult to discover that they are not worth looking for. There is another, rather more positive and optimistic view. The optimistic view is that uncured diseases still require effective vaccines, and that these can be mediated by cellular immunity. This can be addressed through the potent partnership of T cells and antigen presenting cells rather than via antibodies.

Targets still in need of vaccines include: herpes viruses, papillomaviruses, HIV, tuberculosis and malaria. A proper and complete understanding of T cell biology and thus T cell mediated vaccines is a major goal for vaccinology. As this book attempts to show, immunoinformatics can make a major contribution to reaching this objective.

Obviously, the aim of any vaccination is the induction of an effective and appropriate immune response. Yet, for many diseases, what actually constitutes an effective immune response remains unclear. We must look for correlates of protection. For vaccines which work against, say, diphtheria or hepatitis, specific antibody titres are considered to be correlates of protection. For many diseases, correlations of protection are unknown.

## The immune system

The body utilizes the immune system, in both its innate and adaptive guises, to combat and thwart infection, illness and disease, be it the common cold or diabetes or cancer. The ostensive function of immunity – defence against pathogens – manifests itself through a complex system of interacting and cooperating organs, cells and molecules exhibiting behaviour at several characteristic scales. The manifestation of immunology at the whole animal level is, however, an exceedingly complex phenomenon. Cells and molecules involved in mediating immune function are many and varied. The immune system possesses, in totality, a potent combination of anatomical, cellular and molecular mechanisms which allows the repertoire of immune receptors, distributed on cells, to respond to invading pathogens.

The immune system of vertebrates is continually being bombarded at the molecular level by exogenous or foreign material derived from pathogenic micro-organisms – some innocuous, some harmful. Such material may be protein or nucleic acid or carbohydrate or lipid or some complex of two or more. This material will not always be infectious, since we exist in an environment saturated by exogenous material of all kinds. The primary purpose of the immune system is to differentiate exogenous, foreign or non-self, molecules, from endogenous or self molecules. Non-self is always environmental in origin. It can manifest itself as components of organisms, be that pathogenic micro-organisms (viruses, bacteria, fungi or protozoa), quasi-macroscopic multi-cellular organisms, like nematodes or fully macroscopic animals, such as ticks and insects. These components can be part of an organism, as proteins secreted into a host during a bacterial infection for example, or they can be distributed as isolated components, such as air-borne pollen or animal dander. They may also be biological components of manufactured items, such as allergens in latex. Then again, they may be components of the host's own body, as seen in autoimmune disease. Whatever its source, the recognition of non-self by the immune system is a prelude to any response.

Immunity to a pathogen can be inferred from the presence of pathogen-specific host antibodies. Memory cells are also generated. As the strength of an immune response increases, the prevalence of infectious agents is progressively reduced until symptoms diminish. Memory cells remain in circulation, poised to make a fast protective response to subsequent re-infections. Should such infection occur, memory cells respond with such celerity that the resulting immune reaction would rapidly inactivate the disease and typically prevent symptoms. Infection will not develop; the host is immune. Such immunity is usually highly specific for a pathogen.

Since our immune systems constantly face 'natural' challenges, the so-called 'hygiene' or 'jungle hypothesis' has suggested that in our urbanized, technological and increasingly comfortable world, ostensibly beneficial improvements to personal hygiene and public health have, over decades, led to a widespread decrease in our exposure to pathogenic organisms. This has led to a decrease in the breadth and depth of acquired immunity to microbial pathogens and, in turn, to an increase in the prevalence of atopic disease: the increased tendency for individuals to make immediate, and inappropriate, hypersensitivity reactions to otherwise innocuous substances. The exposure to bacterial and viral pathogens early in life plays a significant role in the regulation of allergen-specific immune responses that underlie atopic allergy. Unless we can accept that atopy is the price worth paying for freedom from infection, we must continually train our immune systems so as to prevent allergy.

Active immunity is permanent protection from disease produced by the host immune system, while passive immunity is less permanent or temporary protection offered by transference of immune molecules generated by the immune system of one host into another, different, host organism. Passive immunity is effective, but it is short lived, lasting from a few weeks to a few months. Active immunity is a manifestation of the proper working of the host immune system which is, in turn, comprised of two distinct yet synergistic, sub-systems: the innate immune system and the adaptive immune system. Innate immunity is shared by most multinucleate organisms. Adaptive immunity is, on the other hand, a feature possessed solely by vertebrates. It differs from the innate system by dint of its greater specificity and by its greater memory.

## Innate immunity

The innate and adaptive immune systems are intimately connected and are highly cooperative. The two halves of the overall immune system manifest a much greater and more sustained response to infection, by combining and integrating the optimal features of both systems. Protective immunity thus results from the interplay of the antigen-specific adaptive immune system with an innate response which is not directed specifically at particular antigens. The cells and molecules of the innate system do not exhibit recognition properties which involve the optimization of specificity or selectivity, while the B and T cells characteristic of the adaptive immune system employ receptors which undergo processes of refinement that improve their ability to recognize and discriminate whole antigens or derived peptides.

Most of the operation of the innate immune system is preprogrammed, making use of widely distributed receptors which recognize generic targets: conserved structural motifs or patterns which are characteristic of molecules common to pathogens and microbial life. It does this through the recognition, by 'pattern recognition receptors' or PRRs, of so-called 'pathogen associated molecular patterns' or PAMPs. PRRs detect disturbances to the immune microenvironment (including discrimination of 'non-self') and initiate appropriate innate responses.

It has been said that the crucial feature of PRRs is that they bind multiple ligands by recognizing common PAMPs rather than binding to unique if degenerate epitopes. Attractive though this may appear, it is not wholly accurate. The range of peptides bound by antibodies, and particularly by the MHC-TCR system, is much, much larger than is generally supposed. PRRs engagement of lipopolysaccharide (LPS) or other PAMPs, elicits a response; this is typically pro-inflammatory, involving cytokine generation which activates immune cells. Such reactions are crucial to disease management, but must be controlled since excessive responses are typically pernicious.

Several distinct families of PRRs are known, including the following long list. Arguably the most important, or at least the most prominent, are the so-called toll or toll-like receptors (TLRs). Humans have 10 TLRs; they sense both intracellular pathogens (viruses) and extracellular pathogens (bacteria and fungi). Some bind particular patterns contained in microbial DNA which are absent from vertebrate DNA. More specifically, ssRNA is recognized by TLR7 and TLR8 and dsRNA is recognized by TLR3. TLR2 and TLR6 recognize many ligands: bacterial lipoproteins, peptidoglycan, Zymosan, GPI anchors from *T. cruzi*, LPS and lipoarabinomannanm phosphatidylinositol dimannoside. TLR4 likewise recognizes LPS, Taxol, bacterial HSP60, F protein and fibronectin. TLR5 binds flagellin. TLR9, found on DCs and B cells, detects CpG motifs in DNA. An activated TLR-dependent signalling cascade ultimately induces expression of a variety of response molecules.

dsRNA is also recognized within the cytoplasm by another PRR – RNA helicases such as RIG-I. These are important PRRs, as are the cytosolic NOD-like receptors (NLRs), which play vital roles in innate immunity as intracellular sensors of pathogens and cell damage. This group includes NODs, NALPs, NAIP and IPAF. While TLRs signal from the cell surface or early endosome, NLRs are activated intracellularly by bacterial molecules, such as peptidoglycan, RNA, toxins and flagellin. Whole animal and cell-culture models of bacterial infection suggest a pro-inflammatory role for NLRs, including the regulation of cysteine proteases within the so-called inflammasome. The 700 kDa inflammasome is a multi-protein complex responsible for processing and secreting pro-inflammatory cytokines. Two types of inflammasome are known: NALP1 (comprising NALP1, adaptor protein ASC, caspase 1 and 5) and NALP2/3 (comprising Cardinal protein, ASC and caspase 1).

Other PRRs include FcγRs, which binds opsinized zymogen and serum amyloid P; CD35 and CD11b-CD18, which bind opsinized microbial cells; C-type lectins, such as the mannose receptor (which binds mannosyl and fucosyl moieties) and scavenger receptors (SRs). SRs bind leipoteichoic acid, degradation products from apoptotic cells, and Gram +ve bacteria. Other PRRs include MARCO, MER, PSr, CD36 and CD14.

PRRs are all able to recognize PAMPs, yet each receptor has unique binding properties, cellular expression and engages with different signalling pathways. This diversity within innate immunity protects us from a diverse spectrum of pathogens.

PRRs are encoded by germ line genes, whose structures are inherited. Since the structures of such receptors are inherited, resulting entirely from evolutionary pressure, their specificity is fixed. They evolve relatively slowly by the mechanisms of natural selection through standard processes of point mutation, gene duplication, and so on. The germ line nature of these receptors necessarily limits the eventual repertoire of recognition specificity exhibited by the innate immune system; it does not permit recognition of previously unknown antigens. Yet over long periods it can evolve to ignore self molecules and thus realize some robust discrimination between noninfectious self and infectious non-self.

An advantage to the host of innate versus adaptive immunity is that the innate response is very rapid. Innate immunity is able to respond with considerable celerity to initial infection, acting well ahead of adaptive immunity. The receptors which mediate innate immunity are expressed on a vast array of cells and are thus available for immediate recognition. They are a fast and effective primary defence against invading pathogens. Innate immunity operates within minutes or hours, while the adaptive immune system requires days or weeks.

Innate immunity comprises various cell types; some detect common bacterial products, which then activate the cell causing the release of soluble signalling molecules, such as cytokines and chemokines, or are molecules, such as perforin, which are directly damage invading microbes. Chemokines and cytokines influence the movement and behaviour of other cells. Secretion of such factors can be divided into three classes of interaction: endocrine, paracrine and autocrine. Cytokines involved in long-range interactions can also be divided into three classes: inflammatory mediators, specific immune response regulators and growth and differentiation factors.

## Adaptive immunity

Adaptive immunity uses stochastically-encoded and clonally-distributed sets of receptors. These form a repertoire capable of recognizing any target antigen. This open repertoire is a feature pivotal to proper adaptive immune function: it allows the detection of threats not seen previously as well as responding quickly, effectively and specifically to subsequent antigen encounters. Receptors used are not encoded by fixed, germline genes but arise from a semi-random combinatorial process of protein optimization. This ultimately results in a vast range of receptors which are maintained in clonally distributed cell population.

Adaptive immunity is also characterized by immune memory: initial encounters with an antigen enabling rapid subsequent responses to the same or similar antigen. Of course, the randomly generated nature of this repertoire brings with it problems of discrimination between self and non-self. The specificity evinced by an antibody or T cell receptor is not predetermined by the gene segments generating them. Adaptive immunity must ensure that potentially harmful reactivity against self is mitigated or eliminated. Many mechanisms operate at many levels to facilitate this: first, by shaping the naïve repertoire; secondly, by controlling cell activation by innate immunity; and thirdly, through control by peripheral regulatory cells.

The adaptive immune system can recognize and react to non-self, developing and enhancing its specificity. Adaptive responses are mediated by cells: B and T lymphocytes. B cells produce antibodies able to recognize antigens found on the cell surface or present in the extracellular environment through a variable binding site that binds antigen specifically. B cells are also strongly influenced by CD4+ helper T cells. CD8+ T cells, also known as cytotoxic T lymphocytes or CTLs, together with some other CD4+ T cells, have a direct cytotoxic effect. T cells recognize antigen via cell surface molecules called T cell receptors or TCRs. T cell recognition is more complex than a bimolecular antibody-antigen interaction and involves the formation of a supramolecular complex between self molecules (MHC and TCR) and nonself (antigen-derived peptides). Activated CTLs secrete perforin and granzymes, key mediators of cell lysis.

At a population level, the MHC is very variable; indeed, it is currently thought to be the most variable part of the human genome. Thus different hosts present different peptide sequences depending on the peptide-binding specificity of their particular MHC molecules. Each B cell expresses antibodies with a single specificity and each T cell expresses TCR with a single specificity. The frequency of cells possessing any particular antigen specificity is very low. Thus the population of such antigen-specific cells must be expanded subsequent to any infection or vaccination, which is why adaptive responses can appear slow. It is thought that mainly CTLs, and occasionally helper T cells, clear acute infections. After infection, T and B cells are activated and replicate. Most of these cells die once pathogens are cleared. Regulatory T cells will appear, followed by CTLs and, finally, antibody-secreting B cells.

Immunity is mediated by pattern recognition receptors and adaptive immunity by antibodies and TCR. These two categories form the basis for distinguishing between innate and adaptive immunity, although such a dichotomy is clearly an oversimplification of a very complex reality. As our understanding has deepened so the importance of interactions between innate and adaptive immunity has become ever more obvious. Interactions between the two are many and complex, with innate mechanisms inducing and controlling the adaptive response, as well as being used during adaptive responses.

Within the immune system, components – molecules and cells – build into whole systems. One cannot understand one without understanding the other. At the highest level the whole animal can be thought of as an engine of immunity. At a lower level, the immune system expresses itself through networks of tissues. These include the skin, a largely impermeable barrier to the ingress of pathogenic invaders, and the many mucosal surfaces of the body, such those in the nose and intestines. The gut plays host to the microbiome described above. The degree to which different tissues act as immunological battlegrounds varies enormously.

## The microbiome and mucosal immunity

This microbiome-centred view of host-microbe interactions has led many popular-izers of science to make equivocal and ambiguous statements that some might re-gard as misleading. Statements such as 'are you more microbe than man', or some more gender neutral alternative, have suggested that microbes infest every tissue to the same extent, which is clearly untrue. Muscle, brain, kidneys, fatty tissue and the deep lung have long been believed to be sterile, while it is clear that many organs – the intestines, the buccal cavity, the skin and the mucosal lining of the respiratory tract, which sheds 10 000 tiny bacteria-laden water droplets every minute – are home to a significant microbial population, and there is now evidence that many other tissues – bones, blood, joints and arterial cells – support bacterial populations of varying types.

Of all these locations, the gut is by far the most significant. The total bacterial population, weighing about 1.5 kg, coats the 300 m$^2$ interior lining of the intestine; this population is a complex and dynamic symbiotic living system, and is com-posed of a large and interacting group of bacterial species. Despite comprising few divisions, it is very diverse at the level of strain and subspecies, and is able to help protect the host from pathogenic intruders. During our first year, we humans quickly gain significant, stable microbial intestinal communities. Like the guts of ruminants and termites, our distal intestine (which contains most of our gut microbes) is, in ef-fect, a bacterially programmed anaerobic bioreactor which digests a wide variety of otherwise resistant polysaccharides, such as pectin, cellulose and certain starches.

Our gut microbiome is composed of different cell lineages and is able to com-municate with itself and with us. It consumes, stores and redistributes energy. It can maintain and repair itself through, and it has co-evolved with its host, com-plementing and manipulating human biology for the benefit of both host and mi-crobe. The collective genomes of the microbiome supplement our own genetics and metabolism, providing functionality, such as harvesting otherwise inaccessible nu-trients, which we have not needed to evolve ourselves. The microbiome may be seen as a microbial organ within the host. We are thus all a composite of not one but many species. We possess our own meta-genomes comprising genes from our own host genome and from that of our diverse microbial passengers. The microbiome, which may comprise over 100 times the number of host genes, imbues us with many additional functions. The implications for the human immune system are beginning to emerge, enlarging our picture of self versus non-self to include some or all of this microbial population.

## Cellular components of immunity

At yet another level, the immune system comprises mobile cells freely diffusing or undergoing chemotaxis. At the lowest and most fundamental level, immunity is the outcome of billions of interacting molecules of thousands of types. Much of the emergent behaviour characteristic of immune systems at the organismal level arises from this hierarchy of ascending levels.

The bone marrow is the principal source of adult immune cells, since all blood cells derive from the haematopoietic stem cells present there. Such cells include, amongst many others, B and T lymphocytes, the principal agents of adaptive immunity. Four main kinds of lymphocyte are now known: T cells, B cells, natural killer (NK) cells and regulatory T cells. Phagocytic mononuclear cells, such as macrophages and monocyte, also play a part in mediating immunity, ingesting antigens and becoming 'professional' APCs.

Macrophages and DCs are the main kinds of APC. Together DCs and macrophages form a vital link between innate and adaptive immunity. They can ingest foreign molecules, process them and then present the degraded or isolated products on the cell surface for inspection by T cells. As components of innate immunity, these cells organize and transfer information to adaptive immune cells.

Other, rather less prominent, examples of APC include monocytes, thymic endothelial cells and B cells. Circulating monocytes have the potential to leave the blood and migrate into tissues, where they are recruited to the site of inflammation, differentiating into DCs or macrophages.

Macrophages are one of the prime effector cells of innate immunity. They engulf or phagocytose microbes, secreting TNF alpha to enhance inflammation, destroying the invading pathogen and ultimately presenting the degraded microbial components to helper T cell surveillance. Macrophages typically reside in subepithelial connective tissue and lymph nodes where encounters with antigen are most probable.

Circulating DCs continually sense their environment using several mechanisms: primarily, receptor mediated endocytosis (where ligand bound receptors are internalized via clathrin-coated pits) and macropinocytosis (where surrounding medium is ingested). When a pathogen is encountered, DCs responds generically, triggering activation and maturation. They migrate via afferent lymphatic vessels to lymph nodes where processed microbial components – peptides, carbohydrates and lipids – are presented for immune surveillance by naïve T cells. DCs present degraded material in many ways, as determined by the kind of antigen encountered and the way the antigen interacted with PAMP receptors. This, and the number and variety of cytokines secreted, defines the exact outcome induced by the DC in lymph node B and T cells.

DCs also orchestrate the magnitude and nature of the adaptive response – antibody, cytotoxic T cell or regulatory T cell. This they do in two ways. First, they upregulate cell surface co-stimulatory signalling molecules and, secondly by producing cytokines. Antigen presentation by immature or nonactivated DCs will induce tolerance, while presentation by mature, activated DCs initiates antigen-specific adaptive immunity. We will discuss in greater detail the mechanisms of antigen presentation later.

B and T cells are the principal cellular protagonists of immunity. B cells arise in the bone marrow, have several subtypes and are activated by antigen. B cells are also stimulated by T cells. Once activated B cells proliferate, they move into the blood and rapidly generate large amounts of antibody. T cells recognize protein fragments and other molecules presented by other cells and are activated, proliferate and attack pathogens, as well as activating macrophages and other cells.

There are two types of T cell with distinct cell surface receptor populations: CD4+ and CD8+. CD8+ T cells or cytotoxic T lymphocytes (CTL) or killer T cells induce the lysis of infected cells; they function by seeking, locating and destroying such cells. Helper T cells are induced when naïve CD4+ T cells are stimulated by APCs, proliferating into functionally distinct T helper 1 (Th-1) or T helper 2 (Th-2) cells. Although helper T cell subsets also include Th-0 and Th-17, which preferentially secrete IL-17, the familiar Th-1 versus Th-2 dichotomy remains useful as a paradigm.

Th-1 cells activate macrophages, which are themselves infected or have engulfed microbes. They secrete interferon, cytokines and chemokines, attracting other leukocytes chemotactically, including macrophages and neutrophils, inducing localized inflammation. Th-1 cells induce B cells to manufacture subclasses of IgG antibodies. Th-2 cells secrete many cytokines, including IL-4 and IL-5. These act as B cell growth factors causing B cells to differentiate and produce large quantities of different types of antibodies, such as IgA, IgE and most subclasses of IgG. Th-2 cells also express CD40 ligand, which stimulates B cell proliferation.

Regulatory – or, originally, suppressor – T cells (also called Treg) now constitute an area of intense interest, as their potential importance in the control of immune responses has emerged. Tregs lack unequivocal markers making them hard to identify. For example, CD25, which is used to track Tregs, is also expressed on many other T cell types. Treg control mechanisms are mediated by suppressive cytokines IL-10 and TGF beta.

Natural killer (NK) cells are mainly found in the blood and spleen. NK cells can lyse virus-infected or malignant cells expressing aberrant amounts of MHC. They recognize the absence of molecular self by using inhibitory receptors that detect normal levels of MHC molecules. NK cells also possess activating receptors that recognize molecules that have been up-regulated in other cells. Many pathogens have evolved elegant and sophisticated virulence mechanisms that involve factors able to down-regulate MHC expression. This necessitates the evolution of immune mechanism able to monitor overall MHC expression. Other similar mechanisms include HLA-E, an invariant MHC-like molecule, which binds peptide derived from other MHC: reducing MHC synthesis will thus reduce HLA-E levels and the signals it delivers to its inhibitory receptor. HLA-E and HLA-G may also contact NK cells and inhibit NK-mediated cell lysis. Through recognition of invariant MHC-like proteins, NK cells effectively bridge innate and adaptive immunity.

# Cellular immunity

The binding of peptides presented by MHCs or lipids presented by CD1 by TCRs or the binding of conformational epitopes on whole protein antigens by soluble or membrane-anchored antibodies are the central recognition processes occurring in the adaptive immune response. They are not the only events involved but without them our immune systems would be almost ineffective. We will survey them in what follows. Yet, as we have said, most vaccines protect against disease through the induction of antibodies, yet responses to those target diseases for which we have as yet no effective vaccine are largely or completely mediated by cellular immunity. Thus our discussion here will address, in the main but certainly not exclusively, the biology of the cellular immune response as mediated by T cells. We will leave a more detailed discussion of humoral immunity until later.

An immunogen – a moiety exhibiting immunogenicity – is a substance which can elicit a specific immune response, while an antigen – a moiety exhibiting antigenicity – is a substance recognized by an existing immune response and associated molecules such as T cells or antibodies in a recall response. Immunogenicity is the most important and interesting property for vaccine design and discovery. Put at its most simple, immunogenicity is that property of a molecular, or supramolecular, moiety that allows it to induce a significant response from the immune system. Here a molecular moiety may be a protein, lipid, carbohydrate or some combination thereof and a supramolecular moiety may be a virus, bacteria or protozoan parasite.

As has already been said, cellular immunity is mediated by T cells, which patrol the body constantly seeking proteins originating in pathogens. Their surfaces are enriched by a particular receptor protein: the T cell receptor or TCR. TCRs are able to identify non-self by discriminating size, shape and charge. They function by binding to MHCs expressed on the surfaces of other cells, particularly APCs. MHCs bind small peptide fragments derived by proteolytic cleavage of both host and pathogen proteins.

Formation of this ternary complex lies at the heart of cellular immunity, as it leads to activation of the T cell, which then signals to the wider immune system that a pathogen has been encountered. An activated T cell, which will mature, replicate and enter circulation, is said to be 'primed' and will respond to the same molecular pattern if it encounters the same pathogen, or a similar one, again. T cells can be deceived into recognizing disease-causing organisms if this pattern is presented first as part of a vaccine rather than as part of a pathogen.

# The T cell repertoire

The adaptive immune system is diverse on a vast scale. The clearly combinatorial nature of immunology compounds the immanent problems of receptor specificity. There are some $10^{12}$ T-cells in a human individual. The potential number of amino acid epitopes of length 9, is of the order $10^{11}$. The number of class I alleles of human

MHC molecules exceeds 500 thus allowing for a theoretical $10^{13}$ different class I haplotypes. The number of potentially distinct TCRs within the human T cell repertoire has been estimated to lie somewhere between $10^7$ and $10^{15}$. The vast enormity of the T cell mediated immune system underlies its ability to discriminate between so-called self peptides and those originating in pathogenic microorganisms.

The T cell repertoire is very large, diverse and also, in terms of its dominant recognition properties, highly dependent on environmental factors, particularly infection and vaccination histories. Sir MacFarlane Burnet's 1957 Clonal Selection Theory introduced clonal expansion through proliferation as the means by which the immune system is able to muster vast numbers of diverse antigen reactive cells from a small set of precursors.

T cells have their genesis in the bone marrow and then migrate to the thymus. T cells with receptors recognizing MHC-antigen complexes survive and mature, while T cells without such receptors are destroyed in the thymus. Several mechanisms act to remove potentially damaging self-reactive immune cells: naïve T cells recognize self-MHC molecules (positive selection) but do not recognize complexes between self-peptide and MHC molecules (negative selection). Such mechanisms of themselves offer, at best, a partial and incomplete explanation for repertoire selection. Thymic repertoire selection remains the most crucial component in controlling self-reactivity.

Most T cells produced during gestation and infancy are discarded in childhood. About 1% of initial T cells become part of the mature repertoire – the rest are lost. This prevents the immune system from becoming overly aggressive. Faults in this mechanism may contribute to autoimmune disease. Mature T cells concentrate in the spleen and lymph nodes. Adaptive responses begin in lymph nodes; they are the meeting point for the naïve T and B cell repertoire, which continuously recirculates through the lymphatic system and blood.

Control is also exercised over adaptive immunity by *peripheral tolerance*, which entails generating immunosuppressive regulatory T cells. Alternative mechanisms are labelled 'anergy'; they involve reducing T cell sensitivity to ligand stimulation. Anergy arises when T cells are activated without co-stimulation, which can make them unresponsive to previous active stimuli. Antigen stimulation without co-stimulation can also engender T cell death or regulatory T cell formation.

## Epitopes: The immunological quantum

Immunologists usually refer to the short peptides which are bound by MHC, and are then recognized by the TCR, as epitopes. As the principal components of both subunit and poly-epitopic vaccines, much of immunoinformatics is concerned with the accurate identification of epitopes, the principal chemical moieties recognized by the immune system. Although the importance of nonpeptide epitopes, such as carbohydrates and lipids, is now increasingly well understood, peptidic B cell and T cell epitopes remain the principal goal.

T cell epitopes are short peptides bound by major histocompatibility complexes (MHC) and subsequently recognized by T cells. B cell epitopes are regions of the surface of a protein, or other biomacromolecule, recognized by soluble or membrane-bound antibody molecules. It is the recognition of epitopes by T cells, B cells and soluble antibodies that lies at the heart of the immune response which, in turn, leads to activation of the cellular and humoral immune systems and, ultimately, to the effective destruction of pathogenic organisms. The accurate prediction of B cell and T cell epitopes is thus the pivotal challenge for immunoinformatics.

# The major histocompatibility complex

Epitopes or antigenic peptides are presented by APCs for inspection by T cells via antigen-presenting proteins of the MHC. Humans' MHC are often called HLA, which is commonly assumed to mean human leukocyte antigen, though this attribution is probably erroneous. MHC or HLA genes are located within the somewhat confusingly named MHC region. The MHC region in humans is an approximately 2 centimorgan long, 3.6 Mb region of genomic DNA located on the short arm of chromosome 6 at 6p21.31. The human MHC is believed to be the genomic region with currently the highest known gene density. The MHC is divided into three subregions: class II (centromeric), class III and class I (telomeric). A total of 224 genes has been identified in this region, of which 128 were expected to be expressed. Of these expressed genes, around 40% appeared to have a clear function within the immune system. The human MHC region has six loci encoding class I and II HLA alleles. The first three loci – HLA-DP, HLA-DR and HLA-DQ – encode class II HLA alleles, while the final three loci – HLA-A, HLA-B and HLA-C – encode class I HLA alleles. Six minor loci have also been identified: HLA-E, HLA-F, HLA-G and HLA-H for class I and HLA-DN and HLA-DO for class II. A similar MHC region is found on chromosome 17 in mice. Mouse MHC is about 1.5 centimorgan long and is divided into three loci H-2K, D and L.

Each human class I locus is made of eight exons split by seven introns. Exon 1 encodes the leading sequence, which is cleaved during post-translation modification. The three extracellular domains $\alpha 1$, $\alpha 2$ and $\alpha 3$ are encoded by exons 2 to 4. Exon 5 encodes the transmembrane helix and exons 6 to 8 encode the cytoplasmic tail. Genes on the minor loci produce the so-called nonclassical MHC proteins, which are not involved in CD4 and CD8 T cell activation.

The DP, DR and DQ loci of class II MHC are in pairs, which may come from gene duplication. Each pair encodes one $\alpha$ and one $\beta$ chain of the class II MHC protein. Each major locus of class I MHC encodes a single polypeptide ($\alpha$ chain), which binds to $\beta 2$-microglobulin in the ER and forms the HLA complex. $\beta 2$-microglobulin is encoded separately on chromosome 15. Both class I and II loci are highly polymorphic, with alleles in the thousands. The most polymorphic region is found in the $\alpha$ chains of both class I and II MHC and $\beta$ chains of class II MHC. Some non-MHC proteins are encoded in between the class I and class II regions, such as proteins of the complement system C2, C4 and factor B. These proteins have limited polymorphism and participate in the innate immune system response.

Thus far, the HLA region appears to be the most polymorphic part of the human genome. However, this may simply result from the tendentious nature of scientific enquiry. We look for the things we look for; we often find what we find. This is a rather gnomic way of saying that unless we look systematically at everything everywhere we are likely to miss much of interest and gain a much distorted view of how things actually are. Other regions of the human genome, such as those which encode GPCRs, are known to demonstrate significant levels of allelic variation in their own right. As we shall see, the transplantation of human organs and bone marrow has lead to the typing of MHC genes on a large scale and this has resulted in the accumulation of large registries containing variant MHC gene sequences or alleles. Within a single species an allele is a member of a set of several different yet very similar variant genes at one genetic locus: in principle, within a population, every gene will exist as several alleles.

Compared, say, to a TCR or antibody, the selectivity exhibited by an MHC molecule is determined solely by its inherited structure. As a germ-line gene product, an MHC molecule undergoes no somatic hyper mutation, affinity maturation or thymic selection and is, as part of a restricted set of alleles, an inherited characteristic of individual organisms. However, in humans, as in most other species, the MHC is both polygenic (there are several genetic loci representing MHC class I and class II genes) and polymorphic (there are multiple alleles of each gene). All MHC loci are co-dominant: both maternally and paternally inherited sets of alleles are expressed. When genes on one chromosome are inherited together, like class I and class II MHCs, the linked set is called a haplotype.

An individual will inherit one MHC haplotype from each genetic parent, containing three class I (HLA-A, B and C) and class II (HLA-DP, DR and DQ) loci. Thus an individual will have a maximum of six different class I specificities. An individual heterozygous for all six MHC loci can express 12 HLA molecules per cell. The situation is complicated further for class II HLA, since such alleles consists of an $\alpha$ chain and a $\beta$ chain, one from each parent; thus more than six pairs can be expressed per cell. Occasionally a crossover occurs between the parental chromosomes and this generates new haplotypes with mixed specificity that also contributes to the HLA heterogeneity in the population.

MHCs exhibit extreme polymorphism: within the human population there are, at each genetic locus, a great number of alleles. So far six isoforms of HLA class I molecules have been identified and those include the classical HLA-A, -B and -C, and the nonclassical HLA-E, -F and -G. The classical class I MHC is highly polymorphic, whereas the nonclassical MHC exhibits very restricted polymorphism. For the HLA class II molecules five isoforms have been identified, including the classical HLA-DR, -DQ and -DP, and the nonclassical HLA-DM and -DO. As of January 2007, there are 1633 alleles for the classical human class I MHC: 506 different alleles at the HLA-A locus, 851 alleles for HLA-B and 276 for HLA-C. For the nonclassical MHC: nine HLA-E alleles, 21 alleles for HLA-F and 23 for HLA-G. For the classical human class II MHC there is a total of 826 alleles: three for HLA-DRA, 559 alleles for HLA-DRB, 34 for HLA-DQA1, 81 for HLA-DQB1, 23 for HLA-DPA1 and 126 for HLA-DPB1. For the nonclassical human class II MHC, there are 4 four alleles for HLA-DMA, seven for HLA-DMB, 12 for HLA-DOA and nine for HLA-DOB. Many of these alleles are presented at a significant frequency ($>1\%$) within the human population. The four main mechanisms responsible for creating new MHC alleles are point substitution, allele conversion, gene conversion and recombination.

## MHC nomenclature

The WHO Nomenclature Committee gives each new human allele a name, which is defined using a common template. Each allele will thus have a unique four, six or eight digit number or name. All alleles have at least a four digit name, six and eight digit tags only being assigned where necessary. At the simplest level, the adopted nomenclature takes the following form: HLA-locus*allele. HLA is a prefix which indicates that the gene comes from the HLA region. The locus is one of the restricted set of human MHC loci, such as HLA-A or HLA-DRB1. The first two digits of the allele identifier correspond to the type, which is typically the HLA serotype. The third and fourth digits list the subtype, the individual numbers being assigned in the order in which DNA sequences was submitted. For HLA-A*0101: the HLA-A refers to the HLA locus (the A locus in this case); the first 01 to the serologically-recognized A1 antigen and the final 01 to the individual HLA allele protein sequence. Similarly for class II: HLA-DRB1*0701 is the 0701 allele encoded by the DRB locus. Alleles with differences in the first four digits will have one or more nucleotide substitutions that alter the amino acid sequence of the translated protein product. As many alleles are encoded by the same locus, the allele number varies from 0101 to 8001. For various reasons, MHC alleles are often reported, at least for the purposes of epitope identification, as either a two-digit name or serotype (e.g. HLA-A2) or as a four-digit name (HLA-A*0201). A four-digit HLA name necessarily implies the two-digit serological antigen; a two-digit classification clearly does not imply a specific allele.

The nomenclature has recently been extended to include subsidiary numbers beyond the familiar four-digit code which refer to null sequences, synonymous mutations and mutations outside the coding region. This makes the resulting MHC nomenclature more complex, and includes information on nucleic acid differences in both exons and introns which have no effect on the final amino acid sequence. Alleles that have synonymous, silent or noncoding substitutions within the exons of their coding nucleotide sequence are given an extra fifth and sixth digits, e.g. HLA-DRB1*130102. Alleles that have sequence changes in their introns or in the untranslated regions upstream or downstream of the coding region are annotated through the use of seventh and eight digits, e.g. HLA-DRB1*13010102.

Additional optional suffixes may be added to an allele name to indicate its expression status. Alleles with alternative expression are labelled: 'N', 'S', 'L', 'Q', 'C' or 'A'. Null alleles that are known not to be expressed are given the suffix 'N', e.g. HLA-A*2409N. 'S' denotes an allele which is expressed as a soluble 'secreted' molecule and is absent from the cell surface, e.g. HLA-B*44020102S. 'L' indicates an allele with 'low' cell surface expression compared to normal, e.g. HLA-A*3014L. 'Q' indicates an allele where expression is 'questionable', since its mutation usually down-regulates expression levels, e.g. HLA-A*3211Q. 'C' indicates an allele present in the 'cytoplasm' and not on the cell surface. 'A' denotes 'aberrant' expression where a protein may or may not be produced. No 'C' or 'A' labels have been assigned to date. Data on null sequences and synonymous mutations do not change the amino acid sequence of the expressed MHC molecule and thus do not affect peptide binding and so can be omitted for the purposes of epitope discovery.

## Peptide binding by the MHC

The proteins of the MHC are grouped into two classes on the basis of their three-dimensional structure and biological properties. Class I molecules generally, but not exclusively, present endogenous peptides derived from the cytoplasm of cells. Class I MHCs form a complex population of peptides on the cell surface which is dominated by a combination of self and viral peptides. Class II molecules generally, but not exclusively, present endocytosed exogenous peptides derived from extracellular proteins often of pathogenic origin. However, the overall process leading to the presentation of antigen-derived epitopes on the surface of cells is a long, complicated and not yet fully understood story. We will say more about the interplay between MHC-mediated antigen presentation pathways – so-called cross presentation – below. With the notable exceptions of neuronal and red blood cells, Class I MHCs are expressed by almost all cells in the body. Class I MHCs are recognized by T cells whose surfaces are rich in CD8 co-receptor protein. Class II MHCs are recognized by T cells whose surfaces are rich in CD4 co-receptors and they are only expressed on APCs.

MHCs bind peptides, which are themselves derived through the proteolytic degradation of proteins. MHC class I ligands are derived from endogenous proteins and are typically eight to 11 amino acids long. However, there is now accumulating evidence that longer peptides (13 to 15 amino acids and above) are presented by class I MHCs in many – possibly all – vertebrates including humans, mice, cattle and horses. MHC class II ligands have a more variable length of nine to 25 amino acids and are derived from exogenous proteins. Class I MHC molecules have a binding cleft which is closed at both ends; they are thus constrained to bind shorter peptides. Class II MHC molecules have, on the other hand, a groove which is open at both ends; this allows much larger peptides of varying – indeed potentially unlimited – length to bind. MHCs are not, however, indiscriminate binders, but importantly exhibit a finely tuned yet complex specificity for particular peptide sequences whose sequences are composed of the 20 commonly occurring amino acids.

MHCs also display a wider specificity which is in itself quite catholic in terms of the molecules they can bind; MHCs are not restricted solely to peptides, they also bind a variety of other molecules. Peptides bearing diverse post-translational modifications (PTMs) can also form pMHCs and be recognized by TCRs. Such PTMs include phosphorylation, lipidation and, most importantly, glycosylation. This is especially true for glycopeptides where the carbohydrate chain is short and does not impede peptide–MHC interaction. O-linked glycans survive class II processing, do not interfere with antigen presentation and are presented effectively to T-cells, with carbohydrates forming parts of epitopes recognized by T cells. MHCs also bind other molecules such as chemically modified peptides and synthetically derived peptide mimetics. Even small molecule drug-like compounds bind MHCs; this can mediate pathological effects and has important implications in behaviour-modifying odour recognition.

## The structure of the MHC

Both classes of MHC molecule have similar three-dimensional structures. Class I molecules are composed of a heavy chain in complex with $\beta$2-microglobulin. Class II molecules consist of two chains ($\alpha$ and $\beta$) of similar size (Figure 3.1). The MHC peptide-binding site consists of a $\beta$-sheet, forming the base, flanked by two $\alpha$-helices, which together form a narrow cleft or groove accommodating bound peptides. The principal difference between the two classes is the shape and size of the peptide-binding groove. MHC alleles may differ by as many as 30 amino acid substitutions. Such an uncommon degree of polymorphism implies a selective pressure to create and maintain it. Different polymorphic MHC alleles, of both class I and class II, have different peptide specificities: each allele binds peptides exhibiting particular sequence patterns.

The major part of class I HLA molecules consists of a heavy chain of 44 KD. This is formed from a short intracellular tail of 30–35 amino acids at the C terminus, a single 25 amino acid membrane crossing region and an extracellular region which contains the peptide binding site. In general, MHC crystal structures are produced by expressing soluble constructs that lack the hydrophobic transmembrane region and cytoplasmic tail. The extracellular region is itself divided into three nominal domains: $\alpha$1, $\alpha$2 and $\alpha$3, each of which is around 90 amino acids in length. This particular designation is another example of nomenclature derived from somewhat sloppy thinking.

The three domains defined by sequence analysis do not correspond to the two structural domains apparent in the extracellular region of MHC crystal structures. We are obliged, I am afraid, to retain use of this nomenclature in order to remain

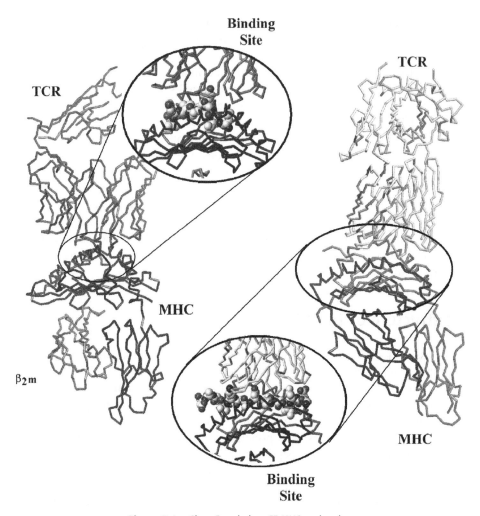

**Figure 3.1**   Class I and class II MHC molecules

consistent, not with what we think to be true and independently verifiable, but with the extant immunological literature. Sequence alignment of MHCs from several species suggests the three $\alpha$ pseudodomains are conserved, but that the transmembrane region and cytopolasmic tail vary greatly.

MHC crystal structures show the true structural-domain: sequence-defined $\alpha1$ and $\alpha2$ domains are connected by a short linker to the $\alpha3$ domain. The heavy chain is attached noncovalently to a light chain, a 12 KD protein called $\beta2$-microglobulin or $\beta_2$m, to form the complete MHC complex. The structures of the $\alpha3$ domain and $\beta_2$m are similar, both possessing an immunoglobulin fold. Both the $\alpha3$ domain and $\beta_2$m consist of two antiparallel $\beta$ sheets, one with four strands and the other with three, linked by a disulphide bond.

# Antigen presentation

Where do MHC-bound peptides originate? This is a simple and straightforward question without a simple, straightforward answer. There are many alternative processing pathways, but we shall concentrate on the two best-understood types: the classical class I and the classical class II. Class I peptides are derived from intracellular sources, and targeted to the proteasome, which cuts them into short peptides. These peptides are then bound by the transmembrane peptide transporter, TAP, which translocates them from the cell cytoplasm to the endoplasmic reticulum where they are bound by class I MHCs. In the class II pathway, following the receptor-mediated endocytosis of exogenous antigens by APCs, presented proteins pass first into endosomes, then into late endosomes, and end up in lysosomes. While in transit, antigens are proteolytically fragmented into peptides by cathepsins. Before final cell surface presentation, peptides are bound by class II MHCs. Crosspresentation, an endogenous route acting via class II and an exogenous one via class I, is an important, if complicating, phenomenon and is beginning to be better understood.

MHC class I ligands are derived primarily from endogenously expressed proteins. Intracellular peptide fragments arise from two sources: self-peptides derived from the host genome and peptides from external sources such as pathogenic microbes. Intracellular proteins, including newly synthesized proteins, are degraded quickly, producing large amounts of short peptides. Nonfunctional proteins, or defective ribosomal products (DRiP), result from errors in translation and processing. They form a significant proportion of newly synthesized proteins, which are rapidly digested by the proteasome. Viruses can invade host cells and generate viral proteins and bacteria can inject protein into the host cell via the type III secretion system; both are also degraded by the host.

# The proteasome

Intracellular protein degradation is mediated by a multiprotein complex called the proteasome. A whole variety of proteins including heat-denatured proteins, incorrectly assembled, mistranslated or misfolded proteins, as well as regulatory proteins with limited half-lives, are targeted by the proteasome. For antigenic proteins, it favours oxidized protein substrates, since about 75% of oxidized intracellular proteins are degraded by proteasomes and the 20S proteasome prefers partially denatured oxidized proteins.

The proteasome is a multimeric proteinase comprising a core of proteolytic enzymes flanked by a complex arrangement of regulatory elements able to recognize, amongst other things, a ubiquitin label. The proteosome has a site with trypsin-like activity (cleavage after basic residues), another with chymotrypsin-like activity (cleavage after hydrophobic residues) and yet another with peptidylglutamyl-peptide hydrolytic activity (cleavage after acidic residues).

There are several different forms of the proteasome found in the cell, including the three most crucial: the most basic form, the 20S core proteasome; the ATP-stimulated 26S proteasome; and the so-called immunoproteasome. Vertebrate immunoproteasomes are assembled from three $\gamma$-interferon-inducible subunits that replace the constitutive subunits of the 20S version. The immunoproteasome has an altered hierarchy of proteosomal cleavage, enhancing cleavage after basic and hydrophobic residues and inhibiting cleavage after acidic residues. This is in accord with C-terminal amino acid preferences for class I MHC binding.

Misfolded, unfolded or short-lived proteins are earmarked for destruction in eukaryotic cells by the attachment of small polymeric chains of ubiquitin, a small, highly conserved protein. The ubiquitin-proteasome system is an essential component of the cell's sophisticated quality control mechanisms necessary for proper maintenance of homeostasis. The ATP driven process of ubiquitination begins by forming a thiol-ester bond between the terminal carboxyl group of ubiquitin and the activated cysteine of the ubiquitin-activating enzyme, usually known as E1. Ubiquitin is then transferred to an ubiquitin-conjugating enzyme, called E2. Ubiquitin protein ligase, also referred to as E3, facilitates the transfer of ubiquitin to a lysine residue on the substrate protein. Additional ubiquitins are then added at lysine 48, again by E3, to form a polymeric chain; a length of four appears to be optimal. Ubiquitin protein ligases impose specificity on the process by bringing together substrate protein and the E2 enzyme. Polymeric ubiquitin chains can be linked not only via lysine 48 but also via other lysine residues. These variant ubiquitins divert protein substrates to fulfil diverse functions: DNA repair, mitochondrial inheritance and also for cell uptake by endocytosis.

The mammalian 20S proteasome is a large, supra-molecular complex consisting of 14 copies of the $\alpha$ subunit and 14 copies of the $\beta$ subunit. This structure is responsible for degrading protein originating in both the cytosol and nucleus. Proteasome crystal structures reveal it to possess a cylindrical structure formed from four rings, one stacked upon another, composed of subunits arranged in an $\alpha7\beta7\beta7\alpha7$ order. The active sites of the proteasome's proteolytic enzymes are found on the $\beta$ subunit on the inner face of the cylinder. The rings of $\alpha$ subunits form a barrier through which unfolded polypeptides enter; they also form the binding site of proteasome activator 28 (PA28). Access to the proteasome's inner compartment is controlled by the 19S regulator, a gatekeeper who only allows ubiquitin-bound protein to enter.

The exact mechanism of proteasome cleavage is unclear, although enzyme-mediated protein cleavage seems to occur via the sliding of unfolded protein through the proteasome. The position of the peptide in the protein and the nature of adjacent sequences determine some of the specificity of proteasome cleavage. In one experiment, a nonameric murine cytomegalovirus epitope was not cleaved when inserted into the hepatitis B virus protein, but was cleaved when a polyalanine peptide was inserted next to it. There is much evidence to suggest that the proteasome is responsible for generating the C terminus but not the N terminus of the final presented peptide. The active sites of the proteasome have different specificities for the P1 residue of the peptide. The mammalian proteasome also cleaves after small neutral residues and after branched amino acids. Analysis of naturally cleaved peptides indicates that the residues on either side of the C-terminus and up to five residues flanking the N terminus can be related to proteasome cleavage.

# Transporter associated with antigen processing

After peptides are degraded by the proteasome, they are transferred into the lumen of the endoplasmic reticulum (ER). The translocation process from cytosol to ER consumes ATP. The so-called transporter associated with antigen processing (TAP) is required for peptide transit. TAP also has the ability to interact with peptide-free class I HLA molecules in the ER. After peptides associate with class I HLA molecules, the resulting complexes are released from TAP and are translocated to the cell surface.

TAP protein is a heterodimer and consists of TAP1 and TAP2. Both proteins are part of a family known as the ABC transporters. TAP is an example of a protein in antigen presentation which is encoded in the class II region. TAP1 and TAP2 associate in the ER and form the TAP heterodimer. The central region of the TAP protein is likely to be the binding site as polymorphic residues in rat TAP2 have been shown to contact the peptide and influence peptide selection and transport. The binding of peptides to TAP does not require ATP, while transport across the ER membrane does.

Immunology dogma suggests that newly synthesized class I MHC molecules are not stable in a peptide-free state and are retained in the ER in a partially folded form. Several chaperone proteins are needed to complete MHC folding. Newly synthesized MHC main chain is associated with a chaperone called calnexin, which is a transmembrane protein. It holds MHC molecules inside the ER. Calnexin may not be an absolute requirement for the assembly of MHC molecules as HLA molecules can be expressed in cell lines lacking calnexin. The immunoglobulin binding protein, or BiP, has a related function to that of calnexin, and may indeed replace it in the cell. When an MHC molecule has bound to $\beta_2$-microglobulin, it is released from calnexin and binds to two other proteins: tapasin and calreticulin (another chaperone which a function related to that of calnexin). After peptide binding, calreticulin and tapasin dissociate from the fully folded MHC molecule. Once complexed to peptide and $\beta_2$-microglobulin, the MHC protein leaves the ER and is transported to the cell surface. The peptide binding process is considered as the rate-limiting step of antigen presentation as only a fraction of peptides can bind to MHC.

# Class II processing

In the MHC class II processing pathway, receptor mediated endocytosis of extracellular protein is followed by targeting to the multi-compartment lysosomal-endosomal apparatus. Within APCs, MHC class II heterodimers are cosynthesized with the so-called invariant chain (Ii): this obligate chaperone controls the intracel-lular trafficking of class II MHC molecules and helps regulate the binding of pep-tides by class II MHC. The repertoire of peptides presented by APCs is contingent upon the stepwise proteolytic degradation of Ii to CLIP, the smallest fragment still able to bind class II-MHC. Another chaperone, HLA-DM, catalyses the exchange between CLIP complexed to MHC and degraded peptides.

Peptide display is also dependent on the processing of proteins into peptides within the endosomal and lysosomal compartments. Here proteins, including those derived from pathogens, are degraded by cathepsins, a particular type of protease. Class II MHCs then bind these peptides and are subsequently transported to the cell surface. The peptide specificity of protein cleavage by cathepsins has also been investigated and simple cleavage motifs are now known. However, more pre-cise investigations are required before accurate predictive methods can be real-ized. Much still remains to be discovered in terms of the mechanism of class II presentation.

## Seek simplicity and then distrust it

However, there are a number of other processing routes that complicate the simple picture outlined above. It is clear that cleavage by the proteasome is not the only proteolytic event in antigen presentation. These include TAP-independent Trojan antigen presentation and the involvement of various other proteases, such as furin. Peptides cleaved by the proteasome are three to 25 amino acids long, while most class I MHC epitopes are less than 15 amino acids long. Only about 15% of those peptides which are degraded by the proteasome are of the appropriate length for class I MHC binding. 70% of peptides are too short and 15% are too long. Long peptides may be trimmed to the correct size by various cellular peptidases. Analyses of peptide generation and T-cell epitopes expression in proteasome-inhibited cells suggest that cytoplasmic proteases other than proteasomes may also be involved in antigen processing pathway.

Peptides are digested in the cytosol by several peptidases such as leucine aminopeptidase (LAP), tripeptidyl peptidase II (TPPII), thimet oligopeptidease (TOP), bleomycin hydrolase (BH) and puromycin-sensitive aminopeptidease (PSA). Tripeptidylpeptidase II (TPPII) was suggested to be a peptide supplier be-cause of its ability to cleave peptides *in vitro* and its upregulation in cells surviv-ing partial proteasome inhibition. Leucine aminopeptidase was found to generate antigenic peptides from N-terminally extended precursors. Puromycin sensitive an-imopeptidase and bleomycin hydrolase were shown to trim the N termini of syn-thetic peptides. Recently, an enzyme located in the ER and named ERAAP (ER aminopeptidase associated with antigen processing) or ERAP1, was proven to be responsible for the final trimming of the N termini of peptides presented by MHC class I molecules. However, currently there are insufficient quantitative data about the role of these proteases to allow a precise bioinformatic evaluation of their

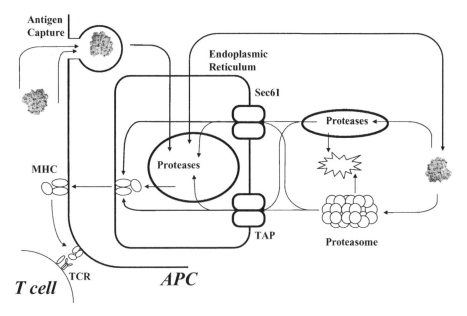

**Figure 3.2**  Class I antigen presentation pathway

impact on the antigen processing pathway. Alternatives to TAP are also now coming to light, such as Sec61, which also effects retrograde transport back into the
cytoplasm from the ER (Figure 3.2).

## Cross presentation

Another complicating feature germane to this discussion is the issue of cross presentation. This is again immunology jargon and really refers to the conceptually
unalarming observation that the class I and class II pathways are not distinct but
are actually interconnected or, at least, leaky, allowing peptides from one pathway
access to the other. In the MHC class I pathway, peptides are generated by various
flavours of proteosome and other major proteases, like TPII, in the cytosol. Recently identified amino-terminal peptidases in both the cytoplasm and the ER then
trim these peptides. This process roughly parallels endosomal processing, in which
endo-proteolysis is followed by amino- and carboxy-terminal trimming. Many peptides can escape from the endosome and pass into the cytoplasm where they enter
the familiar class I pathway comprising the proteasome, TAP and MHC. Likewise,
endogenously expressed cytosolic and nuclear antigens access MHC class II via a
number of intracellular autophagic pathways, including macroautophagy, microautophagy and chaperone-mediated autophagy. Macroautophagy is characterized by
the formation of autophagosomes, double-membrane structures which capture proteins from the cytoplasm, processing them via acidic proteases and eventually fuse

with lysosomes. Microautophagy involves lysosomal invagination which directly sequesters cytoplasmic proteins. During receptor-mediated autophagy, proteases in the cytosol produce peptides that are translocated into lysosomes. These three processes all probably deliver cytoplasmic proteins and/or peptides to endosomal compartments for binding by MHC class II.

# T cell receptor

It is now generally accepted that only peptides that bind to MHC at an affinity above a certain threshold will act as T cell epitopes and that, at least broadly, peptide affinity for the MHC correlates with T cell response. The recognition process itself involves the formation of a ternary complex between an MHC protein, its peptide ligand and a TCR. Like MHCs, TCR molecules are transmembrane glycoproteins. TCR molecules consist of two polypeptide chains, $\alpha$ and $\beta$, although a small percentage of TCRs have $\gamma$ and $\delta$ chains instead. $\gamma\delta$ T cells are mainly expressed in the intestinal epithelium, the skin and the pulmonary epithelium. $\gamma\delta$ T cells function differently; it remains open to debate if they recognize antigens directly.

$\alpha\beta$ T cells can be divided into two groups depending on which glycoproteins – CD8 or CD4 – are expressed on their surface. TCR is associated with the CD3 complex, which consists of four invariant polypeptide chains two $\varepsilon$, one $\delta$ and one $\gamma$. CD3 is coexpressed with the TCR. CD3 helps transport TCR to the cell surface and is involved in intra-cellular signalling when the TCR recognizes MHC-peptide complexes.

While the heterodimeric structure of the T cell receptor appears similar to that of an immunoglobulin Fab fragment, differences in the precise geometry are apparent upon closer inspection. The two variable (V) domains (V$\alpha$ and V$\beta$) and two constant (C) domains (C$\alpha$ and C$\beta$) are similarly situated: each polypeptide chain has a variable (V) region at the N-terminus and a constant (C) region at the C-terminus; the association of the TCR $\alpha$ and $\beta$ chains being reminiscent of the L and H chain pairing of Fabs. $\zeta$ domains are involved in intracellular signal transmission. The TCR proteins are produced by gene rearrangements which are similar to those that generate the immunoglobulins. The $\alpha$ chain is produced by the rearrangement of the variable (V) and the joining (J) segment. The $\beta$ chain is generated by the rearrangement of the variable (V), diversity (D) and joining (J) segments. The rearranged genes are attached to the constant (C) gene to form the complete $\alpha$ and $\beta$ chains.

The constant region is composed of the transmembrane region and the cytoplasmic tail. The two chains are linked by a disulphide bridge at the hinge region connecting the C region and the transmembrane region. Because of low sequence identity, C$\alpha$ domain structure deviates from the established immunoglobulin fold in a number of ways: loss of a conserved tryptophan, different number of amino acids between conserved cysteines, and so on. The net result is that the top strands do not hydrogen-bond into a continuous sheet and may be somewhat pliable facilitating the TCR interaction with CD3. Compared with Fabs, for example, the TCR constant domains have a larger buried surface area and a much more polar interface: charges at the interface are acidic for $C\alpha$ and more basic for $C\beta$. Perhaps the most interesting feature of the $C\alpha$ domains is the large 14-residue FG loop, which extends from both domains and adopts roughly similar conformations in all of the structures, although its actual position varies. This loop appears relatively rigid, owing to a small hydrophobic core, but its exact function has yet to be defined, although it has been proposed to facilitate TCR interaction with co-receptors and CD3. TCR have V regions similar to the Fab part of the antibody, adopting an immunoglobulin fold with two $\beta$ sheets packed tightly against each other. TCR variable (V) domains are highly similar to antibody variable domains. The orientation and buried surface area observed for $V\alpha/V\beta$ interfaces spans a wide range, but correlates well with values seen for known Fab V L /V H pairings. The interface is composed of a core of 24 conserved residues similar to those seen in antibodies but is more symmetrical.

The contact site between the TCR and the MHC complex is in the V region, formed by peptide loops. TCR binding sites for peptide-MHC complexes are formed from three hypervariable regions on $\alpha$ and $\beta$ chains; these so-called complementarity-determining regions (CDRs) resemble those of immunoglobulins. These hypervariable complementarity-determining regions (CDR1, CDR2 and CDR3) form the contact site between TCR and pMHC complex. The combining sites of TCRs are quite flat, similar to antiprotein antibodies and consistent with the TCR's function of binding the relatively flat surface of the peptide-MHC complex. CDR3 is the most variable and is considered to be responsible for TCR specificity. CDR3 has contact with P5 to P8 of the peptide in the crystal structure. Mutations on the CDR3 loops can abolish MHC-peptide recognition. CDR1 loops contact the N terminus residues of the peptide and CDR2 loops cover the C terminus of the peptide. The positions of the CDRs within the TCR binding site are all similar to antibodies except for CDR2, which undergoes a strand switch in $V\alpha$ and occasionally in $V\beta$. Analysis of the known structures of $V\alpha$ and $V\beta$ domains indicates that their first and second hypervariable regions have one of three or four different main-chain canonical structures: approximately 70 % of $V\alpha$ segments and 90 % of $V\beta$ segments have hypervariable regions with a known canonical structure. Six of these canonical structures have the same conformation in isolated V domains, the free receptor or in peptide-MHC complexes. The conformation of the first two hypervariable regions is one drawn from a small subset of canonical structures. It is well defined and is conserved on complex formation.

TCRs recognize class I MHC and class II MHCs and form distinct tertiary structures in each case. Currently a wider range of complexes are available for class I while complexes with class II complexes are a more recent development. TCRs make a diagonal footprint on the surface of the class I peptide-MHC complex. This enables the TCR to interact with the relatively conserved MHC molecule and discriminate between antigenic peptides. The $V\alpha$ domain contacts the amino-terminus of the peptide and the $V\beta$ domain contacts the carboxy-terminus of the peptide and certain surrounding MHC residues. Changes in CDR loop conformation are an important mechanism expanding TCR specificity. The range of $V\alpha/V\beta$ pairings is an additional mechanism of expanding the TCR recognition repertoire. For class I complexes, TCR–MHC binding is not parallel, but is about 20–30° towards the diagonal. A hydrophobic pocket is formed above the binding site between residue 93–104 of the $\alpha$ chain and 95–107 of the $\beta$ chain, which could accommodate a side chain of the peptide. The more genetically diverse regions of the TCR – CDRs 3 and 4 – interact in a direct manner with the peptide bound by the MHC. The other CDRs interact with the surface helices of the MHC molecule. The orientation of the footprint does vary considerably, but is distinct from class II MHC–TCR, where the orientation is more orthogonal and conserved. Bound peptide side chains that face out of the MHC groove are likely to make similar interactions with TCRs. The MHC helices dominate the TCR–MHC interface allowing discrimination between bound peptides. $V\alpha$ is predominant in steering the TCR–peptide–MHC orientation, as known structures have very similar locations for the footprint of $V\alpha$ on the MHC.

The TCR repertoire is comparable to that of antibodies, at least in terms of the scale of how extensive and diverse it is. Moreover, it is coupled to an MHC polymorphism that alters the size and diversity of antigenic peptides presented for inspection by the TCR. However, although assembled by genetic recombination of V, D, J and C segments, TCRs do not undergo the same affinity maturation experienced by antibodies. Thus with affinities usually in the low micromolar range, TCR–MHC binding is much weaker than that of antibody complexes, yet great specificity arises from the small differences in peptide structure compared to the relatively conserved, yet polymorphic, surface of the MHC.

## T cell activation

The activation of the T cell which results from formation of the MHC–peptide–TCR complex is enhanced by other protein–protein interactions between cells. These involve a whole array of other molecules both on the cell surface and inside the cell, including CD3, CD45, CD28, CD8 or CD4 co-receptors, different lipid rafts, components of the cytoskeleton and a whole tranche of intracellular signalling molecules. TCR recognition of class I MHC-peptide complexes depends on several invariant co-receptors, such as CD8. CD8 increases the affinity of TCR for MHC 10-fold by interacting directly with the $\alpha 3$ domain of the MHC. Likewise, class II MHC-TCR interaction is stabilized by CD4. However, all TCR–peptide–MHC complex structures are monomeric and there is no evidence of higher order oligomerization in these structures, despite the importance of clustering in TCR function. Moreover, no large-scale conformational changes occur that might mediate signal transduction.

TCR-pMHC recognition activates the tyrosine kinase cascade involving various enzymes such as lck and fyn of the src family. The cascade activates other cellular processes leading to cell proliferation and differentiation. For example, lck induces the phosphorylation of immunoreceptor tyrosine-based activation motifs (ITAM) on CD3. Several accessory molecules are involved in signal transduction, such as CD28 and CD45. CD28 molecules interact with signal molecules on the antigen presenting cell and activates the T cell. CD45 catalyses and activates tyrosine protein kinases by dephosphorylation.

## Immunological synapse

The spatio-temporal organization of this wide variety of molecules – TCRs, MHCs, CD8 or CD4, CD3, CD45, and so on – leads to the formation of a supramolecular complex – now known as the immunological synapse (IS) – a communication nexus between APC and T cell. Here TCR–MHC complexes are greatly concentrated and other molecules, such as CD45, are excluded. The IS is a specialized cell-to-cell junction characterized by its relative stability, sustained signalling and by the ordered series of complex coordinated events on both cells.

The canonical structure of the IS involves formation of an interface between an APC and a T cell. Rings form around a central cluster consisting of pMHC–TCR complexes and protein kinase C-$\theta$. These rings are composed of talin, together with intercellular complexes formed between Leukocyte function-associated antigen 1 (LFA-1) and intercellular adhesion molecule 1 (ICAM-1). LFA-1 is an important co-receptor which recognizes ICAM-1. Binding of LFA-1 to ICAM-1 stops T cell migration and initiates TCR engagement. After several minutes, the TCR-pMHC complexes translocate to the centre of the interaction area, where they are surrounded by LFA-1/ICAM-1 complexes.

The mature IS consists of two functional domains: a central cluster of TCR–pMHC complexes and a surrounding ring of adhesion molecules. Segregation of adhesion molecules and TCRs is thought to be primarily due to size. The TCR region is about 15 nm in length and the LFA-1-rich region is much longer, at 30–40 nm. The IS is no empty lacuna, but is densely populated by signalling and adhesion molecules. The differences in length between these regions create a functionally important supramolecular structure on the mesoscale and beyond. Indeed, the IS can be visualized using a light microscope. This dynamic supramolecular complex remains stable for hours, during which time peptide recognition occurs and a signal is transduced, triggering activation of the T cell. The structure of the mature IS appears to differ significantly between different cell types. The previously-described classical bull's eye pattern formed with B cells, or with supported planar bilayers, exhibits a central focus of interacting TCR-pMHC complexes. Dendritic cells, on the other hand, display an IS with multiple foci of interaction with the T cell.

## Signal 1, signal 2, immunodominance

Within naïve T cells, a threshold controls the adaptive response. If this is exceeded, the cell is activated, generating memory and effector T cells. This activation is contingent upon the simultaneous stimulation of TCRs by pMHC or lipid-CD1 complexes (known as *signal 1* amongst the immunological cognoscenti) and other receptors triggered by the innate response (known as *signal 2* or the co-stimulatory signal). APCs express co-stimulatory cell-surface molecules able to activate T cells directly. These also secrete cytokines, which induce T cells to proliferate and differentiate into CTL, killing other infected cells. Secretion of IL-2 down-regulates TCR, CD8 and CD3, reducing unintended activation of non-specific T cells. Some APCs express co-stimulatory molecules weakly; these only activated CD8+ T cells in the prescence of CD4+ T cells, which activate CD8+ T cells directly or induce their proliferation by secreting IL-2.

The focusing of cellular immunity toward one, or just a few, epitopes, even during an immune response to a complex micro-organism or antigen, is usually referred to as immunodominance. Although described in many systems, the underlying molecular mechanisms that determine immunodominance are only now beginning to be properly appreciated, especially in relation to the interplay between T cells of differing specificities and the interactions between T cells and APCs. It certainly remains difficult, if not impossible, to predict which peptides will become immunodominant based solely on the sequences of potential antigens.

T cell recognition is by no means a simple process, and remains poorly understood. Even simple questions, such as how many peptide–MHC complexes are required to trigger T cells is not known with any unequivocal certainty. Likewise, central mechanistic questions regarding the basis of immunogencity have not been greatly illuminated by the many pMHC–TCR structures that are now extant. Exotic mechanisms, such as proofreading similar to that exhibited by DNA replication, have been invoked to explain both immunogenicity and the initiation of the T cell response. The involvement of accessory molecules, although essential, is not properly understood, at least from a quantitative perspective. Ultimately, the accurate modelling of all these complex processes will be required to gain full and complete insight into the process of epitope presentation.

## Humoral immunity

Having said all that about T cell mediated immunity, and much there is to say on the subject, it is nonetheless sobering to realize that, with the notable exception of BCG, the antituberculosis vaccine, the protection offered by all vaccines is mediated completely or predominantly through the induction of antibodies, which act mostly in infection at the bacteremic or viremic stage. Humoral immunogenicity, as mediated by soluble or membrane-bound cell surface antibodies through their binding of B cell epitopes, is of prime importance for most existing vaccines. It can be measured in several ways. Methods such as enzyme-linked immunosorbent assay (ELISA) or competitive inhibition assays yield values for the antibody titre, the concentration at which the ability of antibodies in the blood to bind an antigen has reached its half maximal value. This is a well-used measure of antibody mediated immunity, and it is also possible to measure directly the affinity of antibody and antigen, using, for example, equilibrium dialysis.

Both transmembrane cell-surface expressed and soluble antibodies are monomeric dimers of dimers, consisting of two identical light (L) chains (25 kD each) and two identical heavy (H) chains (50–75 kDa). Antibody variable domains confer the ability to bind antigen, while heavy chain constant domains confer on it effector functions, which include the capacity to recruit help from complement molecules and immunological cells. Inter-chain H–L disulphide bonds help give antibodies a characteristic 'Y' shape. Depending on its isotype, heavy chains consist of an equal number of three or more constant domains (designated $C_{H1}$, $C_{H2}$, $C_{H3}$, etc.) and one variable domain ($V_H$). Each L chain consists of a variable domain ($V_L$) and a constant ($C_L$) domain. An antibody thus has three functional regions: two variable regions, one per arm of the molecule, containing identical antigen-binding sites, and a single constant region, which confers an effecter function allowing other immune components to recognize the antibody–antigen complex.

The sequences of $V_L$ and $V_H$ domains are the basis for antibody–antigen recognition. The antigen-binding site of most antibodies is formed from six 'hypervariable loops' or 'complementarily determining regions' (CDRs): three from the $V_L$ domain (L1, L2 and L3) and three from the $V_H$ domain (V1, V2 and V3). Framework regions between CDR loops help determine the overall topology of the antibody paratope. The lengths of the six CDRs partly define its shape: long CDR-L1, CDR-L2, CDR-H1 and CDR-H2 with short CDR-L3 and CDR-H3 confer a groove, while a long CDR-L1 and CDR-L2 with a medium-to-long CDR-H2 and short CDR-L3 results in a pocket, and CDRs of more equivalent length confer a planar site.

B cell exposure to antigen may initiate isotype switching. This somatic recombination results in permanent alteration of the cell in which specific C domain genes are chosen for expression. After isotype switching, B cells may differentiate into plasma cells which secrete soluble antibodies. There are five main human antibody isotypes: IgM, IgD, IgG, IgE and IgA. IgM and IgA form mutimeric complexes. IgM forms pentamers. IgA forms monomers and dimers. IgG is the most numerous antibody isotype in blood.

Before exposure to antigen, during early lymphoid development, gene rearrangement generates a diverse repertoire of B-lymphocytes each expressing a different antigen-binding antibody. C domain genes reside upstream from V, D and J genes, and determine the isotype of the expressed antibody. Naïve B cells express the first two C domain genes producing surface IgM and IgD molecules. Antibodies are thus encoded by segments designated V, D, J and C, deriving from both maternal and paternal chromosomes. $D_H$ and $J_H$ segments initially undergo rearrangement on both chromosomes of the pre-B cell, followed by recombination of the newly formed $DJ_H$ segment and $V_H$ segment. If this event results in a viable gene with a correct reading frame and stop-codon, it is repeated. The expressed antibody is a product of $VDJ_H$ and $C_H$ segments. Antibody signalling suppresses further rearrangement. Gene rearrangement of $V_L$ and $J_L$ gene segments then begins. If this fails, rearrangement is redirected again. Transcription of surface IgM now proceeds, and further rearrangement is prevented. V, D and J segment joining can be inaccurate with extra nucleotides inserted at the edges of V–D–J segments. These many processes combine to increase antibody structural diversity.

The primary antibody repertoire contains a few million distinct structures, resulting in low-affinity encounters with antigen. The probability of high affinity antibodies arising naturally from the initial V, D and J genes is low, yet an effective response to antigen depends on the repertoire containing specific, high-affinity antibodies. From this initial repertoire, B cells able to recognize antigen with low affinity are selected for colonel expansion. This is an iterative process of directed hypermutation and antigen-mediated selection which can produce antibodies with high affinity and antigen-specificity. This rapid, quasi-evolutionary process can raise affinity by 10- to 100-fold over the course of an immune response, with concomitant efficacy enhancements to host defense. Though antigen alone may activate B cells, high-affinity antibodies require CD4+ helper T cells. Antigen presented to the B cell must be internalized, processed and potential T cell epitopes presented to helper T cells via the MHC–peptide complex.

There is a relationship between the convexity of an antigen binding site and the curvature of the corresponding antigen, resulting from the nature of both surfaces and the observation that the antibody-combining site always buries a significant proportion of the antigen epitope on complex formation. Somatic mutations of combining-site residues increase affinity by forming extra hydrogen bonds and improved intermolecular interactions. The maturation process may not enhance van der Waals' contacts or hydrogen bonds, but improve the network of apolar interactions and surface complementarity resulting in augmented affinity, while the overall interface remains fairly constant. Antibodies in free and bound forms undergo conformational rearrangements in the binding site, and this may be mirrored by conformational change within the antigen.

## Further reading

In this chapter we have barely scratched the surface of one of the most complex and demanding disciplines in contemporary science. To dig a little deeper, try one of the many excellent textbooks currently available: *Janeway's Immunobiology* by Murphy, Travers and Walport (ISBN 0815341237); *Immunology* by Kuby, Kindt, Osborne and Goldsby (ISBN 0716767643); *Roitt's Essential Immunology* by Delves, Martin, Burton and Roitt (ISBN 1405136030).

# 4
# Vaccines: Data and Databases

*In science there is only physics, all the rest is stamp collecting.*

—Attributed to Lord Rutherford (1871–1937)

## Making sense of data

A clear distinction between information and the understanding built upon it has existed in science since at least the era of Copernicus and Newton, and probably long before. Much of science is now based upon acquiring and utilizing data. In the high throughput era – be that astronomical, metrological or post-genomic – data generation is no longer the principal and overwhelming bottleneck; instead it is the ability to interpret data usefully that limits us. After a century of empirical research, immunology and vaccinology, amongst a plethora of other disciplines, are poised to reinvent themselves as genome-based, high-throughput sciences. Immunology, and indeed all biological disciplines in the post-genomic era, must address a pressing challenge: how best to capitalize on a vast, and potentially overwhelming, inundation of new data; data which is both dazzlingly complex and delivered on a hitherto inconscionable scale. Though many might disagree, I feel that immunology can only do so by embracing fully computation and computational science.

However, to be useable and useful, data that we wish to model, understand and predict must be properly accumulated and archived. Ideally, this accumulated and archived data should be easily accessible, and transparently so. Once this would have meant card indexes and an immeasurable proliferation of paper; now we can automate this process using computers. This is the role of the database, and biological databases are the subject of this chapter. Once we have stored our data, we must

---

*Bioinformatics for Vaccinology*   Darren R Flower
© 2008 John Wiley & Sons, Ltd

analyse it. This is the province of data-mining. We explore this issue separately in Chapter 5.

# Knowledge in a box

If we look back into history, we find many, many forerunners of the modern database: the library, the single-author history, the multi-author encyclopedia, the museum and many more. Indeed, well before the Industrial Revolution and the mechanization of human action, the kind of systematic data items found in databases – often called records – existed as sales receipts, accounting ledgers and other collections of data related to the mercantile endeavour. Thus we can certainly trace the database, as it is conceived of today, at least as far as the inception of double-entry bookkeeping first recorded by Italian mathematician Louis Pauli in 1479. Two precursors in particular prefigure the modern database: the cabinet of curiosities (or wonder rooms) and the museums that arose from them, and the idea of an encyclopedia. Indeed, in many important ways databases are simply the modern reification of a long-cherished ambition: to encompass in a single place all knowledge of any value or utility. This is indeed a lofty goal and one which began early. Antiquity is littered with so-called universal histories. Probably the best known was the seven volume *Historia naturalis* written by Gaius Plinius Secundus (23–79), better known as Pliny the Elder. The determination to concentrate all knowledge into a single work found its greatest expression during the European enlightenment and the work of the encyclopedists. Pierre Bayle's *Dictionnaire Historique et Critique* (1696), the *Encyclopédie* (1751–1772) of Jean le Rond d'Alembert (1717–1783) and Denis Diderot (1713–1784) and Smellie's *Encyclopaedia Britannica* (1768–1771) are perhaps the three best known.

Biological databases, immunological or otherwise, are only starting their journeys to completeness. As we shall see below, they need to be expanded and integrated. Many projects are attempting to do these things and much more besides, but things are only just beginning. Most notably, the desire to systematically integrate existing data of diverse and divergent kinds which are spread across countless sources both formal (existing archives, peer-reviewed books and journals, etc.) and informal (websites, laboratory notebooks, etc.). Traditionally, the kind of data found in biological database systems was almost exclusively nucleic acid and protein sequences. Today, things are very, very different. Now the data contained within databases can be anything related to the functioning of biology. This may include, but is in no way limited to, the thermodynamic properties of isolated enzyme systems, or the binding interactions of proteins, or the expression profiles of genes, or, indeed, anything. As a consequence, biological databases are now proliferating, necessitating a database of their own just to catalogue them.

# The science of -omes and -omics

Nonetheless, and no doubt for a long time to come, the most important biological databases will continue to focus on sequence data. Genomics has seen to that. Genomics is the science of genome analysis. The words genome and genomics have spawned countless other '-omes', and the last 10 years or so has seen an explosion of '-omes' and their corresponding '-omics'. There are literally hundreds of different '-omes'. New ones are coined with monotonous regularity. Some of these are abstract or fanciful or are of little merit and interest. Some are germane to the study of immunology and thus to immunoinformatics. We can isolate two in particular: the genome and the proteome.

The genome is the DNA sequence of an organism. Part of the genome codes directly for genes which make mRNA which make proteins, which in turn do more or less everything in the cell. Part of the genome is involved with regulating and controlling the expression of DNA as mRNA and proteins. The number of sequenced genomes is now large and ever increasing. Yet currently, and despite the enormous quantity of time and money expended in developing the science of genomics, even quite simple questions remain unanswered. How many genes are there? The answer to this should, in the genomic era, be relatively straightforward, at least at the conceptual level, but is it? Let us look at the best characterized complex genome: the human one. The putative size of the human genome has presently been revised down from figures in excess of 100 000 first to about 40 000 genes and then down to only 20 000. A recent and reliable estimate from 2006 puts the number of human protein coding genes at or about 25 043; while, a 2007 estimate places the value at about 20 488 with, say, another 100 genes yet to be found.

Remember that this human genome is a composite derived from at least five donors. In 2007, the first individual human genomes were sequenced and published. Thus, James Watson and J. Craig Venter became the first of thousands – perhaps in time millions – to know their own DNA. Clearly, the size of the human genome and the number of immunological molecules remain simply estimates. Both will change we can be certain. For other genomes, the situation still lags some way behind in terms of annotation and the identification of immunological molecules. Distinct proteins have different properties and thus different functions in different contexts. Thus the genomic identification of genes is therefore the beginning rather than the end. As the hype surrounding the sequencing of the human genome begins to abate, functional genomics is now beginning to take centre stage. Elaborating the functions of countless genes, either by high throughput methods or by the hard graft of traditional biochemistry, will be a much more refractory, but infinitely more rewarding, task.

# The proteome

Proteome is a somewhat loose term encompassing the protein complement analogous to the genome and deriving in part from it. The proteome is very complex and involves, at its broadest definition, both degraded and proteolytically processed protein products and post-translationally modified proteins. The proteome is in part a product of itself, processing and acting on itself. From an immunological perspective, one of the most interesting aspects of the wider proteome is the peptidome: this is the complex and dynamic set of peptides present in a cell or organism. Unlike the genome, transcriptome, proteome and metabolome, the peptidome has received little or no attention until relatively recently. The peptidome can be thought of as a key example of how a single gene can be diversified through the transcriptome and proteome to affect innumerable functionalities at different points in space and time. Given the complexity of the peptidome and its highly dynamic nature there is a pressing requirement for improved peptide discovery that seamlessly combines the identification of peptide sequences with the spatio-temporal profiling of peptides. Standard proteomic techniques are not up to the job, since they are typically inadequate at low molecular mass. The emergent discipline of peptidomics seeks to analyse and visualize comprehensively small peptides, and thus bridge the worlds of proteomics and metabolonomics. Apart from its role in discovering biomarkers, peptidomics is a key component of discovery in immunology and vaccinology. The mapping of the peptidome will, for example, have profound implications for the experimental and computational discovery of T cell epitopes.

## Systems biology

Many of these '-omes' are at both a practical and at a conceptual level highly interlinked. They are, to some extent at least, layered one upon another. Proteins, acting as enzymes, catalyse the creation of the peptidome, metabolome and glycome; while their creation is, in part, regulated by the metabolome's interaction with the transcriptome and genome. The apotheosis of post-genomic research is embodied in the newly emergent discipline of systems biology, which combines molecular and system-level approaches to bioscience. It integrates many kinds of molecular knowledge and employs the synergistic use of both experimental data and mathematical modelling. Importantly, it works over many so-called length scales from the atomic, through the mesoscale, to the level of cells, organs, tissues and whole organisms. Depending on the quality and abundance of available data, many different modelling approaches can be used. In certain respects, systems biology is trying to wrestle back biology from those happy to describe biological phenomena in a qualitative way and to make it once more a fully quantitative science. Long, long ago, when biochemistry was young, this was very much the intention of the discipline but the advent and ultimate victory of gene-manipulating molecular biology very much effaced these early good intentions. It shares with disciplines as diverse as engineering and cybernetics the view that the ultimate behaviour of a system, be that biological or mechanical or psychological, is independent of its microscopic structure with behaviour emerging at various levels of scale and complexity. Implicit within systems biology is the tantalizing hope of truly predictive, quantitative biology. Two fundamentally different approaches to systems biology have emerged. The Top-down approach characterizes biological systems by combining mathematical modelling with system-wide data delivered by high-throughput post-genomic techniques. The bottom-up approach begins not with data but rather with a detailed molecular-scale model of the system. Top-down systems biology is often seen as phenomenological but can give real insights into a system nonetheless.

Immunology can also be studied using system biology techniques. Indeed, for many, immunology is a prime example of systems behaviour in biology. How immunology behaves and how this behaviour arises from its constituent parts is of enormous interest to both clinician and computer scientist alike. For system immunology, however, read immunomics. This is the study of immunology using genome-based high-throughput techniques within a conceptual landscape borne of systems biology thinking. Clearly, all of the '-omes' and '-omics' we have discussed or alluded to above are of direct relevance to the study of immunology, since genes, proteins and glycoproteins, and small molecules too, all play their part in the enumeration and elaboration of the immune response.

## The immunome

Finally, though, let us discuss another '-ome' – the immunome. There are several definitions of the immunome. One defines it as the set of antigenic peptides, or possibly immunogenic proteins, within a micro-organism, be that virus, bacteria, fungus or parasite. There are alternative definitions of the immunome that also include immunological receptors and accessory molecules. It is thus also possible to talk of the self-immunome, the set of potentially antigenic self-peptides. This is clearly important within the context of, for example, cancer (the cancer-immunone) and autoimmunity (the auto-immunome), which affect about 30% and 3% of the global population respectively.

The immunone, at least for a particular pathogen, can only be realized in the context of a particular, defined host. The nature of the immunome is clearly dependent upon the host as much as it is on what we shall, for convenience, call the pathogen. This is implicit in the term antigenic or immunogenic. A peptide is not antigenic if the immune system does not respond to it. A good example of this is the major histocompatibility complex (MHC) restriction of T cell responses. A particular MHC allele will have a peptide specificity that may, or may not, overlap with other expressed alleles, but the total specificity of an individual's alleles will not cover the whole possible sequence space of peptides. Thus peptides that do not bind to any of an individual's allelic MHC variants cannot be antigenic within a cellular context. The ability to define the specificity of different MHCs computationally, which we may call *in silico* immunomics or *in silico* immunological proteomics for want of a more succinct term, is an important, but eminently realizable, goal of immuninformatics, the application of informatics techniques to immunological macromolecules. However, immunomics argues that for immunoinformatics identifying immunological molecules and epitopes is not an end but only a beginning.

In part, bioinformatics' goal is to catalogue the postgenomic world. It is crucial to drawing meaning and understanding from the poorly organized throng of information that still constitutes biology. Immunology has, for example, developed its own obfuscating ways of describing familiar biological events. There has been much reinventing of the wheel. New discoveries in one discipline are merely the independent reinvention of ideas or tools well known in another. The days are long gone of the renaissance scholars able to hold the whole of human knowledge in their head. The most we can now hope to hold in our minds is but a tiny fraction of the whole. The only way to make full use of this burgeoning diversity of information is computational; the best reification of this desire is the database.

## Databases and databanks

Within the discipline of computer science a database is defined variously, but a useful and general definition runs along these lines: a database is a structured collection of itemized information contained within a computer system, particularly combining storage with some kind of software – such as a database management system (DBMS) – that can retrieve data in response to specific, user-defined queries. The word database can also mean just the data. Others make a distinction between the organized data, which they refer to as a data bank, and the software-enabled manifestation of this, which they call a database. Outside the strictures of database theory, and often by people without a computer science education, these words are used ambiguously and without precision: a database can then refer to the data, the data structure and the software system which stores and searches it. I am certainly guilty of using lax terminology. In doing so, I am motivated by my interest not in the data structure or the software but the data and what it can tell me about biology. To the biologist, and indeed to many bioinformaticians, a database is no more than a tool. At a fundamental level, we are interested not in what a database is or how it works, only in what it can do. We are concerned by how best we can use the tool and how to get the most from it.

A database is of a set of pieces of information, often known as 'records'. For a particular set of records, within a particular context, there will be a particular description of the kind of information held within a database. This is known as a schema, which describes both the nature of the information archived and any explicit relationships between such data. There are several ways of organizing a schema, and thus modelling the database structure: these are known as data models.

The simplest form of database is the flat file. This can be parsed using handcrafted software. The Protein Data Bank was in this form until quite recently. Indeed, my own experience suggests that this is the format in which most bioinformaticians want their data, rather than being buried and inaccessible within a database. A flat file is likewise distinct from a flat data structure. Such a structure – also known as the table model – comprises a two-dimensional array of data items.

Each item in a column and each item in a row will be related implicitly to every other item in their column or row.

Other types of database and data model include *inter alia*: the hierarchical model, where information is nested into a dependent tree with items linked vertically to mother and daughter nodes; the distributed model; the functional data model; and the object-orientated model, which enjoys success with complex, intrinsically-structured data. However, two types of database dominate computer science applied to life science: the relational database and databases based on XML. Of the two competing technologies, the relational database is the more mature and is thus the more prevalent.

## The relational database

The relational model was first proposed explicitly by the English computer scientist Edgar Frank Codd (1923–2003) in his 1970 paper 'A Relational Model of Data for Large Shared Data Banks'. The first practical implementations of the relational model followed 6 years later with Michael Stonebraker's Ingres and the System R project at IBM. The first commercially successful relational databases were Oracle and DB2, which appeared in or about 1980, while dBASE was the first successful relational database for personal computers. Today, the principal relational database management system is ORACLE, which is the commercial standard; it runs the sophisticated query language or structured query language (SQL). In the last decade or so, ORACLE has increasingly faced competition from open source query languages and database implementations. Notable amongst these are PostgreSQL (www.postgresql.org/) and MySQL (www.mysql.com/), which mimic the features of SQL but, shall we say, in a more cost-effective manner.

Like the flat data model, the basic underlying structure of the relational model represents data items as tables. Such tables are composed of rows (or *records*) and columns (or *fields*). A single, unique data item sits at the intersection of a record and a field. An entity is any object about which data can be stored and forms the 'subject' of a record or a table. A database may contain many, many related tables. Despite decades of activity, relational databases still exhibit certain inherent limitations. They can be seen as inflexible, as all data types must be predefined. Once created, revising a database is by no means a trivial undertaking. The database may need to unpick its internal structure necessitating significant outage. In response to these limitations, XML databases – which seek to circumvent some of this by removing the traditional divide between information and the documents that store and present it – have become fashionable.

## The XML database

XML is a data description language designed to foment the exchange of complex, nonheterogeneous information. XML is an acronym for extensible markup language. In many ways, XML is a tool for the storage and transmission of information that is independent of hardware and software, much as HTML is a way to control the display of text and graphics that is ostensibly independent of software and hardware. Platform independence is a great strength of HTML and also a great strength of XML.

XML is a mark-up language similar to, yet different from, HTML. The mark-up tags used in XML are not predetermined and the creator of an XML document must define their own – XML is thus said to be extensible. XML gives structure to the data it stores. An XML document may contain a wide variety of data types, yet itself does nothing. It is simply information wrapped by XML tags. Like HTML, software is required to process or display this information. However, XML is not intended to replace HTML, or even to supercede it; the two were devised with quite different goals in mind. XML has certainly developed with considerable celerity, and has been widely adopted. Some say that XML will yet become the commonest means of manipulating and transmitting data.

XML is certainly seen by many as the natural choice for biological databases, at least small ones. XML handles irregularity of data well and is highly suited to developing databases which are likely to change and expand rapidly over time. Speed is an issue, however. When databases are relatively small, any lack of speed probably passes unnoticed. Such a dearth of celerity is anyway often compensated for by a concomitant gain in flexibility and use of use. However, as the quantity of data grows, the innate celerity achievable by XML increasingly becomes a concern. Although history suggests that growth in processor speed will always greatly exceed growth in the demand made by applications, this issue may make XML seem unattractive for very large-scale database projects.

There was a time, not so long ago, when the volume of data within biological sequence databases was considered a challenge, despite the observation that transactional database systems used for finance and stock trading and the like had dealt with data on a comparable scale for a long time. Generally, and particularly in the nascent era of petascale computing, this is no longer a concern. The human genome project and its progeny, not to mention the Hubble Space Telescope, medical imaging, satellite weather forecasting and an unrestrained plethora of other applications, have generated data on a previously unimagined and unimaginable scale – databases do exist which can deal with this level of information and then some.

## The protein universe

Whatever we can say about the origins of life on earth – distant and totally inaccessible and unknowable though such origins may be – today we live in a protein universe. To many, such an assertion is tantamount to heresy. Long has biology been thrall to the hegemony of the gene, the dominance of genetics and the relegation of much else in biology to rather poor also-rans. Clearly, while genetics plays its part, it is the interactions of proteins and lipids and membranes that mediate immunogenicity. Thus we focus, but not exclusively, on proteins here rather than nucleic acids – the engine rather than the blueprint.

The proteins which comprise the immune system and the peptides that are recognized by them are composed of amino acids. The archiving and comparison of protein sequences is of vital importance in the postgenomic era. This is particularly true of immunology. When dealing with entire genome sequences, the need for software tools, able to automate the laborious process of scanning millions of sequences comprising million upon million of nucleotides or amino acids, is both obvious and essential. One of the aims of bioinformatics is to identify genes descended from a common ancestor and to characterize them by identifying similarities between them at the global (whole sequence) and local (motif) levels. Such similarities imply a corresponding structural and functional propinquity. The assumption underlying this is an evolutionary one: functionally-similar genes have diverged through a process of constrained random mutation resulting in sequences being increasingly dissimilar to each another. Inferences connecting sequence similarity to common function are complex, confusing and can be confounding. Successful functional assignment necessitates significant biological context. Such context is provided by databases: implicit context present as archived sequences and explicit context present as annotation.

Genomes and the databases that seek to encapsulate our knowledge of them are composed of sequences of nucleotides. The proteome and the databases that seek to encapsulate our knowledge of them are composed of sequences of amino acids. To a crude first approximation, genomes are subdivided into genes and the ultimate products of genes are proteins. Proteins and fragments thereof are, by and large, those moieties which the adaptive immune system recognizes and to which it responds. Peptides within the cell are derived from a variety of sources and as the result of a multitude of mechanisms. Many peptides are encoded specifically within the genome. Some are generated specifically through an enzyme-mediated manner. Others still are generated by a more stochastic and less explicitly regulated process through the proteolytic degradation of proteins by a complex network of over 500 proteases. As is obvious, the peptidome is intimately linked mechanistically to the state of proteome. The peptidome acts both within and beyond the cell and is regulated, at least in part, by the subtle interplay of protease inhibitors and proteases.

Much of computational immunology is thus concerned with protein databases and their contents. T cell epitope prediction methods, which we will describe subsequently, attempt to convert the sequences of exogenous or endogenous proteins into ordered lists of high-affinity peptide epitopes. Likewise, attempts to predict B cell epitopes and antigens work primarily with protein sequences. The molecular products arising from the metabolome of pathogens, such as carbohydrates, lipids and exotic nucleotides, which are in turn the recognition targets of PRR etc., are rather less well understood and are, generally speaking, currently not well served by databases. Thus attempts to predict successfully molecules such as carbohydrates and lipids lag some way behind attempts to predict proteinacious epitopes. It is thus unsurprising that attention has mainly focused on protein rather than nonprotein epitopes, since the corresponding volume of data is vastly greater.

## Much data, many databases

There is an interesting distinction to be drawn between linear sequences (nucleic acids and proteins), branched sequences (carbohydrates) and discrete small molecules (lipids, metabolites). Linear biopolymer sequences are today much easier to deal with, both experimentally and computationally, at least in terms of experimental characterization, data storage and searching. Biologically interesting carbohydrates are seldom linear sequences but rather multiple branched structures necessitating a more complex and ambiguous nomenclature compared with that used to represent nucleic acid and protein sequences. Small molecule structures, particularly synthetically complex natural products, are the most difficult by some distance. As nonpolymers they must be represented explicitly on an atom-by-atom basis and likewise computational searching of small molecules relies on complex graph theory rather than text processing.

From the perspective of immunogenicity and *in silico* immunology, the most important and prevalent kinds of basic biological molecules are the amino acids and proteins built from them. As far as we can tell, throughout the whole tree of life and with currently very few exceptions, a tiny handful of amino acids form a small set of components from which are constructed the workhorses of the cell – proteins. Proteins abound in nature and the diversity of function exhibited by proteins is both extraordinary and confounding.

## What proteins do

Arguably, the most fundamental property of a protein is its ability to bind other molecules with tuneable degrees of specificity. Proteins are responsible for the binding and transport of otherwise water insoluble compounds, such as retinol, or small, indiscriminately reactive molecules such as oxygen or nitric oxide or the ions of heavy metals. The consequences of a protein's ability to form complexes manifest themselves in many ways, not least when they act as enzymes. Enzymes catalyse most, but not all, naturally occurring chemical reactions within biological systems. Secondary metabolism is littered with reactions which proceed, wholly or partly, without help from enzymes. For example, levuglandins and isolevuglandins (also referred to as neuroketals or isoketals) are generated by rearrangements of prostanoid and isoprostanoid endoperoxides which are not catalysed by enzymes. The levuglandin pathway is part of the cyclooxygenase pathway, and the isolevuglandin pathway is part of the isoprostane pathway. In cells, prostaglandin H2 undergoes a nonenzymic rearrangement to form levuglandin even when prostaglandin binding enzymes are present. Isolevuglandins, on the other hand, are formed through a free radical-mediated autoxidation of unsaturated phospholipid esters.

The other well known example of nonprotein mediated catalysis is the ribozyme. Most natural ribozymes concern themselves with RNA maturation. Ribozymes catalyse the activation of either a water molecule or a ribose hydroxyl group for nucleophilic attack of phosphodiester bonds. Although ribozymes have a limited repertoire of functional groups compared to those possessed by protein catalysts, they are able to utilize a variety of mechanisms: general acid-base catalysis and metal ion-assisted catalysis, amongst others. Several varieties of these RNA catalysts are now know: the hammerhead ribozyme, the hairpin ribozyme, hepatitis delta ribozymes and self-splicing introns. The largest ribozyme currently known, however, is the ribosome; it is also the only naturally occurring RNA catalyst with a synthetic activity. As we all know, the ribosome effects protein synthesis. It has emerged recently that the principal active site responsible for peptide bond formation (also called the peptidyl-transferase centre) of the bacterial ribosome – and, by inference, that of all ribosomes – is formed solely from rRNA.

Enzymatic catalysis can be largely, if not quite completely, explained in terms of binding. The classical view of how enzymes enhance the celerity of reactions within biological systems holds that an enzyme binds to the transition state reducing the activation barrier to kinetic reaction rates in either direction. This enhancement can be very significant. Enzymes such as catalase (which catalyses the degradation of hydrogen peroxide $H_2O_2$) can enhance reaction rates by as much as $10^6$. The catalytic efficiency of catalase is so great that the overall rate of reaction is, essentially, diffusion limited; that is to say, the observed reaction rate is limited by diffusion of the peroxide substrate into the active site. Other than catalase, a few enzymes approach this thermodynamic perfection, including acetylcholine esterase and carbonic anhydrase. Compared to the uncatalysed reaction, hydrolysis of phosphodiester and phosphonate esters by a dinuclear aminopeptidase from streptomyces griseus exhibits a rate enhancement of $4 \times 10^{10}$ at neutral pH and room temperature. However, even this vast augmentation of reaction rates pales in comparison to orotidine 5′-phosphate decarboxylase. This enzyme, which catalyses the decarboxylation of orotidine 5′-monophosphate to uridine 5′-monophosphate, can enhance the rate of this reaction by $1.7 \times 10^{17}$ or over a billion billion times. At room temperature and neutral pH, uncatalysed orotic acid decarboxylation in aqueous solution has a half-life estimated at 78 million years. In order to effect this staggering level of rate enhancement, orotidine 5′-phosphate decarboxylase is thought to bind its transition state with a $K_d$ of approximately $5 \times 10^{-24}$ M.

Proteins also act as conformational sensors of altered environmental pH or the concentrations of cellular metabolites. Proteins are responsible for coordinated motion at both the microscopic scale, as mediated by components of the cytoskeleton, and at the macroscopic scale where the sliding motion of myosin and actin mediates muscle contraction. Cell surface receptors maintain and marshal intercell communication and the interaction between cells and their immediate milieu, effecting signal transduction. Proteins are involved in the regulation and control of growth, cell differentiation, DNA expression and diverse cell functions. The geometry and structural integrity of cells are maintained by fibrous and globular structural proteins, such as those involved in forming the cytoskeleton.

## What proteins are

Proteins are macromolecular heterobiopolymers composed of linear chains of amino acids polymerized through the formation of peptide bonds. Short chains of amino acid polymers are called peptides. Longer chains are sometimes distinguished as oligopeptides or polypeptides. As epitopes, peptides are exceptionally important in immunology, as they are elsewhere in biology as signalling molecules or degradation products. Proteins are typically much longer amino acid polymers. As ever, terminology is imprecise; there is no universally accepted, exact demarcation between peptide and oligopeptide and protein. How large a polypeptide must be to fall into a particular category is largely a matter of personal choice. A chain of between, say, 20 and 100 amino acids, some would call an oligopeptide, others would class it as a protein.

## The amino acid world

Generally, when we think of biologically important amino acids, we think first of the 20 standard amino acids, as listed in Figure 4.1. They consist of at least one acidic carboxylic acid group (COOH) and one amino group (NH2). These two groups are attached to a central carbon atom, known as the $\alpha$ carbon. This is also attached to a hydrogen atom and a side chain. In chemistry, an amino acid is any molecule containing both amino and carboxyl functional groups. In biochemistry, the term 'amino acid' is usually reserved for $\alpha$ amino acids, where the amino and carboxyl groups are directly attached to the same carbon. However, as any synthetic organic chemist knows, these 20 amino acids are just the tip of the iceberg. Within the fundamental pattern common to all L-$\alpha$-amino acids the potential for structural diversity is enormous. Potentially any organic molecule could be modified to contain the core $\alpha$ amino acid functionality and thus be combined with others to make a protein.

The 20 amino acids encoded by the standard genetic code are called biogenic or proteinogenic or 'standard' amino acids. More complex, rarer amino acids are often referred to as 'nonstandard'. In what follows, we generally limit our discussion to amino acids that have an $\alpha$ amino group and a free $\alpha$ hydrogen. While these features are held in common by all standard amino acids they do not, in themselves, apply constraints, in terms of protein engineering or evolution, on possible biochemistries. Consider 2,5-diaminopyrrole, an amino acid derivative from the Murchison meteorite: it contains no free carboxyl group; it and its coevals are thus of limited interest to us here.

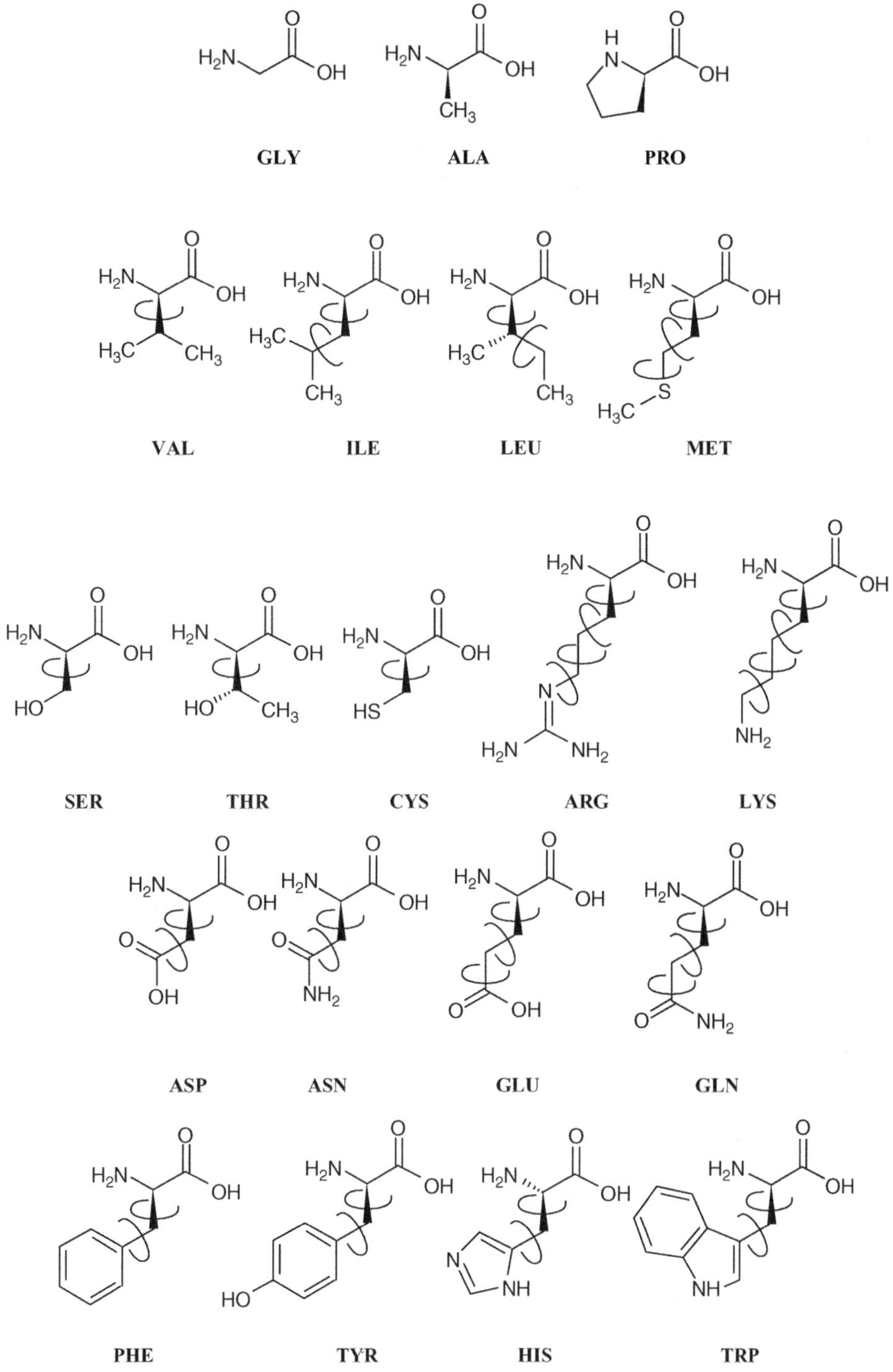

**Figure 4.1** The chemical structures of the 20 compound amino acids (arrows indicate rotatable bonds)

Although in most organisms only 20 amino acids are coded for genetically, over 80 different kinds of amino acids have thus far been discovered in nature. Of these naturally occurring amino acids, 20 (or more strictly 22) are currently considered to be the precursors of proteins. These amino acids are coded for by codons: triplets of nucleotides within genes in an organism's genome, which is itself a sequence of nucleotides segregated into chromosomes and plasmids. All or, more usually, part of the genome will code for protein sequences. The alphabet of DNA is composed of only four letters. These correspond to four different nucleotides: adenine (symbolized as A), cytosine (or C), guanine (G) and thymine (T). Three nucleotides are needed to specify a single amino acid, since one nucleotide (and thus four possibilities) or two nucleotides (giving 16 possibilities) are not enough; only three nucleotides (64 possibilities) can code for 20 amino acids. A group of three successive nucleotides is usually known as a codon. The set of all possible codons is often called the genetic or triplet code. The code is not overlapping nor does it contain systematic punctuations, such as spacer codons. Three of the 64 possible codons – UAA, UAG and UGA – each act as a 'stop' signal, terminating protein synthesis. UAG is sometimes called *amber*, UGA is called *opal* (or occasionally umber), and UAA is called *ochre*. The *amber* codon was so named by its discoverers – Charley Steinberg and Richard Epstein. The name honours their colleague, Harris Bernstein, whose last name is the German rendering of 'amber'. The remaining 61 codons each encode one of the 20 different biogenic amino acids. The codon AUG acts as a start signal, and also codes for methionine.

All other amino acids are not encoded by codons, but are post-translational modifications (PTMs): that is they result from the chemical modification of one or other of the 20 biogenic amino acids. Such modifications occur in an enzyme-mediated process subsequent to ribosome-mediated protein synthesis. Post-translational modifications are often essential for proper protein function.

The structural – and thus functional – diversity exhibited by amino acids is exemplified well by two databases which contain information on amino acids: ResID and AA-QSPR. As of August 2007, the AA-QSPR database (www.evolvingcode.net:8080/AA-QSPR/html/) contained details of 388 amino acids. These amino acids derive from many sources and comprise both natural biological and synthetic abiotic amino acids. The natural amino acids are composed of the standard 20 biogenic amino acids, plus 108 that are produced by enzymatic post-translational modification and 177 other amino acids found in natural systems. These 177 include a plethora of amino acids which act as intermediates in main metabolic pathways, as well as neurotransmitters and antibiotics. The non-natural group of amino acids includes 69 thought to be synthesized in various abiotic processes and 58 which have been created specifically by synthetic chemists. Engineered artificial amino acids never seen in nature are now commonly incorporated into biological systems. Abiotic amino acids included in AA-QSPR include those produced by chemical degradation, or ones which result from chemical simulations of the prebiotic earth, or have been identified from examination of the Murchison meteorite. RESID (www.ebi.ac.uk/RESID/), in its turn, documents the 23 $\alpha$-amino acids known to be genetically encoded – including N-formyl methionine, seleno-cysteine and pyrrolysine – and over 300 other residues which arise through natural, co- or post-translational modification of amino acids. The database includes artificially produced modifications encountered in mass spectrometry.

The most obvious role for amino acids is in the synthesis of proteins: to all intents and purposes amino acids make peptides and peptides, as they grow, become proteins. Proteins, as they exist within and outside the cell, are not composed solely of amino acids – post-translational modifications see to that – but without them proteins would simply not exist. Beyond their role in making proteins, and making proteins work, amino acids also have many important roles to play in diverse biological systems. Some amino acids function as intermediates within metabolic pathways. For example, 1-aminocyclopropane-1-carboxylic acid (ACC) is a small disubstituted cyclic amino acid and a key intermediate in the production of the plant hormone ethylene. Other amino acids fulfill roles as neurotransmitters (glycine, glutamate and GABA, for example). Other amino acids include carnitine (with its role in cellular lipid transport), ornithine, citrulline, homocysteine, hydroxyproline, hydroxylysine and sarcosine. As natural products or secondary metabolites, plants and micro-organisms, particularly bacteria, can produce very unusual amino acids. Some form peptidic antibiotics, such as nisin or alamethicin. Lanthionine is a sulphide-bridged alanine dimer which is found together with unsaturated amino acids in lantibiotics (antibiotic peptides of microbial origin).

## The chiral nature of amino acids

These amino acids, or residues as they are often called, at least when incorporated in proteins, differ in the nature of their side chains, sometimes referred to as an *R-group*. An amino acid residue is what remains of an amino acid after the removal of a water molecule during the formation of a peptide bond. In principal, the side chain of an amino acid can have any chemically tractable structure that obeys the laws and rules of chemistry. The use of the term R-group derives again from organic chemistry, where it is a common convention within the study of structure-activity relationships in congeneric series: here the terminology usually refers to molecules built around multiple substitutions of a common core, each such substitution being a seperate R-group ($R_1$, $R_2$, $R_3$, etc.). The R-group varies between amino acids and gives each amino acid its distinctive properties. Proline is the only biogenic amino acid with a cyclic side chain that links back to the $\alpha$-amino group, forming a secondary amino group. In times past, proline was confusingly labelled as an imino acid.

Chirality is a fundamental and pervasive, yet not necessarily appropriately appreciated, characteristic of all biology. Chirality manifests itself at both the molecular and the macroscopic level. The overwhelming preference for one of two possible mirror image forms is called biological homochirality. It is a puzzling, and not properly understood, phenomenon. Except for glycine, which has no chiral centre, amino acids occur as two possible optical isomers. These are labelled D and L in the relative configuration system of Fischer, and R and S in the Cahn-Ingold-Prelog system. All life on earth is, in the main, comprised of L-amino acids and D-sugars.

D-amino acids are, however, found within proteins produced by exotic marine organisms, such as cone snails; they can also be found in the cell walls of bacteria. Thus the existence, not to mention the function, of D-amino acids prompts questions of some note. D-amino acids are thought to be formed primarily by nonenzymatic racemization from L-amino acid during ageing. *In vivo* enzyme-mediated quality control will edit out D-amino acids from certain proteins; yet, as tissue ages, and particular after death, D-amino acids accumulate.

D-aspartic acid, in particular, has been found in numerous human proteins. Sources are all of geriatric origin; they are principally tissues in which metabolism, particularly protein metabolism, is practically inert or, at least, proceeds slowly. Examples of such tissue include the lens of the eye, the brain, bone and the teeth, as well as the skin and the aorta. The Asp-151 and Asp-58 residues in aged lens alpha A-crystallin are particularly stereochemically labile and the ratios of D and L amino acids for these residues are found to be greater than unity. This was the initial observation that the chiral inversion of amino acids occurs *in vivo* during natural ageing. A particularly well-known example of this phenomenon is the proportion of D-aspartic acid in human dentin which is known to rise gradually with age. Somewhat similar to bone, dentin is a hard calcareous component of teeth and placoid scales. Dentin sits between the pulp chamber and the enamel layer in the crown or the cementum layer in the root of the tooth. Ivory from elephants is solid dentin. It is a yellow, porous connective tissue with a 70% inorganic component composed mainly of dahllite. Dentin has a complex structure built around a collagen matrix: microscopic channels with a diameter of 0.8 to 2.2 $\mu$m – known as dentinal tubules – ramify outward from the pulp cavity through the dentin to its exterior interface with the cementum or enamel layer, often following a gentle helical course. Dentin exposed by abrasion or gingivitis causes so-called sensitive teeth in humans; treatments include plugging tubules with strontium.

Racemization observed in fossil bones, teeth and shells allows dating of ancient material comparable to that offered by radiocarbon dating and dendrochronology, since the D to L ratio varies with time. In forensic medicine, for example, D-aspartate in dentin has been used to estimate post-mortem age. Rates of racemization vary between different amino acids. L-alanine converts to D-alanine more slowly than the equivalent transformation of aspartic acid: a half-life (at room temperature and pressure and a pH of 7.0) of 3000 years versus 12 000. Amino acid racemization is also very temperature dependent: the half-life for conversion of aspartic acid rises to 430 000 years at 0°C.

Chiral and chirality, as words, derive from the Greek for handedness; it comes from the Greek stem for hand: $\chi \varepsilon \iota \rho \sim$. Chirality is the asymmetric property of being one hand or the other: objects both real (snail shells or staircases) and abstract (coordinate systems) can – in three dimensions – be either right-handed or left-handed. Something, such as a molecule, is said to be chiral if it cannot be superimposed on its mirror image. An object and its mirror image are enantiomorphs (Greek for 'opposite forms'). When referring to molecules, enantiomer is used instead. Enantiomers are completely nonsuperimposable mirror images of each other. They have, at least in a symmetric environment, the same physical and chemical properties except that they rotate plane-polarized light equally but in opposite directions. Objects lacking the property of chirality are termed achiral (or, rarely, as amphichiral).

A single chiral or asymmetric or stereogenic centre or stereocentre always makes a whole molecule chiral. Molecules with two or more stereocentres may or may not be chiral. Such stereochemical isomers or stereoisomers can be enantiomers or diastereoisomers. Diastereoisomers (or diastereomers) are stereoisomers which are not simple mirror images, and have opposite configurations at one or more chiral centres; they often have distinct physical and chemical properties. If a molecule has two centres, up to four possible configurations are possible: they cannot all be mirror images of each other. The possibilities continue to multiply as the number of stereogenic centres increases. Isomers of achiral molecules, possessing two or more chiral centres, are also sometimes known as meso-isomers or superimposable stereoisomers.

Several elements are common chiral centres. The most prevalent chiral centre in organic chemistry is the carbon atom, which has four different groups bonded to it when sp3 hybridized. Other common chiral centres include atoms of silicon, nitrogen and phosphorous. They may be tetrahedral (with four attached atoms) or trigonal pyramidal molecules (with a lone pair as one of the different groups).

Three systems describe the chirality of molecules: one based on a molecule's optical activity, one on the comparison of a molecule with glyceraldehyde and the current system based on the absolute configuration. The relative system is now deprecated, but is still used to label the amino acids. Why should this be? Apart from the understandable desire of the specialist to make his arcane knowledge as recondite as possible, and because sloth and lethargy inhibit the change from a familiar system to one which is more sensible and logical, there are also good reasons. The D/L system remains convenient, since it is prudent to have all amino acids labelled similarly: i.e. as L (as opposed to D). The so-called 'CORN' rule is a simple way to determine the D/L form of a chiral amino acid. Consider the groups: COOH, R (i.e. the amino acid side chain), NH2 and H arranged around the central chiral carbon atom. If the groups are arranged counter-clockwise then the amino acid is the D but if it is clockwise, it is L.

The current, and most logically self-consistent, system is the R/S or absolute configuration system owing to Cahn–Ingold–Prelog and their priority rules. This system allows for an exact labelling as S or R of a chiral centre using the atomic number of its substituents. This system is not related to the D/L classification. If a substituent of a chiral centre is converted from a hydroxyl to a thiol, the D/L labelling would not change, yet the R/S labelling would be inverted. Molecules with many chiral centres have a corresponding sequence of R/S letters: for example, natural $(+)$-$\alpha$-tocoperol is R,R,R-$\alpha$-tocoperol. However, in the R/S system most amino acids are labelled S although cysteine, for example, is labelled R.

## Naming the amino acids

It is possible to use different nomenclature to identify each amino acid since each has many names. The commonly used name for the smallest residue is glycine. The IUPAC name for glycine is 2-aminoacetic acid. As molecules get bigger and more complex, ways of naming them also proliferate. In 1968, the International Union for Pure and Applied Chemistry (or IUPAC to its friends) introduced a one-letter code for the then 20 naturally occurring amino acids, which was complementary to the earlier three-letter code (Table 4.1). The use of this code is now so prevalent as to be nearly universal; we cannot easily imagine using any other. The IUPAC nomenclature evolved from an original proposal formulated during the 1950s by Frantisek Sorm (1913–1980). When Sorm selected the letters to represent the different amino acids he chose to omit B, O, U, J, X and Z. At this time, Sorm's coding was not widely known, and many – the Chemical Society included – were sceptical that it might allow the spelling out of obscene words and offensive phrases. Sorm asserted that the then extant world of proteins contained no obscenities. He inferred from this the wholesale wholesomness of nature. Because of the dominance of English as the international language of science, Latin letters have been used for both the one- and the three-letter codes.

Mindful, no doubt, of obscenities, a number of authors have nonetheless searched sequence databases for words formed from the 20 letters – corresponding to the biogenic amino acids – which exist in languages that make use of Latin letters. Gonnet and Benner searched in English: the longest words they obtained were HIDALGISM (the practice of a hidalgo) and ENSILISTS (plural of ensilist). Jones extended this search to include words of other languages, including Esperanto. He identified the words ANSVARLIG (Danish for liable), HALETANTE (French for breathless), SALTSILDA (Norwegian for salted herring), STILLASSI (Italian for to drip), SALASIVAT (Finnish for to keep hidden), and ANNIDAVATE (to nest). Simpson, amongst several others, has also searched the sequence databases in a similar fashion. He found SSLINKASE in the sequence of oat prolamin and also PEGEDE, which is Danish for to point.

However, the present amino acid nomenclature, particularly in its one letter form, is actually fairly arbitrary. The long names given to the standard amino acids, and thus the three- and one-letter codes derived from them, arose as an historical accident. Science could easily have chosen a quite different coding. The different amino acids were discovered during a 130 year period between 1806 and 1935. The first amino acid to be discovered was asparagine. It was isolated in 1806 by French chemist, Louis-Nicolas Vauquelin, from the juice of asparagus shoots, hence the name. In 1935, the American biochemist William Rose, finalized the list when he isolated threonine, the last essential amino acid to be discovered. If we choose, we could map Latin letters to an arbitrary choice of different amino acid symbols. The IUPAC one-letter code offers one alternative but there are more. One might choose to compare the frequency of letters in English, or other languages, to the frequency of the different amino acids.

**Table 4.1** Amino acids listed in alphabetical order

| Amino acid | 3 letter code | 1 letter code | Codons encoding amino acid | MW | Rot. bond | #O | #N | #S | #HBD | #HBA |
|---|---|---|---|---|---|---|---|---|---|---|
| Alanine | *Ala* | A | GCA GCC GCG GCU | 89.1 | 0 | 0 | 0 | 0 | 0 | 0 |
| Arginine | *Arg* | R | CGA CGC CGG CGU | 174.2 | 4 | 0 | 3 | 0 | 3(4) | 1 |
| Asparagine | *Asn* | N | AAC AAU | 132.1 | 2 | 1 | 1 | 0 | 1(2) | 1 |
| Aspartate | *Asp* | D | GAC GAU | 133.1 | 2 | 2 | 0 | 0 | 1(1) | 2 |
| Cysteine | *Cys* | C | UGC UGU | 121.2 | 1 | 0 | 0 | 1 | 1(1) | 1 |
| Glutamine | *Gln* | Q | CAA CAG | 146.2 | 3 | 1 | 1 | 0 | 1(2) | 1 |
| Glutamate | *Glu* | E | GAA GAG | 147.1 | 3 | 2 | 0 | 0 | 1(1) | 2 |
| Glycine | *Gly* | G | GGA GGC GGG GGU | 75.1 | 0 | 0 | 0 | 0 | 0 | 0 |
| Histidine | *His* | H | CAC CAU | 155.2 | 2 | 0 | 2 | 0 | 1(1) | 1 |
| Isoleucine | *Ile* | I | AUA AUC AUU | 131.2 | 2 | 0 | 0 | 0 | 0 | 0 |
| Leucine | *Leu* | L | UUA UUG CUA CUC CUG CUU | 131.2 | 2 | 0 | 0 | 0 | 0 | 0 |
| Lysine | *Lys* | K | AAA AAG | 146.2 | 4 | 0 | 1 | 0 | | 0 |
| Methionine | *Met* | M | AUG | 149.2 | 3 | 0 | 0 | 1 | 0 | 0 |
| Phenylalanine | *Phe* | F | UUC UUU | 165.2 | 2 | 0 | 0 | 0 | 0 | 0 |
| Proline | *Pro* | P | CCA CCC CCG CCU | 115.1 | 0 | 0 | 0 | 0 | 0 | 0 |
| Serine | *Ser* | S | UCA UCC UCG UCU AGC AGU | 105.1 | 1 | 1 | 0 | 0 | 1(1) | 1 |
| Threonine | *Thr* | T | ACA ACC ACG ACU | 119.1 | 1 | 1 | 0 | 0 | 1(1) | 1 |
| Tryptophan | *Trp* | W | UGG | 204.2 | 2 | 0 | 1 | 0 | 1(1) | 0 |
| Tyrosine | *Tyr* | Y | UAC UAU | 181.2 | 2 | 1 | 0 | 0 | 1(1) | 1 |
| Valine | *Val* | V | GUA GUC GUG GUU | 117.2 | 1 | 0 | 0 | 0 | 0 | 0 |

*Key* MW: molecular weight. Rot. bond: rotateable bond, see Figure 4.1. #O: number of oxygen atoms. #N: number of nitrogen atoms. #S: number of sulphur atoms. #HBD: number of hydrogen bond donors. Bracketed numbers indicate the number of available hydrogens. #HBA: number of hydrogen bond acceptors.

There are thus 26!/6! different ways to map the 26 letters in the English alphabet to the 20 chemical distinct amino acids. 26!/6! works out to be 560 127 029 342 507 827 200 000, which is approximately 560 127 029 343 trillion. This is clearly a rather large number. In fact it is so large a number as to render it almost meaningless. Even a trillion is difficult to comprehend. About 50 000 pennies would fill a cubic foot, while a trillion pennies would fill a volume greater in capacity than two St Paul's Cathedrals. A million seconds is about 11.5 days, while a billion seconds would last roughly 32 years; a trillion by comparison is 32 000 years. A 2003 study in the journal *Science* estimated that the age of the universe lay somewhere between 11.2 billion and 20 billion years. Assuming you could write one of the different 26!/6! encodings every second – which is, to say the least, an optimistic assessment of the celerity of my handwriting – then it would take you 127 000 times longer than the lower bound and 200 000 times longer than the upper bound on the history of the universe to fully enumerate the list of all possible mappings between amino acids and English letters.

If we allow for the free substitution of letters representing the different amino acids, we can quickly find much longer words than HIDALGISM or ENSILISTS: words such as *dichlorodiphenyltrichloroethane* or *cyclotrimethylenetrinitramine*. These words would obviously map to utterly different looking sequences using the conventional coding, but the underlying pattern of permutation would be the same.

## The amino acid alphabet

Two new standard biogenic amino acids other than the standard 20 were discovered rather more recently; they are incorporated into proteins during translation rather than as a result of post-translational modification. Selenocysteine, the 21st amino acid, was discovered in 1986 and arises through the modification of serine after its attachment to tRNA; most other non-standard amino acids result from post-translational modification of standard amino acids with whole protein chains subsequent to ribosomal processing. The identification of selenocysteine was followed 16 years later by the discovery, reported in May 2002, of the 22nd amino acid: pyrrolysine. Pyrrolysine is encoded directly by the DNA of methanogenic bacteria found in the alimentary canal of cattle, where it is used catalytically by methane-manufacturing enzymes. It is a modified form of lysine, coded for by the codon UGA, which acts as a stop codon in other species. Like selenocysteine, pyrrolysine has its own codon, UAG, which it somehow also managed to appropriate from one of the three standard stop codons. Like other DNA encoded biogenic amino acids, it makes use of a specialized tRNA.

Protein sequences are today stored in the form of their one-letter codes. Those who work with such sequences should try to learn, either by rote learning or by assimilation, the one letter codes for each amino acid. As one letter codes, the 20 standard amino acids form an alphabet, from which protein sequences are constructed.

The sequences of biological macromolecules – at least those of DNA, RNA and proteins – are linear. There is thus a similarity between protein sequences and texts written in a language using the Latin alphabet. We saw a moment ago that even real words can be found buried away in protein sequences. Some people have sought to extend this analogy to higher levels of abstraction, equating, for example, functional domains to words. While this works well at the level of metaphor, like all analogies it breaks down under close inspection. Nonetheless, it is interesting to explore amino acid sequences in terms of alphabets.

Most alphabets contain 20–30 symbols, although the varying complexities of different sound systems leads to alphabets of different lengths. The shortest seems to be Rotokas, from the Solomon Islands, with 11 symbols. The longest is Khmer with 74 letters. Protein sequences written using the one-letter code show clear similarities to Latin texts. Latin is an Indo-European language, which was particularly influenced by Greek and Etruscan. Originally, Latin had 21 letters; two more, Y and Z, were added during Cicero's lifetime: these were reserved for loan-words taken from Greek. K survives only in the words kalendae and the praenomen kaeso. The alphabet comprises 20 main letters – A, B, C, D, E, F, G, H, I, L, M, N, O, P, Q, R, S, T, V and X – and three minor letters: K, Y and Z. The vast majority of Latin utilized an alphabet of 20 letters.

Latin texts were written without word separations or punctuation or differential capitalization. The grammatical structure implicit within sentences in classical texts was meant to be inferred from context. Having said that, there are from the first century BC onwards a few Latin texts of the classical epoch where words were, like certain monumental inscriptions, divided by a point after each word. Word division in Latin did not become prevalent until the Middle Ages. Latin was written solely in majuscule – capital or uncial – lettering, with lowercase, or miniscule, lettering only being introduced in the early medieval period. English began to use a capital letter to begin a sentence in the thirteenth century, but this practice did not gain near universality until the sixteenth century.

However bald, bare, and bland classical Latin might appear, it still only bears at best an incomplete resemblance to printed amino acid texts: some letters are different, and the order and prevalence of the common letters is very different. As we shall see later, the frequency and usage of different amino acids, although clearly governed by rules (which are in themselves rather unclear), are nonetheless very different to those adopted when writing extant written languages.

There have been several attempts to increase and decrease the size of the available amino acid alphabet. Augmenting the alphabet is a current focus of synthetic biology; it seeks to expand the number and diversity of the encoded amino acids by enlarging the base genetic code though the introduction of extra nucleotides. Others have tried to answer related questions: what is the fewest amino acid types required for a protein to fold? How does this reduced amino acid alphabet affect the stability of the structure and the rate of folding? Many studies demonstrate that stable proteins with native, topologically-complex conformations can be coded by sequences with markedly less than 20 biogenic amino acids. In an early, landmark study,

Riddle *et al.* showed that the SH3 domain, a compact $\beta$-sheet fold, can be coded for by only five amino acids but not by three.

## Defining amino acid properties

The properties of the 20 different amino acids differ. The capacity of an enzyme to catalyse a reaction or for an MHC to recognize a peptide will arise as a consequence of the structure of these proteins. The structure of a protein is a consequence of its sequence, which is composed of amino acids. Changing the sequence will change the functional characteristics of a protein. To understand the hows and the whys of such changes we need to gain a proper understanding of the properties of different amino acids. A tacit assumption underlying much of our thinking about proteins is that these properties, singly or in combination, determine the structure, and thus the biological role, of a whole protein sequence. Differences between sequences manifest themselves as differences in function exhibited by the native protein. Convergent evolution aside, similar sequences will exhibit more similarity at the function level than will greatly divergent or unrelated sequences. Or so we believe. It is the task of experiment to catalogue these similarities and it is the job of theory and computation to give meaning to such data and to predict the effects of differences in protein sequences. To say this task is challenging is to define understatement. Some such properties are important in some contexts and not in others. The functionalities important when amino acids are buried in the core of a protein are not necessarily the same as those of amino acids within a binding site.

Amino acids are often classified on the basis of the physico-chemical characteristics of their side chains. One categorization divides them into four groups: acidic, basic, hydrophilic (or polar) and hydrophobic (or nonpolar). This is one amongst many ways to reduce the common biogenic amino acids into some smaller and more easily comprehended set of groups. Such classifications are important. One can also categorize amino acids into those with aliphatic side chains and those with aromatic side chains. Aliphatic side chains contain saturated carbons, while aromatic side chains contain delocalized aromatic rings. It is fairly clear cut which residues fall into either class, despite the lack of an unequivocal definition of aromaticity. Most definitions begin with benzene and work from there. To a synthetic chemist, aromaticity implies something about reactivity; to a biophysicist interested in thermodynamics, something about heat of formation; to a spectroscopist, NMR ring currents; to a molecular modeller, geometrical planarity; to a cosmetic chemist, a pleasant, pungent smell. My own definition is similar to that used in the SMILES definition. To qualify as aromatic, rings must be planar – or nearly so – all atoms in a ring must be sp2 hybridized and the number of available 'shared' p-electrons must satisfy Hueckel's 4n+2 criterion. Such definitions become important in discussions of amino acids when we talk about histidine, that most perverse and mercurial residue. Neutral histidine contains an aromatic ring (although, obviously, it is not benzene). The imidazole ring of histidine is a heterocycle having two nitrogen atoms. Only one of the nitrogen's nonbonding electron pairs partakes in the aromatic $\pi$-electron sextet. The other electron pair has more characteristics in common with a lone pair. Through the hybridization of nitrogen to a $sp^2$ state, a p-orbital is created which is occupied by a pair of electrons and oriented parallel to the carbon p-orbitals. The resulting ring is planar and thus meets the initial criteria for aromaticity. Moreover, the $\pi$-system is occupied by six electrons, four from the two double bonds and two from the heteroatom, thus satisfying Hückel's Rule. A protonated HIS will behave differently, however, and have different properties.

## Size, charge, and hydrogen bonding

As we shall see later, the potential number of different properties associated with the 20 amino acids is extraordinarily large. There is nonetheless a seeming consensus – that is to say at least a partial agreement, which is as close to a consensus as one is likely to reach in such a diverse area – that thinking about amino acids is rightly dominated by a limited number of broadly-defined characteristic properties, among which the most important are hydrophobicity, hydrogen bonding, size and so-called electronic properties. The category of electronic properties is something of a catch-all. This category includes things as straightforward as formal charge, as well quasi-intuitive qualities such as polarity, as well as more recondite attributes like polarizability, electronegativity or electropositivity.

Size and formal charge are relatively straightforward things to think about. For size, we can look at the molecular weight of different amino acids, or their surface area or their molecular volume. For charge, the side chains of arginine and lysine are positively charged (or cations) while the side chains of glutamic acid and aspartic acid are negatively charged (or anions); all others are uncharged, except for histidine. However, even seemingly straightforward properties can be measured or calculated in many ways, producing subtly different or significantly different scales.

The capacity for hydrogen bonding is another vitally important property. Hydrogen bonds are believed by many to be the most important and most easily understood property, possibly because they can be visualized so easily. Hydrogen bonds are highly directional and, as we shall see in a later chapter, particularly important in a structural context. As a discriminatory property able to differentiate between molecules, and thought of in its simplest terms, hydrogen bonding is often interpreted as the count of hydrogen bond donors and hydrogen bond acceptors that molecules – amino acids in the present case – possess. A hydrogen bond acceptor is a polar atom – an oxygen or a nitrogen – with a lone pair. A hydrogen bond donor is a polar atom – an oxygen or a nitrogen – with a hydrogen atom it can donate.

Obviously, there are much more rigorous, much more chemically meaningful ways to describe hydrogen bonds. Consider an ester and an amide. A very naïve chemist might look at the two-dimensional structure of an amide and assume that it contains a carbonyl oxygen which acts as a hydrogen bond acceptor and a nitrogen atom which is able to both donate and accept a hydrogen bond. However, amides are planar, delocalized structures where the nitrogen acts solely as a donor. Again, a chemist might assume that both oxygen atoms in an ester would be acceptors. Analysis of small molecule crystal structures suggests otherwise. While the ester carbonyl is an effective hydrogen bond acceptor, inductive effects reduce the accepting capacity of the ether oxygen to virtually nothing. Different atoms in different chemical environments have very different hydrogen bonding capacities.

## Hydrophobicity, lipophilicity, and partitioning

Hydrophobicity is a property of great importance in understanding amino acids, the protein structures to which they give rise and the interactions a protein makes with membranes and other molecules. However, in determining the relative hydrophobicity of different amino acids there is an absolute requirement for assessing their individual structures and the interactions they can make with other amino acids (i.e. within a folded protein) or with a bulk phase. By assessing the lipophilicity of an amino acid one may hope to disentangle different and competing types of interaction. Highly specific and directional interactions dominate in the folded protein where the degrees of freedom for an individual residue are constrained compared to those seen in a bulk phase.

For small molecules, partitioning between water and some hydrophobic phase has been measured experimentally. The problem is that bulk partitioning is itself a complex and involved phenomenon which results from many types of interaction rather than a single, easily understood one. Hydrophobicity is not a property obviously separable from others, such as hydrogen bonding. Some amino acids partition as fully nonpolar molecules and others as molecules possessing both regions of polarity and nonpolarity. This has lead many to seek a bioinformatics solution instead and analyse experimental protein structures for a measure of residue hydrophobicity.

The partition coefficient, denoted $P$, is the ratio of the concentration of a molecule in two phases: one aqueous and one organic. Traditionally, experimental measurement involves dissolving a compound within a biphasic system comprising aqueous and organic layers and then determining the molar concentration in each layer:

$$P = \frac{[drug]_{organic}}{[drug]_{aqueous}}. \tag{4.1}$$

The value of $P$ can vary by many orders of magnitude: octane, for example, has an ethanediol:air partition constant of only 13 yet its hexane:air partition constant is 9300. However, for most, but not all, studies the organic solvent used is 1-octanol. $P$ can range over 12 orders of magnitude, and is usually quoted as a logarithm: $\log_{10}(P)$ or $\log P$. The partition constant is distinct from the distribution constant, denoted $D$, which is dependent upon pH. It is usually quoted as $\log D$. The distribution or 'apparent' partition coefficient results from the partitioning of more than one form of a molecule – be that neutral or charged – which alters with pH. The ionization of a molecule in the aqueous phase decreases its unionized form in the organic phase.

A $pK_a$ value defined as $-\log_{10}(K_a)$; where $K_a$ is the ionization constant, a measure of a titratable group's ability to donate a proton:

$$K_a = \frac{[H^+][A^-]}{[HA]} \qquad (4.2)$$

The $pK_a$ value is therefore equal to the pH when there is an equal concentration of the protonated and deprotonated groups in solution. For an acidic site, if the pH is below the $pK_a$ then the hydrogen or proton is on, but if the pH is greater then the hydrogen is off. The opposite holds for basic sites. For an amino acid without an ionizable side chain, such as glycine or alanine, at high pH (solution is basic) it will be a carboxylate ion, at low pH it will be an ammonium ion, at an intermediate point it will have two equal but opposite charges.

The distribution coefficient of an amino acid when calculated at its isoelectric point (or p*I*) is equal to log*P*. Each amino acid will have a different isoelectric point, hence its partitioning between phases will be different. At the pI, the concentration in the organic phase of an amino acid will be greatest, likewise for a whole peptide. For an amino acid, the isoelectric point is the point where its net charge is zero. For amino acids lacking an ionizable side chain, this point is midway between the two principal $pK_a$ values. For ionizable side chains, the p*I* approximates to the average of the two $pK_a$ values either side of the electrically-neutral, dipolar species.

As we have said, it can generally be assumed that the log*P* of a neutral species will be 2–5 log units greater than that of the ionized form; this is sufficiently large that the partitioning of the charged molecule into the organic phase can be neglected. For singly ionizeable species, log*P* and log*D* are related through simple relations, which correct for the relative molar fractions of charged and uncharged molecules.

For monoprotic acids:

$$\log D_{pH} = \log P - \log[1 + 10^{(pH - pK_a)}]. \qquad (4.3)$$

For monoprotic bases:

$$\log D_{pH} = \log P - \log[1 + 10^{(pK_a - pH)}]. \qquad (4.4)$$

However, where molecules possess two or more ionizable centres, the equivalent relationships will become ever more complex. For example, ampholytes, or amphoteric compounds, have both acidic and basic functions; ampholytes fall into two main groups: ordinary and zwitterionic, which are distinguished by the relative acidity of the two centres. In ordinary ampholytes, both groups cannot simultaneously ionize, since the acidic $pK_a$ is greater than the basic $pK_a$. However, for zwitterions, the condition that the acidic $pK_a$ is less than the basic $pK_a$ holds and so both can be ionized at once. Thus a zwitterion is an electrically-neutral internal salt. Dipolar ion is another term used for a zwitterion. The zwitterionic nature of amino acids is consistent with their salt-like character, since they have relatively low solubilities in organic solvents and unusually high melting points when crystallized: glycine, for example, melts at 506 K.

For ordinary ampholytes

$$\log D_{pH} = \log P - \log[1 + 10^{(pH - pK_a^1)} + 10^{(pK_a^2 - pH)}]. \tag{4.5}$$

For zwitterions, however, the situation becomes complicated. It is most straightforward to express $\log D$ formally based on molar fractions:

$$\log D_{pH} = \log[f_N P_N + f_Z P_Z + f_C P_C + f_A P_A] \tag{4.6}$$

where $P$ is the partition coefficient and $f$ the molar fraction; subscript N refers to neutral, Z to zwitterion, C to cation, and A to anion. Thus, neglecting the monocharged forms, which are present in negligible amounts, the following is obtained

$$\log D_{pH} = \log\left[P_N\left(\frac{1}{1 + K_T}\right) + P_Z\left(\frac{K_T}{1 + K_T}\right)\right], \tag{4.7}$$

where $K_T$ is the tautomeric constant that describes the equilibilibrium between the zwitterionic and uncharged forms. It is also possible to express this in terms of the hydrogen ion concentration:

$$\log D_{pH} = \log P - \log\left[1 + \frac{1}{k_1^0[H^+]} + \frac{k_2^0}{k_2^{\pm}} + k_2^0[H^+]\right]. \tag{4.8}$$

For polyprotic molecules with three of more ionizable groups, the situation is more complex. Consider the protic equilibrium between microstates of a triprotic molecule. For such systems, $\log D$ is given by:

$$\log D_{pH} = \log P - \log\left[1 + \frac{1}{k_1^0 k_S^S[H^+]^2} + \frac{k_S^S}{k_S^s k_S^s[H^+]} + \frac{1}{k_S^s[H^+]}\right.$$
$$\left. + \frac{1}{k_S^s[H^+]} + \frac{k_2^0}{k_2^{\pm}} + \frac{k_S^s}{k_S^s} + k_2^0[H^+]\right] \tag{4.9}$$

Consideration of ion-pairing leads to even more complex relations. The necessary correction due to ionization required for distribution coefficients is thus not trivial in the general case of a multiply protonatable molecule.

# Understanding partitioning

Understanding the equilibrium partitioning of a molecule between two distinct phases is not facile. Several empirical rules of thumb (i.e. subjective and intuitive) are available to help understand these phenomena. For example, like dissolves like, and thus polar molecules prefer polar phases and nonpolar molecules prefer nonpolar phases. This idea is often misconstrued as like only dissolves like. This is not true. Descriptions of molecules as being polar or nonpolar provides an inaccurate, all-or-nothing binary classification which short-changes the more sophisticated and nuanced truth. It is the hydrogen-bond polarity, rather than polarity based on permanent dipole moments, that control a large part of partitioning. In bulk phases, dipole–dipole interactions are small in magnitude compared to other intermolecular interactions. It is simplistic to discriminate between hydrogen-bonding or polar molecules and nonhydrogen-bonding or nonpolar molecules. Hydrogen bonds are very directional and do not occur between the totality of a pair of polar molecules; only between individual hydrogen bond donors and acceptors.

Another explanation of partitioning is that repulsive forces exist between nonpolar and polar molecules, such as water; or that attractive interactions occur only between nonpolar molecules and not between polar and nonpolar ones. Similar conjectures are used to explain many aspects of hydrophobicity either on the bulk, macrosocopic level or on the microscopic, molecular level. The language used to describe hydrophobicity, and the ideas that such language embodies, is confusing and confused. This arises partly because our understanding of the microscopic – atomic and mesoscale – level is polluted by ideas drawn from macroscopic interpretations. Thus intuitive ideas of 'greasy stuff' depoting into other 'greasy stuff' is contrasted with the specificity exhibited by the world of atoms and molecules – a world dominated as much by quantum mechanics as it is by conventional, traditional, large-scale physics.

A hydrophobic force can not be measured; hydrophobicity does not exist in isolation: rather it exists as a property of a complex system. No new 'vital force' is necessary to explain it. Like hydrogen bonds, which can be adequately explained solely by electrostatics, hydrophobicity is the result of conventional atomic interactions. Ideas of repulsive interactions between polar and nonpolar molecules completely fail to explain the behaviour seen at interfaces and surfaces. Instead, the hydrophobic effect is a very complicated, even counter-intuitive, phenomenon which is entropic in nature, arising not from direct enthalpic interactions between molecules or groups, but from the relative energetic preferences of solvent–solute interactions. More specifically, one of the major driving forces is the high free energy required for cavitation within the aqueous phase.

Account must be taken of real interactions – van der Waals and hydrogen bonding – and we must consider both cavity formation and interactions between partitioning molecules and the bulk phase solvent. Partitioning into an aqueous phase is unfavourable for nonpolar molecules because they are unable to make interactions with water that compensate for the loss of water to water hydrogen bonds.

Hydrophobicity results from interactions between water molecules being more attractive than those between nonpolar molecules and water, which can be attractive, albeit less so. There are other, as yet unmentioned, factors which complicate matters still further. Hydrophobic and hydrophilic ions exhibit different transfer mechanisms. 1-octanol is actually a poor choice for a nonpolar phase. It is said to be 'wet', since it contains much dissolved water. Thus it fails to effectively separate hydrophobic from other intermolecular phenomena. However, the presence of water in the octanol phase is not necessarily a bad thing. Relatively hydrophobic ions transfer directly into low-polarity phases via unassisted, one-step reactions. Such reactions do not need organic electrolytes to be present, and to a great extent are not dependent on the concentration of water in the organic phase. Hydrophilic ions, on the other hand, will only transfer into clusters of water molecules already dispersed within the nonpolar phase. Strongly hydrophilic ions also require hydrophobic counter-ions to be present in the organic phase: a so-called shuttling mechanism. For more polar and hydrophilic ions, therefore, the rate and magnitude of transfer will depend on the relative 'wetness' of the organic phase.

While it would be desirable to work with $\log D$ rather than $\log P$ values, unfortunately for amino acids and peptides $\log P$ values are often the only data available in any quantity. For several reasons, it is not practical to arbitrarily adjust $\log P$ values, and thus generate $\log D$ values, unless we have access to reliable $pK_a$ values for the molecules in question, which will have two or more protonatable groups. Moreover, the relevance to the definition of hydrophobicity of partitioning into 1-octanol remains open to question. Many have suggested that the measurement of partitioning into phospholipid bilayers or micelles is more appropriate.

A closely related way to assess the hydrophobicity or lipophilicty is to look at chromatographic retention times. The retention times can be used directly or an approximate partitition coefficient calculated using an equation such as

$$\log D/P = \log \left[ \frac{U(t_R - t_o)}{V_t - t_o U} \right].$$ (4.10)

In this particular equation $U$ stands for the rate of flow of the mobile phase, $t_R$ is the solute retention time, $t_0$ is the retention time of the solvent front, and $V_t$ is the total capacity of the column.

## Charges, ionization, and pKa

Generally speaking, peptides, as opposed to amino acids, can be multiply charged polyprotic ampholytes, with both N- and C-terminal and several side chain charges. While one can measure multiple $pK_a$ values using modern spectrophotometric and potentiometric methods, this has yet to be undertaken systematically for peptides. Thus measured peptide $\log D$ values are not widely available. Measured $pK_a$ values of ionizable groups in both proteins and peptides differ significantly from values measured for model compounds. Why is this? Hydrogen bonds are a key determinant of a side chain's $pK_a$ value. If we know the $pK_a$ of a particular group then its protonation state can be determined at a given pH. $pK_a$ values determine important properties such as protein solubility, protein folding and catalytic activity. Ionizable groups may be divided into acidic, which are neutral in their protonated state, and basic, which are positively charged in their protonated state. The protonated and the nonprotonated forms of a residue can be very different chemically. In the case of His, the protonated form is hydrophilic and positively charged while the nonprotonated form has a hydrophobic and aromatic character. Consequently, the interactions made by ionizable groups differ significantly above or below the $pK_a$. Each titratable group has a model or 'intrinsic' $pK_a$ value, defined as the $pK_a$ value when all the other groups are fixed in their neutral state.

In real protein-solvent systems, interactions between a residue and its environment will significantly alter $pK_a$ values for a titratable group. The intrinsic $pK_a$ value ($pK_{Model}$) combined with an environmental perturbation ($\Delta pK_a$) equate to a group's real $pK_a$ value:

$$pK_a = pK_{Model} + \Delta pK_a \qquad (4.11)$$

It can be difficult to quantify $pK_a$ shift caused by the environment. This is particularly true of ionizable active-site residues which differ markedly from the intrinsic $pK_a$. Three main factors mediate environmental perturbation: intermolecular hydrogen bonding, desolvation and charge–charge interactions. Hydrogen bonding is the predominant determinant of altered $pK_a$ values. Since the strength of hydrogen bonding varies with both distance and orientation, the degree of perturbation is contingent on the relative disposition of interacting residues. Desolvation takes a residue from a fully solvated state to one buried in a protein core. It increases the energies of negatively-charged, basic forms, thus increasing the $pK_a$ value. In the case of His, Lys and Arg, desolvation increases the energy of positively-charged acidic forms, decreasing the $pK_a$ values. The size of the shift depends on the relative burial of the residue within the protein. The third main factor is coulombic or charge–charge interactions between ionizable groups. The pair-wise interactions are dependent on the charges of the respective groups, but also on their location as only residues that are buried produce significant charge–charge interactions.

Table 4.2 is a list of 'textbook intrinsic' $pK_a$ values and the average values from the protein $pK_a$ database (PPD) database. Certain residues, such as aspartate or lysine, have relatively narrow $pK_a$ value distributions, while other residues, such as cysteine, have a wider distribution, though this may only reflect the much reduced quantities of data available for these residues. While the mean values approximate to model values, the corresponding standard deviations are high, reflecting the wide distribution of residue ionization states in proteins. As data for each residue increases in volume, trends will become ever more evident.

To a crude first approximation, amino acid properties can be roughly divided into characteristic properties and preferences. Characteristic properties, which generally

**Table 4.2** Amino acid $pK_a$ values

| Name | $pK_{a1}$ | $pK_{a2}$ | pI | Warshal | Forsyth | Edgecoombe | Average in protein (PPD) |
|------|-----------|-----------|-----|---------|---------|------------|--------------------------|
| Arg | 2.17 | 9.69 | 10.8 | 12.0 | - | - | - |
| Asp | 2.02 | 8.84 | 3.0 | 4.0 | $3.4 \pm 1.0$ | - | $3.60 \pm 1.43$ |
| Cys | 1.71 | 10.78 | 5.0 | 9.5 | - | - | $6.87 \pm 2.61$ |
| Glu | 2.19 | 9.67 | 3.2 | 4.4 | $4.1 \pm 0.8$ | - | $4.29 \pm 1.05$ |
| His | 1.82 | 9.17 | 7.6 | 6.3 | - | $6.6 \pm 0.9$ | $6.33 \pm 1.35$ |
| Lys | 2.18 | 8.95 | 9.7 | 10.4 | - | - | $10.45 \pm 1.19$ |
| Tyr | 2.20 | 9.11 | 5.7 | 10.0 | - | - | $9.61 \pm 2.16$ |
| N term | - | - | - | 7.5 | - | - | $8.71 \pm 1.49$ |
| C term | - | - | - | 3.8 | - | - | $3.19 \pm 0.76$ |
| Gly | 2.34 | 9.60 | 6.0 | | | | |
| Ala | 2.34 | 9.69 | 6.0 | | | | |
| Asn | 2.02 | 9.04 | 5.4 | | | | |
| Gln | 2.17 | 9.13 | 5.7 | | | | |
| Ile | 2.36 | 9.68 | 6.0 | | | | |
| Leu | 2.36 | 9.60 | 6.0 | | | | |
| Met | 2.28 | 9.21 | 5.7 | | | | |
| Phe | 1.83 | 9.13 | 5.5 | | | | |
| Pro | 1.99 | 10.60 | 6.3 | | | | |
| Ser | 2.21 | 9.15 | 5.7 | | | | |
| Thr | 2.63 | 9.10 | 5.6 | | | | |
| Trp | 2.38 | 9.39 | 5.9 | | | | |
| Val | 2.32 | 9.62 | 6.0 | | | | |

Notes: Forsyth et al reviewed 212 experimental carboxyl pKa values (97 glutamate and 115 aspartate) from 24 structurally characterized proteins. Overall average pKa values for ASP were $3.4 \pm 1.0$; for basic (pI > 8) proteins, the average pKa value was $3.9 \pm 1.0$; and for acidic (pI < 5) proteins, average pKa was $3.1 \pm 0.9$. Overall average pKa values for GLU were $4.1 \pm 0.8$, while average pKa values for glutamates are ~4.2 in both acidic and basic proteins. Likewise, Edgcombe and Murphy recently reviewed the literature values of pKa's for titratable histidines: average pKa values for titratable HIS were $6.6 \pm 0.9$.

correspond to properties of individual residues, can be divided between derived or calculated values (such as accessible surface area or molecular volume or electronegativity) and measured values (such as partition into membranes or lipid-like solvent). Preferences can also be measured or calculated, though calculations tend to predominate; these refer, in the main, to statistical tendencies or predilections, such as for forming protein secondary structures or being involved in binding sites.

## Many kinds of property

We have described measured properties at length above. The other principal forms of amino acid property are the calculated preference values, which are usually defined through computational analysis of large numbers of protein structures. The difference between a preference and a measured property is largely semantic. The difference can again be illustrated by reference to $pK_a$ values. A model or intrinsic $pK_a$ value is a measured property, but an average or mean $pK_a$ value is a preference since it is derived from ensemble properties measured over many, many instances. Other illustrative examples are solvent accessible surface areas or amino acid frequencies.

Amino acid frequencies are important. In the current genomic age, it is straightforward to analyse large numbers of protein sequences. Counting the frequency of different residues we see that the distribution of letters in the amino acid alphabet is not uniform, any more than the distribution of letters in English or, indeed, any other language. The most frequent residue is alanine ($f = 0.13$); the least frequent is trytophan ($f = 0.015$). The frequency of dipeptides and higher tuples do not reflect the base frequencies. When compared to what is expected, the tripeptide CWC is five times over-represented while CIM is under-represented by a factor of 10. This indicates that there is structure in the pattern of residues reflecting constraints imposed by the genetic code, by the need for structural stability, by the need for a protein to fold, by functional constraints imposed by chemistry and the need for solubility, amongst many others.

In the final analysis, however, individual properties, whether characteristic or preference values, become little more than a scale or index: a series of numbers, each number associated with an individual amino acid. Let us assume, for the moment at least, that each amino acid has a different value associated with it. This gives us 20! different ways of ordering the set of amino acids. As we have said before, this number is large: 2 432 902 008 176 640 000. If we allow an arbitrary number of amino acids to have the same value – i.e. to form equivalent nonempty subsets – we see that the total number of possible combinations of 20 amino acids is vastly greater.

At this point, we should perhaps ask how many ways are there to partition the 20 biogenic amino acids into one or more nonempty subsets? Assuming that the subsets are unordered, then there is one way to partition 20 amino acids into 20 subsets and there is one way of partitioning 20 amino acids into one subset. This is very logical and very simple. For other numbers of subsets, the result is equally logical but rather more complicated. For example, for 19 subsets we need only calculate the number of ways of pairing two amino acids: 20 times 19 divided by two, or 190. As the number of groups increases the calculation rapidly becomes somewhat tiresome.

Fortunately these results were worked out long ago and can be conveniently calculated using Stirling numbers of the second kind. Stirling numbers of the first kind describe the partitioning of sets into sets of cycles or orbits. While interesting in their own right, they are not germane to the present discussion. However, Stirling numbers of the second kind – which are written $s(n, k)$ where $n$ is the size of the set and $k$ the number of partitions – directly address the partitioning of sets into a number of nonempty subsets. They can be calculated recursively, but there are also more explicit formulae, of which the following is the most direct:

$$s(n, k) = \frac{1}{k!} \sum_{j=1}^{k} (-1)^{(k-j)} \left( \frac{k!}{j!(k-j)!} \right) j^n.$$
(4.12)

There are many other ways to enumerate these quantities; indeed, one of the most pleasing aspects of combinatorics is that correct answers can be arrived at via different paths (Table 4.3). Clearly, the number of ways to reduce the amino acid alphabet or group residues is very large; far too large for us to properly comprehend. To calculate the total number of ordered partitions, such as is required by a scale of properties, we need only multiply each set of possible partitions by the number of ways of ordering said partitions. In short, to multiply the number of $k$ possible subsets by $k!$ (Table 4.3). The total number of possible scales is thus: 2 677 687 796 244 380 000 000. This number is very large indeed. Even if we allow for the symmetry between a scale and its inverse, this only reduces this large number by a factor of two. If we then factor in the possibility of the same ordering of amino acids but with variable separations between the values associated with each group – even after normalization of a scale to have a mean of 0.0 and a standard deviation of 1.0 – then we can quickly see that the number of combinations is truly astronomic.

Within the enormous number of possibilities are a limited number of scales which correlate well with the observable features exhibited by proteins and their sequences. It is one of the tasks of the bioinformatician to try to identify and properly use those scales which are useful descriptors of biologically important features of amino acid sequences, whether this is exhibited in terms of structure, action or function. Putting the multiplicity of possible scales to one side, the usefulness or validity of a scale is found in its utility not in its ability to be rationalized. People want to explain these data in terms of poorly understood biophysical properties, such as hydrophobicity, but in reality scales are just numbers and they can be understood as such.

There is an understandable yet vast and perplexing gulf in our knowledge and understanding of the plethora of nonstandard amino acids when compared with our

**Table 4.3** Ways of arranging partitions of the 20 amino acids into ordered subsets

| K (number of subsets) | Ways of dividing 20 amino acids into K subsets | Ways of arranging K subsets | Total number of ordered subsets |
|---|---|---|---|
| 1 | 1 | 1 | 1 |
| 2 | 524287 | 2 | 1048574 |
| 3 | 580606446 | 6 | 3483638676 |
| 4 | 45232115901 | 24 | 1085570781624 |
| 5 | 749206090500 | 120 | 89904730860000 |
| 6 | 4306078895384 | 720 | 3100376804676480 |
| 7 | 11143554045652 | 5040 | 56163512390086100 |
| 8 | 15170932662679 | 40320 | 611692004959217000 |
| 9 | 12011282644725 | 362880 | 4358654246117810000 |
| 10 | 5917584964655 | 3628800 | 21473732319740100000 |
| 11 | 1900842429486 | 39916800 | 75875547089306800000 |
| 12 | 411016633391 | 479001600 | 196877625020902000000 |
| 13 | 61068660380 | 6227020800 | 380275818414396000000 |
| 14 | 6302524580 | 87178291200 | 549443231303980000000 |
| 15 | 452329200 | 1307674368000 | 591499300737946000000 |
| 16 | 22350954 | 20922789888000 | 467644314338353000000 |
| 17 | 741285 | 355687428096000 | 263665755136143000000 |
| 18 | 15675 | 6402373705728000 | 100357207837286000000 |
| 19 | 190 | 121645100408832000 | 23112569077678100000 |
| 20 | 1 | 2432902008176640000 | 2432902008176640000 |
| Total: | 51 724 158 235 372 | 2 561 327 494 111 820 000 | 2 677 687 796 244 380 000 000 |

knowledge and understanding of the 20 biogenic amino acids. This gulf is largely, if not completely, a consequence of the practical limitations imposed by the logistics – i.e. the cost, labour and time – involved in measuring the chemical and physical properties of nonstandard amino acids experimentally.

## Mapping the world of sequences

There have now been several decades of experimental sequencing. This effort has seen an ever-escalating degree of sophistication. This focused first on the sequencing of individual proteins and genes followed by the analysis of whole genomes and proteomes. Beginning with painstaking chemical dissection of proteins – the era of Edman degradation – followed in turn by hand-crafted gene sequencing and now by the full flowering of automated genome sequencing. Protein derives from the Greek word *protas*, meaning 'of highest importance'. The word *protein* was first used by the great Swedish chemist Jöns Jakob Berzelius (1779–1848), who was also the first to use the words isomerism, polymerization and catalysis. The first and greatest mystery of proteins, their primary structure, was finally resolved when Fred Sanger (1918–2003) successfully sequenced insulin in 1949. Sanger later received the first of his two Nobel prizes for this work; he later received a second one for gene sequencing. Sanger's work was itself a pivotal discovery, leading to the development of modern gene manipulation and genomics. Since then sequence data has accrued unceasingly, resulting first in the accumulation of vast numbers of text files and then by the staggering growth of a whole host of databases, each of which is ever larger and ever more sophisticated. These contain macromolecular sequences – DNA and protein – represented as strings composed of a small set of characters: four for DNA and 20 for protein. This much we know.

The accessibility of data is critical for proper characterization and analysis of host–pathogen interaction. Vast quantities of sequence information and related data have been collated from the literature, and stored in a bewildering variety of database systems. Yet sequence databases are not overly important in themselves. Nothing is. It is only as part of a wider system able to capitalize on and utilize their contents that they gain importance. Meanwhile, genomics moves on apace. In 2007, James Watson and J. Craig Venter became the first to know their own DNA. Such self-knowledge will, many hope, be a significant component driving the development of personalized medicine. At the same time Venter's ocean survey has mapped the genomes of thousands of marine bacteria, opening up the era of the environmental genomics of biodiversity.

Thus, in the space of a few years the sequencing of a genome has gone from a transcendent achievement capable of stopping the scientific world in its tracks to the almost mundane, worthy of only a minor mention in a journal of the second rank. In future times, genomic sequencing may simply become a workaday laboratory technique. Within a few years it may become the stuff of a postgraduate student's thesis. Within a decade an undergraduate might need to sequence a dozen genomes to complete their final year project. Certainly within a short period, the $1000 genome will become a medical mainstay. Slightly further off, micro-automation may render single nucleotide polymorphisms and gene indels in the human genome sequence routine markers much as a dip-stick test is today.

# Biological sequence databases

Having said that, however prevalent readouts of the human genome become, and however wide the ecological net of the sequencer may become, we will continue to need databases to store and disseminate the information that arises from their efforts. Likewise, the availability of different kinds of biologically meaningful data means that the total number of databases is now huge. To say that catalogues which simply list biological databases now run into thousands of entries would be an exaggeration, but as exaggerations go, not a huge one. Over 100 new biological databases are added each year to the Molecular Biology Database Collection, for example. Having said that, it would also be fair to say that despite the legion of available databases the majority of effort and resource goes into a few major se-quence and structures databases.

Most databases in current use were neither conceived nor designed initially as databases, but grew haphazardly to expedite particular pieces of research. Indeed, databases continue to emerge from local research projects in a similar fashion. When such resources grow large enough, they are often made accessible via the Web. Many databases start by storing data as so-called flat files containing data as text, but evolve quickly into relational or XML databases. The principal aim of such endeavours is to benefit the scientific community at large. This is easy for small databases, as they require only a minimal outlay of resources. Attempting to create usable, flexible databases of true depth is rather more difficult. Properly maintaining them over time is even more difficult. Keeping a database operational is not trivial. Software must be maintained and updated. Databases must evolve as the areas of knowledge they try to encapsulate evolve, expand and diversify. Such expansion must be guided, necessitating input from biological as well as computa-tional perspectives.

How much does this cost and where do the funds come from? A financial study of several biological databases at the end of the last century revealed that they had ap-proximately 2.5–3.5 full-time employees and cost around $200 000. These figures are little changed today. For an academic database, costs pay for hardware mainte-nance, software upgrades and the salaries of several technicians or students under-taking data entry as well as programmers, postdoctoral annotators and knowledge-domain experts. The vast majority of database funding still originates from governmental research agencies, nonprofit organizations and charities; relatively little comes from industry or directly from users. It is a deep frustration to those who maintain and develop databases that such funding covers the initial development but seldom supports on-going maintenance. Other well-funded databases exist only as an extension of various experimental programmes. They may be a bespoke database for a particular genome or microarray experiment. Such databases have lifespans which are unlikely greatly to exceed the projects they serve.

## Nucleic acid sequence databases

Beginning during the 1980s and lasting well into the 1990s, bioinformatics was dependent upon protein annotation generated through the Sisyphean labours of a small number of enthusiastic, skilled and highly experienced human annotators spread through a small set of key sequence databanks, such as GenBank, PIR and Swiss-Prot. Their work involved scouring the experimental literature, the parsing of individual research papers and the careful analysis of experimental facts, deductions and hypotheses, all coupled to and supplemented by more systematic, if ultimately less reliable, bioinformatics analysis and prediction. All this effort has resulted in the creation and dissemination of invaluable data-sets. These form the core of current gene and protein knowledge bases.

It is not a little futile to regale the reader with long and uninteresting accounts of all of these different and competing systems, but it would be equally pointless to ignore them altogether. Thus we will content ourselves with a brief review of the really well-established players.

There are three main nucleic acid databases: EMBL, GenBank and the DNA Data Bank of Japan (DDBJ). Long ago, these databases began to cooperate, seeking to cope with burgeoning sequence data being created globally: Genbank and EMBL joined forces in 1986 to form the International Nucleotide Sequence Database or INSD. DDBJ joined INSD in 1987. The three databases famously synchronize their records daily. Each member of INSD feeds – and is fed by – its partners. They all receive data from individual research groups around the world, and from patent offices, including the European Patent office (EPO), the Japanese Patent Office, and the US Office of Patents and Trademarks (USPTO). However, an increasing proportion of sequence data is now submitted directly from research groups and, increasingly, factory-scale sequencing centres. This component is beginning to dwarf other routes of submission. However, with this come problems. Thus, the ultimate responsibility for the verity and veracity of deposited sequences rests with submitting authors. Moreover, nucleic acid databases can only provide very basic annotation.

The EMBL database was the world's first nucleic acid sequence database, coming into being in 1982 when it comprised 568 entries. Europe's primary repository of gene and genomic sequences, EMBL is now maintained by the European Bioinformatics Institute or EBI. DDBJ began life in 1986 at the National Institute of Genetics at Mishima, Japan. GenBank is a general-purpose nucleotide database, covering coding, genomic, EST and synthetic sequences. GenBank opened for business in December 1982 when it contained 606 entries.

GenBank is currently part of the impressive and evolving collection of different databases offered by the National Centre for Biotechnology Information (NCBI). They are the purveyors of PUBMED and PUBCHEM, for example, which are open-access databases addressing the biological literature and chemical structure. Protein sequence databases at NCBI originate as nucleotide database translations, and also come from PIR, SWISS-PROT, Protein Research Foundation, the Protein Data Bank and USPTO.

## Protein sequence databases

In addition to these three vast collections of nucleic acid data, there are two main protein sequence databases: PIR and Swiss-Prot. The Protein Identification Resource (or PIR) grew out of the 1965 book by Margaret Dayhoff: *Atlas of Protein Sequence and Structure*. The atlas expanded during the late 1960s and 1970s and, by 1981, it contained 1660 sequences. In 1984, Dayhoff's Atlas was released in a machine-readable format renamed the Protein Sequence Database (PSD) of the Protein Identification Resource (PIR). It continues today at the Georgetown University Medical Center. PIR had an initial size of 859 entries. PIR is a low-redundancy database of annotated protein sequences. It encompasses structural, functional and evolutionary annotations of proteins and classifies protein sequences into superfamilies, families and domains. PIR entries are extensively cross-referenced to other major databases.

First appearing in the early 1980s, Swiss-Prot is a protein sequence and knowledge database maintained by Amos Bairoch and Rolf Apweiler. Its first official release was 1986, when it contained in excess of 4000 sequences. It is widely regarded as the key repository of high-quality annotation. Expert, manually-curated annotations, with minimal redundancy and high integration, are the hallmarks of Swiss-Prot. Each entry contains two types of database record: fixed and variable. Fixed records are always present. Such data includes: protein name, taxonomic data, citation information, the protein's amino acid sequence, and so on. Variable records may or may not be present. Such data includes: protein function, enzyme activity, sequence or structural domains, functional sites, post-translation modifications, sub-cellular location, three-dimensional structure, similarities to other proteins, polymorphisms and disease-associations. Entries are often cross-referenced to other relevant data sources. The number of sequences in Swiss-Prot is at best a small fraction of all available protein sequences, due to the prodigious difficulties involved in maintaining quality. TrEMBL (for translated EMBL) greatly extends the scope of Swiss-Prot. It contains translations of all EMBL nucleotide sequences not present in Swiss-Prot, and provides automatically derived annotations which propagate Swiss-Prot entries to new sequences.

Together, PIR and Swiss-Prot form part of the Universal Protein Resource or UniProt. UniProt is a collaboration between the European Bioinformatics Institute (EBI), the Swiss Institute of Bioinformatics (SIB) and PIR. It is comprised of four databases: the UniProt Knowledgebase or UniProtKB; the UniProt Reference Clusters or UniRef; the UniProt Archive or UniParc; and UniProt Metagenomic and Environmental Sequences or UniMES. UniProtKB is a compilation of extensively annotated protein data, and is built from the Swiss-Prot, TrEMBL and PIR-PSD databases. It comprises two parts: a fully manually annotated set of records and another containing computationally analysed records awaiting full manual annotation. These sections are known as the Swiss-Prot Knowledgebase and TrEMBL Protein Database, respectively. The UniProt Reference Clusters within UniRef amalgamate sequences (at various levels of similarity) from the UniProt Knowledgebase and selected UniParc entires into single records aiming to accelerate sequence searching. Three cluster levels are available: 100% (UniRef100), greater than 90% (UniRef90) and greater than 50% (UniRef50), providing coverage of sequence space at different resolutions. In UniRef100, identical sequences and subfragments are placed into a single cluster, hiding redundant sequences but not their annotation. UniParc is a comprehensive protein sequence compendium solely containing unique identifiers and sequences, which reflects the history of all protein sequences. UniMES has been developed to address nascent metagenomic and environmental data.

## Annotating databases

More important perhaps than enumerating databases per se is the need to discuss some of the vital and unresolved research issues in maintaining, populating and extending modern sequence databases.

In themselves, sequences arising from genomics and proteomics are all but incomprehensible and all but useless. To render them comprehensible and useful requires associating with them some context in the form of meaningful biological facts. This is the purpose of genomic and proteomic annotation. According to the dictionary, annotation is 'the action of making or adding or furnishing notes or is a note added to anything written, by way of explanation or comment'. In molecular biology databases, such notes typically contain information about the cellular role and mechanism of action of genes and their products. In the distant past, biological databases simply stored the sequences and structures of genes and proteins. Initially, that was enough. Soon, however, databases such as Swiss-Prot began to supplement sequence entries with biological context; currently as little as 15% of Swiss-Prot is sequence, the remainder is annotation: references to the literature and experimental data and the like.

When confronted by a novel sequence, there are three principal means of obtaining information on function. First, based on unequivocal similarity, function, in the form of associated annotation, can be inherited from one or more other sequences. Secondly, a predictive computational technique can 'forecast' function. Thirdly, we can use phylogenetic techniques to 'infer' more generic, less specific, functional information such as the identity of function-critical residues. No technique is ever absolutely reliable so it is advisable to combine the results of many strategies. The initial stage in function identification using homology is to find the protein group to which a sequence belongs. Defining such a group involves an iterative procedure of similarity searching in sequence, structure and motif databases to create a sequence corpus. This corpus is representative of the whole sequence set comprising the family.

Annotation is thus often inferred from the observed similarities between sequences. This can lead to errors, particularly when similarity is ambiguous. Thus within commonly-used databases there are now substantial numbers of inaccurate and thus misleading annotations. This problem is further compounded by 'error percolation', whereby annotations of similar proteins may have been acquired through chains of similarity to other proteins. Such chains are seldom archived explicitly, rendering it impossible to determine how a particular database annotation has been acquired.

Such a situation leads to an inevitable deterioration of quality, and poses an ongoing threat to the reliability of data as a consequence of propagating errors in annotation. Although curators continually strive to address such errors, users must be constantly on their guard when inferring function from archived data.

However, rationalizing biological data is today beyond the scope of the individual and requires large-scale effort and some kind of automation. Two views exist, and these views are strongly polarized. One contends that manual annotation is dead and must be replaced – and replaced with the utmost celerity – by unsupervised methods. The other and opposing view holds that only rigorous and highly labour-intensive manual annotation can generate high-quality databases. These are clearly caricatures, gross simplifications, yet capture something of the essential dialectic dichotomy here.

While both pragmatism and bitter experience support the veracity of the second view, the first view, despite being couched in pessimistic language, is nonetheless that of an optimist. In many ways it echoes the desire, and ostensive failure, of theoreticians to create methods able to predict protein structure from sequence – despite the 30 years of effort, an effective and efficient system still eludes us. What seems an easy – almost facile – task is, in reality, difficult to the point of being confounding; so too with text mining and the other attempts to automate annotation. Asking a computer truly to understand and manipulate meaning is currently asking the impossible.

# Text mining

This kind of reasoning has led to the development of alternative paradigms providing other directions that database development might follow. Text mining is perhaps the more obvious avenue, while others place their faith in ontologies. Text mining is, superficially at least, abstracting data from the literature in an automated manner. A principal impediment to effective text mining is variation in terms. This is why text mining often fails to even identify genes or proteins within text: this is, arguably, its simplest and most mundane task. Term variation can include both morphological variation ('transcriptional factor SF-1' versus 'transcription factor SF-1') and orthographic variation ('TLR-9' versus 'TLR9' versus 'TLR 9'). This is compounded by switching between arabic and roman numerals ('IGFBP-3' versus 'IGFBP III' or 'type 1 interferon' versus 'type I interferon') or between Greek symbols and Latinized equivalents ('TNF-$\alpha$' versus 'TNF-alpha'), the haphazard use of acronyms ('Toll-like receptor 9' versus 'TLR-9'), and the use of new versus older nomenclature ('B7' versus 'B7.1'). Even the insertion of extra words (e.g. 'Toll Receptor' versus 'Toll-like receptor') or the different possible ordering of words ('Class I MHC' versus 'MHC Class I') can pose problems.

Even worse, of course, and certainly more confusing, is that many proteins have been named independently many times over: consider S100 calcium-binding protein A8 or Protein S100-A8 alias P8 alias Leukocyte L1 complex light chain alias cystic fibrosis antigen or CFAG alias Calgranulin A alias Migration inhibitory factor 8 or MRP-8 alias 60B8AG alias CAGA alias Calprotectin L1L subunit alias CGLA alias CP-10 alias L1Ag alias MA387 alias MIF alias NIF alias Urinary stone protein band A. As many readers will know, this is by no means an exceptional case. For example, Neutrophil gelatinase-associated lipocalin or NGAL is also known as lipocalin 2 and siderocalin and 24p3 protein and human neutrophil lipocalin (HNL) and superinducible protein 24 kD or SIP24 and uterocalin and neu-related lipocalin (NRL) and $\alpha_2$-microglobulin associated protein. Such examples are legion. It reflects biology's proclivity to rediscover the same protein in innumerable different contexts. Biochemical nomenclature is generally a mishmash of systematic nomenclature (such as the CD antigen system), alternate naming conventions and so-called trivial nomenclature; all of which are applied in a haphazard and almost random fashion when viewed on a large scale. No wonder mindless computers struggle.

There are various simple tricks, such as normalizing terms (e.g. deleting hyphens, spaces and other symbols; converting all text to be upper or lower case, etc.), to obviate these problems, yet these are seldom effective. In addition to normalization, soft string-matching, which scores the similarity of text strings, can also be used. This permits nonidentical terms to be associated and provides multiple candidate associations ranked by similarity.

Much of the data that goes into sequence and structure databases is, due to the requirements imposed by journals and the largesse of publicly-funded genome sequencing projects, deposited directly by their authors. However, much of interest – the results of tens of thousands of unique experiments stretching back over the decades – is still inaccessible and hidden away, locked into the hard copy text of innumerable papers. As the scientific literature has moved inexorably from paper to a fully electronic and online status, the opportunity to interrogate it automatically has likewise arisen. However, and notwithstanding the effort expended and the establishment of text-mining institutes, the results have yet to be impressive. The goal is doubtless a noble and enticing one, but so far little of true utility has been forthcoming. People – indeed people in some number – are still an absolute necessity to parse and filter the literature properly.


# Ontologies

Research into so-called ontologies is also currently very active. Ontologies can be used to characterize the principal concepts in a particular discipline and how they relate one to another. Many people believe they are necessary if database annotation is to be made accessible to both people and software. Others feel it is crucial to facilitating more effective and efficient data retrieval. Thus a formal ontology can be crucial in database design, helping to catalogue its information and to disseminate the conceptual structure of the database to its users.

A dictionary might define an ontology as: '1. A study of being: specifically, a branch of metaphysics relating to the nature and relations of being. 2. A theory or conception relating to the kinds of entities or abstract entities which can be admitted to a language system.' The well-known 'Gene Ontology' consortium, or GO, defines the term ontology as: '. . .specifications of a relational vocabulary'. Others define it as 'the explicit formal specification of terms in a domain and the relationships between them'. Thus an ontology is a group of defined terms of the kind found in dictionaries; terms which are also networked. An ontology will define a common vocabulary for information sharing which assists separation of operational knowledge from domain knowledge. Terms will likely be restricted to those used in a given domain: in the case of GO, all are biological.

GO is a restricted vocabulary of terms used to annotate gene products. It comprises three ontologies: one describing proteins in terms of their subcellular location or as a component of a protein complex (cellular component ontology); one describing binding or enzymatic activity (molecular function ontology); and one which describes cellular or organismal events undertaken by pathways or ordered biological processes (biological process ontology). The assignment of terms proceeds based on direct experimental validation or through sequence similarity to an experimentally validated gene product.

Should one wish to find all major histocompatibility complexes in an annotated database, genome or other sequence set then one could search with software agents able to recognize proteins labelled 'MHC' or 'HLA' or 'major histocompatibility complex' or even as 'monotopic transmembrane protein' as an aid to finding all possible targets. This rather trivial example illustrates both the potential utility and the potential pitfalls of an ontology. For example, 'monotopic transmembrane protein' would include all MHCs but many other proteins besides. Synonyms can be used to identify the same core entity: 'MHC' = 'major histocompatibility complexes' = 'HLA' and so on. Relationships within an ontology relate concepts in a hierarchical fashion: thus 'HLA-A*0201' is a form of 'MHC'. More serious ontologies require sophisticated semantic relations which form some kind of network specifying how terms are related in meaning.

Thus an ontology should specify a concept explicitly, defining a set of representations which associate named entities (classes or functions) with human-readable text describing the associated meaning. An ontology is often composed of four components: classes, a hierarchical structure, relations (other than hierarchical) and axioms. The heart of an ontology is an 'entity hierarchy' which groups together entities with similar properties. Its overall structure is a tree or directed acyclic graph. Often, such a hierarchy will comprise terms related by two sorts of relationship: parthood (i.e. 'part of') or subsumption (i.e. 'is a'). A useful ontology should describe the application domain, define all entities, catalogue characteristic properties describing these entities and allow meaning-rich reasoning based on the relationships between terms. Ontologies can be dismissed as simply controlled vocabularies, but the point is that an ontology should be either useful or interesting or both. How one distinguishes between a good ontology and a poor ontology is a difficult question to answer.

There are now many biological ontologies: FuGO (the Functional Genomics Investigation Ontology), which details the key concepts and relations in functional genomics experiments and FMA (Foundational Model of Anatomy), which details the ideas and interrelations of vertebrate anatomy, are examples. Ontologies have even been introduced into immunology. There are three main complementary immunological ontologies available: the IEDB ontology (which addresses epitopes), the IMGT-Ontology and the Gene Ontology (GO). The IMGT-Ontology, probably the first ontology of its kind, provides an exceptional ontological framework for immune receptors (antibodies, T cell receptors, and MHCs). It has a specific immunological content, describing the classification and specification of terms required in immunogenetics. What the IMGT ontology lacks is information on epitopes. GO provides broad vocabularies which are controlled and structured vocabularies and, as we intimated above, cover several biological knowledge domains including immunololgy. Recently, Diehl et al. [1] have extended existing immunological terms found in GO. GO again does not cover epitopes specifically. IEDB has developed an ontology framed in terms of immunoinformatics: it is specifically designed to capture information on immune epitopes.

## Secondary sequence databases

Another, rather more unambiguously useful, area of database development, again intimately connected with annotation, is the so-called secondary sequence database. Also known as motif or protein family databases, such databases, when compared to primary sequence databases, such as NCBI or Swiss-Prot, are fruitful areas of research in bioinformatics. They depend on robust diagnostic sequence analysis techniques able to identify and group proteins into meaningful families. Many analytical approaches form the basis of such discriminators: regular expressions (PROSITE), aligned sequence blocks (BLOCKS), fingerprints (PRINTS), profiles (ProDom) and hidden Markov models or HMMs (Pfam). Each approach has different strengths and weaknesses, and thus produces databases with very different characters. However, all rely on the presence of characteristic and conserved sequence patterns.

There are many ways to discover such motifs: through human inspection of sequence patterns, by using software such as PRATT to extract motifs from a multiple alignment or by using a program like MEME to generate motifs directly from unaligned sequences. The resulting set of one or more motifs becomes the input into a motif database. Motif databases thus contain distilled descriptions of protein families that can be used to classify other sequences in an automated fashion.

PROSITE (www.expasy.ch/prosite/) is perhaps the first example of such a secondary protein database. It is very much a motif database being composed of a collection of patterns characterizing functional sites (i.e. glycosylation sites) and protein family membership. Other databases include BLOCKS (http://blocks.fhcrc.org/), PRINTS (www.bioinf.manchester.ac.uk/dbbrowser/PRINTS/) and PFAM (www.sanger.ac.uk/Software/Pfam/). These are high quality endeavours: while PRINTS focuses on exceptionally high-quality annotation at the expense of coverage, the semi-automated creation of PFAM can be said to have the opposite characteristics. Another database – TIGRFAMs (www.tigr.org/TIGRFAMs/) – was introduced in 2001 as a group of protein families and associated HMMs. Originally it included more than 800 families of two classes. There are now 2946 in release 6.0 of TIGRFAMS. A derived or combined (or, more accurately, metaprediction) database system, such as SMART (http://smart.embl-heidelberg.de/) or InterPRO (www.ebi.ac.uk/interpro/), can then be built on top of one or more individual motif databases.

## Other databases

However, bioinformatics is never still and databases, like other aspects of the discipline, have moved on. Biologically focused databases now encompass entities of remarkable diversity and they continue to proliferate; indeed they now require their own database just to catalogue them. Again we will explore this area briefly, highlighting the validity and utility of data integration, without any attempt to be exhaustive or encyclopedic in our coverage.

The scientific literature itself is fast becoming a searchable database. The emergence of PUBMED – and, to a lesser extent, ISI – coupled to the recent development of open- access journals (such as BIOMED CENTRAL and PLOS), time-delayed access and user pays open-access scenarios increasingly used by major publishers and accessible over the internet, has created a wholly unprecedented situation compared, say, with that which existed only 20 years ago. If one also takes on board the fact that Google has scanned a large proportion of all books published in English, the potential for searching all of recorded human knowledge is not too distant a prospect. If we replace searching with text mining then the possibility exists of automatically parsing all that humankind has ever known. These two potent possibilities are on a collision course with as yet undreamed potential.

We have already alluded to databases comprising whole genome sequences, transcriptomic and proteomic experiments, yet there are also many other kinds of information available within databases that impact data-set creation for the prediction of immunogenicity or the identification of antigens. Another whole area is also now emerging: databases that catalogue experimental thermodynamic and kinetic measurements.

## Databases in immunology

Databases in immunology, and thus in vaccinology, have a long history. Such databases, which tend to focus on molecular immunology, do no more than apply standard data warehousing techniques in an immunological context. There is nothing very exceptional about them in terms of what they do or how they do it. What makes them interesting to us is their focus – their focus on immunology and the immune system (see Table 4.4).

## Host databases

We begin by looking at host databases, which have made the analysis of important immunological macromolecules their focus for many years, and have concentrated on the compilation and rigorous annotation of host side sequences and structures. Following the sequencing of the first antibody during the mid 1960s, Elvin A. Kabat and Tai Te Wu began compiling and aligning all published complete and partial human and mouse immunoglobulin light chain sequences. The Kabat database became properly established in the early 1970s, when it contained 77 sequences. At its height, the database was the most complete compilation of sequences of proteins of immunological interest and contained in excess of 19 382 sequence entries – including immunoglobulins (Ig), TCRs, MHCs and other immunological molecules – from 70 species. The Kabat database has its own nomenclature and analysis tools including keyword searching, sequence alignment and variability analysis. The Kabat database is amongst the oldest of biological databases, and was for some time the only database containing sequence alignment information. Today, noncommercial access to the database is limited.

Another important host database is VBASE2, which stores germline sequences of human and mouse immunoglobulin variable (V) genes. VBASE2 replaced the now defunct VBASE, which comprised germline variable regions of human antibodies. Established in 1997, it offered the usual search facilities, as well as maps of the human immunoglobulin loci, numbers of functional segments and restriction enzyme cuts in V genes. ABG is another legacy database archiving germline variable regions from mouse antibody kappa and heavy chains.

**Table 4.4** A list of bioinformatics and immunoinformatic databases

| Database | | | |
|---|---|---|---|
| Host | IMGT/TR | Annotated T cell receptor sequences and sequences | http://imgt.cines.fr/textes/IMGTrepertoire |
| | IMGT/HLA | Annotated HLA sequences | http://www.ebi.ac.uk/imgt/hla/allele.html |
| | IPD Database | Annotated sequences for non-human MHC | http://www.ebi.ac.uk/ipd/index.html |
| | VBASE2 | Database of human and mouse antibody genes | http://www.vbase2.org/ |
| | V BASE | Database of human antibody genes | http://vbase.mrc-cpe.cam.ac.uk/ |
| Pathogen | APB | Airbourne Pathogen Database | http://www.engr.psu.edu/ae/iec/abe/database.asp |
| | ARS | Database of sequences from viral, bacterial, and fungal plant pathogens | http://www.ars.usda.gov/research/projects/projects.htm?accn_no=406518 |
| | BROP | Resource of Oral Pathogens | http://www.brop.org/ |
| | EDWIP | Database of the World Insect Pathogens | http://cricket.inhs.uiuc.edu/edwipweb/edwipabout.htm |
| | FPPD | Fungal Plant Pathogen Database (FPPD) | http://fppd.cbio.psu.edu |
| | ORALGEN | Database of bacterial and viral oral pathogens | http://www.oralgen.lanl.gov/ |
| | ShiBASE | Database of Shigella pathogens | http://www.mgc.ac.cn/ShiBASE/ |
| Virulence Factor | VFDB | Reference database for bacterial virulence factors | http://zdsys.chgb.org.cn/VFs/main.htm |
| | CandiVF | Database of C. albicans virulence factors | http://research.i2r.a-star.edu.sg/Templar/DB/CandiVF/ |
| | TVfac | Toxin & Virulence Factor database | http://www.tvfac.lanl.gov/ |
| | ClinMalDB-USP | Database containing virulent determinants | http://malariadb.ime.usp.br/malaria/us/bioinformaticResearch.jsp |
| | Fish Pathogen database | Database of virulence genes | http://dbsdb.nus.edu.sg/fpdb/about.html |
| | PHI-BASE | Integrated Host-pathogen database | http://www.phi-base.org/ |
| T cell | AntiJen | Comprehensive Molecular Immune database | http://www.jenner.ac.uk/antijen/aj_tcell.htm |
| | EPIMHC | Database of MHC Ligands | http://bio.dfci.harvard.edu/epimhc/ |
| | FIMM | Integrated Functional IMMunology database. | http://research.i2r.a-star.edu.sg/fimm/ |
| | HLA Ligand Database | Legacy Repository of MHC binding data | http://hlaligand.ouhsc.edu/index_2.html |
| | HIV Immunology | CD8+ and CD4+ T cell HIV epitopes, proteome epitope maps | http://www.hiv.lanl.gov/immunology |

**Table 4.4** (*Continued*)

| Database | | | |
|---|---|---|---|
| | HCV Immunology | CD8+ and CD4+ T cell HCV epitopes, proteome epitope maps | http://hcv.lanl.gov/content/immuno/immuno-main.html |
| | IEDB | T cell epitope database | http://epitope2.immuneepitope.org/home.do |
| | JenPep | Legacy Repository of MHC binding data | http://www.jenner.ac.uk/jenpep2/ |
| | MHCBN | Repository database of Immune Data | http://www.imtech.res.in/raghava/mhcbn |
| | MHCPEP | MHC-presented epitopes | http://wehih.wehi.edu.au/mhcpep |
| | SYFPEITHI | MHC-presented epitopes, MHC-specific anchor and auxiliary motifs | http://www.syfpeithi.de |
| B cell | AntiJen | Quantitative binding data for B cell epitopes | http://www.jenner.ac.uk/antijen/aj_bcell.htm |
| | BCIPEP | B cell epitope database | http://www.imtech.res.in/raghava/bcipep |
| | CED | Conformational Epitope Database | http://web.kuicr.kyoto-u.ac.jp/~ced/ |
| | EPITOME | Database of Structurally inferred Antigenic Epitopes in Proteins | http://www.rostlab.org/services/epitome/ |
| | IEDB | B cell epitope repository | http://epitope2.immuneepitope.org/home.do |
| | HaptenDB | Databse of Haptens | http://www.imtech.res.in/raghava/haptendb/ |
| | HIV Immunology | B cell HIV epitopes | http://www.hiv.lanl.gov/immunology |
| | HCV Immunology | B cell HCV epitopes | http://hcv.lanl.gov/content/immuno/immuno-main.html |
| Allergen | ALLALLERGY | Database of specific allergens | http://www.allallergy.net/ |
| | ALLERDB | Allergen database | http://sdmc.i2r.a-star.edu.sg/Templar/DB/Allergen/ |
| | Allergen Database | Information on allergens and epitopes | http://allergen.csl.gov.uk/ |
| | Allergome | Repository of allergen molecules | http://www.allergome.org/ |
| | AllerMatch | Database of allergenic food proteins | http://www.allermatch.org/ |
| | BIFS | Database of food and foodbourne pathogens | http://www.iit.edu/~sgendel/ |
| | FARRP | Database of known and putative allergens | http://www.allergenonline.com/ |
| | IMGT | International Immunogenetics Information System | http://imgt.cines.fr/ |
| | InformALL | Database of allergenic foods | http://foodallergens.ifr.ac.uk/ |
| | IUIS Allergen Nomenclature | Repository of recognised Allergens | http://www.allergen.org |
| | SDAP | Structural database of allergenic proteins | http://fermi.utmb.edu/SDAP/ |

First established in 1989, the ImMunoGeneTics Database (IMGT), which specializes in vertebrate antigen receptors (immunoglobulins, MHCs and T cell receptors), is an international collaboration between groups run by Marie-Paul LeFranc and Steve Marsh. IMGT is really two databases – IMGT/LIGM-DB (a comprehensive system of databases covering vertebrate antibody and TCR sequences and structures for over 80 species) and IMGT/HLA (a less ambitious yet definitive database of human MHC). Much of IMGT has a rich, some might say daunting, complexity that separates it from other databases. Data is available for nucleotide and protein sequences, alleles, polymorphisms, gene maps, crystal structure data, primers and disease association. Tools allow for production of sequence alignments, sequence classification and direct sequence submission.

MHCDB, founded in 1994, is a database utilizing ACeDB. Like IMGT/HLA, it comprises a compendium of data concerning human MHC molecules, containing physical maps of over 100 genes and other markers, the location of YAC and cosmid clones, annotated genomic sequences and cDNA sequences of class I and class II MHC alleles.

Current databases, including IMGT, omit a murine MHC database with a sound nomenclature. The mouse is, after all, the premier model organism for vaccine development. However, compilation of such a database, or construction of such a nomenclature, has made scant and exiguous progress in the last 20 years. The Immuno Polymorphism Database (IPD) system, a set of databases facilitating the analysis of polymorphic immune genes, has recently emerged from the long shadow cast by IMGT. IPD focuses on a variety of data and importantly looks at nonhuman species, such as nonhuman primates, cattle and sheep, and thus extends work in nonprimates beyond laboratory model animals into commercially important farm livestock. IPD currently comprises four databases: IPD-MHC which contains MHC sequences from different species; IPD-HPA containing human platelet alloantigens antigens; IPD-KIR, which contains alleles of killer-cell immunoglobulin-like receptors; and IPD-ESTDAB, a melanoma cell line database.

The Hybridoma Data Bank (HBG), established in 1983, is another legacy database. Like IPD-ESTDAB, it comprised information about hybridomas and other cloned cell lines, as well as their immunoreactive products, such as mAbs. The database used standardized terminology to archive and transfer data, and contained a wealth of data on each cell line, including: origin, methodological details, reactivity profile, distributors and availability.

## Pathogen databases

Host databases are complemented by others which focus on microbial life. Microbial genomes are now legion: 200+ from bacteria, 1200+ from viruses, 600+ from plasmids, 30+ eukaryotes and over 500 from organelles – such counts will be superceded long before this book is published. Pathogens form a small but exceptionally important subset of these genomes, leading to the development of the specialist pathogen database. Apart from databases devoted to HIV and HCV, oral pathogens are particularly well served. Other representative examples are listed in Table 4.4. Currently, there is no question that sequence data should not be made freely available. Such largesse is seen as a necessity, helping the research community as a whole, since today molecular biology research is largely, though far from completely, contingent on publicly available data and databases. There are, however, cogent counter arguments to this. Free access to the genomes of pathogenic microbes could help facilitate experimental tampering with disease virulence, potentially opening the way to the development of bespoke bioweapons of unprecedented severity. While such fears are doubtless overblown, such possibilities remain a cause of concern. In truth, however, terrorists would find sufficient minatory capabilities in extant zoonotic infections.

Positioned between databases that concentrate on host or pathogens separately are resources which focus on host–pathogen interactions. The best example is the so-called virulence factor, which enables pathogens to successfully colonize a host and cause disease. The analysis of pathogens, such as *Streptococcus pyogenes* or *Vibrio cholerae*, has elucidated defined 'systems' of proteins – toxins and virulence factors – which may comprise in excess of 40 distinct proteins. Virulence factors have been thought of as mainly being secreted or outer membrane proteins. They have been classified as adherence/colonization factors, invasions, exotoxins, transporters, iron-binding siderophores and miscellaneous cell surface factors. Another definition partitions virulence factoirs into three groups: 'true' virulence factor genes; virulence factors associated with the expression of 'true' virulence factor genes; and virulence factor 'lifestyle' genes required for microbes to colonize the host.

There is an interesting commonality between virulence factors and certain natural products or secondary metabolites. Primary metabolites are intermediates – ATP or amino acids – in the key cellular metabolic pathways. At least in the context of potentially pathogenic micro-organisms, many secondary metabolites seem to be compounds without an explicit role in the metabolic economy of the microbe cell. Some, but not all, of such compounds have a signalling role, being implicated in quorum sensing and the like. One argument posits an evolutionary rationale for the existence of many such molecules: secondary metabolites enhance the survival of the organisms that produce them by binding specifically to macromolecular receptors in competing organisms with a concomitant physiological action. The complexity and intrinsic capacity for making specific interaction with biological receptors make secondary metabolites generally predisposed to macromolecular complex formation. This may, in part, explain why a diversity of PRRs has evolved, as part of the host–pathogen arms race, to recognize microbial metabolic products and evoke a concomitant immune response.

The Virulence Factors Database (VFDB) contains 16 characterized bacterial genomes with an emphasis on functional and structural biology and can be searched using text, BLAST or functional queries. TVFac (Los Alamos National Laboratory Toxin and Virulence Factor database) contains genetic information on over

250 organisms and separate records for thousands of virulence genes and associated factors. *Candida albicans* Virulence Factor (CandiVF) is a small species-specific database that contains VFs which may be searched using BLAST or a HLA-DR Hotspot Prediction server. PHI-BASE is a noteworthy development, since it seeks to integrate a wide range of VFs from a variety of pathogens of plants and animals. The Fish Pathogen Database, established by the Bacteriology and Fish Diseases Laboratory, has identified more than 500 virulence genes. Pathogens studied include *Aeromonas hydrophila*, *Edwardsiella tarda* and many *Vibrio* species.

## Functional immunological databases

Functional databases – which focus on the mechanics of cellular and humoral immunology – are now multiplying (Table 4.4). Historically, databases which look at cellular immunology came first: these look primarily at data relevant to MHC processing, presentation and T cell recognition. Such databases are now becoming increasingly sophisticated, with a flurry of new and improved databases that deal with T cell data. B cell epitope data, and thus B cell epitope databases, have also started to proliferate after a long lag period.

A relatively early, extensive and extensively used database is SYFPEITHI, founded in 1999. It contains a current and useful compendium of T cell epitopes. SYFPEITHI also contains much data on MHC peptide ligands, peptides isolated from cell surface MHC proteins *ex vivo*. SYFPEITHI purposely excludes data on synthetic peptide 'binders', which are often unnatural or are of uncertain provenance in regard to cellular processing. Thus their approach reduces our potential understanding of MHC specificity yet avoids clouding our perception of the whole presentation process. Moreover, it holds hundreds of MHC binding motifs, as extracted from the literature, which covers a diversity of species though it focuses on human and mouse. SYFPEITHI has both search tools (including searching by anchor positions, peptide source or peptide mass) and a prediction component based on motif scoring.

EPIMHC is a relational database of naturally occurring MHC-binding peptides and T cell epitopes. Presently, the database includes 4867 distinct peptide sequences from various sources, including 84 tumour antigens. MHCBN is another cellular immunology database, which contains 18 790 MHC-binding peptides, 3227 MHC nonbinding peptides, 1053 TAP binders and nonbinders and 6548 T cell epitopes.

Several now-defunct databases exist in this area. Probably the first database of its kind having been established in 1994, MHCPEP archived over 13 000 human and mouse T cell epitopes and MHC binding peptides in a flat file format. Each database record contained the peptide sequence, MHC specificity and, if available, experimental details, activity or binding affinity, plus source protein, anchor positions and literature references. Subsequently a full Web version became available, albeit transiently. More recently, Brusic and colleagues developed a more complex and sophisticated database: FIMM. This system was an integrated database, similar to ones to be described below. In addition to T cell epitopes and MHC-peptide binding data, FIMM archived numerous other data, including MHC sequence data together with the disease associations of particular alleles. The HLA Ligand Database is another system again comprising T cell epitope data. It included information on HLA ligands and binding motifs.

## Composite, integrated databases

Three databases in particular warrant special attention, albeit for different reasons: the HIV Molecular Immunological Databases, AntiJen and IEDB. They are so-called composite databases, which seek to integrate a variety of information, including both B cell and T cell epitope data.

The HIV Molecular Immunology database is one of the most complete of all immunological databases. It focuses on the sequence and the sequence variations of a single virus, albeit one of singular medical importance. Nonetheless, the database's scope is, at least in terms of the type of data it archives, broader than most. Thus its obvious depth could be argued to be at the expense of breadth and generality. It contains information on both cellular immunology (CD4+ and CD8+ T cell epitopes and MHC binding motifs) and humoral immunology (linear and conformational B cell epitopes). Features of the HIV database include viral protein epitope maps, sequence alignments, drug-resistant viral protein sequences and vaccine-trial data, responses made to the epitope including its impact on long-term survival, common escape mutations, whether an epitope is recognized in early infection and curated alignments summarizing the epitope's global variability. Currently, its CD8+ T cell epitope database contains 3150 entries describing 1600 distinct MHC class I epitope combinations. Perhaps, one day all immunological databases will look like this.

The same group has recently added the HCV database, which contains 510 entries describing 250 distinct MHC class I epitope combinations.

AntiJen is an attempt to integrate a wider range of data than has hitherto been made available by other databases. Implemented as a relational postgreSQL database, AntiJen is sourced from the literature and contains in excess of 24 000 entries. AntiJen, formerly called JenPep, is a recently developed database, which brings together a variety of kinetic, thermodynamic, functional and cellular data within immunobiology and vaccinology. While it retains a focus on both T cell and B cell epitopes, AntiJen is the first functional database in immunology to contain continuous quantitative binding data on a variety of immunological molecular interactions, rather than other kinds of subjective classifications. AntiJen also holds over 3500 entries for linear and discontinuous B cell epitopes, and includes thermodynamic and kinetic measures of peptide binding to MHCs and the TAP transporter and peptide–MHC complex interactions with TCRs, as well as more diverse immunological protein–protein interactions, such as the interaction of co-receptors, interactions with superantigens and so on.

Data on T cell epitopes is currently limited to an annotated compilation of dominant and subdominant T cell epitopes. While there are many different ways to identify T cell epitopes, including T cell killing, proliferation assays such as thymidine uptake and so on, the quantitative data produced by such assays is not consistent enough to be used outside particular experimental conditions. Linear B cell entry fields include the mapped epitope sequence, the name of the epitope's host protein, information on its respective antibody, including host species where possible, and details of the experimental method and immunogenic properties.

Epitope sequences can be submitted to an in-house BLAST search for identification of similar epitopic sequences in other protein and gene sequences. AntiJen also contains quantitative specificity data from position specific peptide libraries, and biophysical data on MHCs and other immunological molecules, such as cell surface copy numbers and diffusion coefficients. For MHC binding, AntiJen records a number of alternative measures of binding affinity which are currently in common use. These include radiolabelled and fluorescent $IC_{50}$ values, $BL_{50}$ values calculated in a peptide binding stabilization and $\beta$2-microglobulin dissociation half-lives. For each such measurement, it also archives standard experimental details, such as pH, temperature, the concentration range over which the experiment was conducted, the sequence and concentration of the reference radiolabelled peptide competed against, together with their standard deviations. As it is rare to find a paper which records all such data in a reliable way, standardization remains a significant issue. Although the breadth, depth and scope of the data archived within AntiJen sets it apart from other databases in immunology, there is still some overlap between it and other databases.

As stated, AntiJen is built upon the remnants of JenPep, which was composed of three relational databases: a compendium of quantitative affinity measures for peptides binding to class I and class II MHCs; a list of T cell epitopes; and a group of quantitative data for peptide binding to the TAP peptide transporter. The database, and an HTML graphical user interface (GUI) for its interrogation, remain available via the Internet.

The Immune Epitope Database and Analysis Resource or IEDB has recently become available. It is an NIH funded database that addresses issues of biodefence, such as potential threats from bioterrorism or emerging infectious diseases. The database is on a much grander scale than others existing hitherto. It benefits from the input of 13 dedicated epitope sequencing products which exist, in part, to populate the database. IEDB may yet eclipse all other efforts in functional immune databases.

## Allergen databases

Dedicated allergen databases form another distinct strand among immunologically-orientated database systems. Like antigens, allergens are recognizable and distinct immunological entities and are thus straightforward things to collect and collate.

They are present in general sequence databases – as of June 2007, for example, 338 protein allergens are available in Swiss-Prot – and also in specialist, allergen-focused databases. Thus, a number of such focused databases are now available, covering general and food-borne allergens.

Several databases have been developed for food and foodstuffs. The Biotechnology Information for Food Safety (or BIFS) data collection was probably the first allergen database. BIFS contains three types of data: food allergens, nonfood allergens and wheat gluten proteins. The June 2007 update comprises data for 453 food allergens (64 animals and 389 plants), 645 nonfood allergens and 75 wheat gluten proteins. It also contains a nonredundant listing of allergen proteins, which is designed to help assess the potential allergenicity of foods allergens.

The Central Science Laboratory (CSL) allergen database contains both food and inhalant and contaminant allergens. The Food Allergy Research and Resource Programme (FARRP) Protein Allergen database contains 1251 unique protein sequences of known, and suspected, food, environmental and contact allergens and gliadins which may induce celiac disease. The InformAll database, formerly the PROTALL database, is maintained by a European consortium and archives information on plant food allergens involved in IgE-induced hypersensitivity reactions. It contains general, biochemical and clinical information on 248 allergenic food materials of both plant and animal origin. ALLALLERGY is a database that can be queried by food type and lists all chemical allergens. It contains over 4500 allergenic chemicals and proteins as well as information on adverse reactions, cross-reactivity and patient assessment, background information, synonyms and functions of each archived allergen.

The International Union of Immunological Societies (IUIS) database lists clinically relevant allergens and isoallergens. The Allergen Nomenclature database of IUIS serves as a central resource for ensuring uniformity and consistency of allergen designations. To maintain data integrity, the database is curated by committee members and includes only allergens able to induce in humans IgE-mediated allergy (reactivity $> 5\%$). IUIS is arguably one of the most widely-used and authoritative sources of allergen data. As of June 2007, IUIS contains more than 779 allergens and isoallergens originating from 150 species.

The Allergome database lists allergen molecules and their biological functions, and additionally contains allergenic substances for which specific allergen proteins have yet to be identified. It emphasizes allergens causing IgE-mediated disease. The database currently holds information from 5800 selected scientific literature.

A number of criticisms have been levelled at available allergen databases, particularly concerning the consistency, accuracy and availability of allergen data derived from public databases. Difficulties in sequence annotation are further compounded when post-translational modifications are the source of allergenicity rather than the protein itself. Ultimately, it may not be possible to integrate all available allergens databases completely; yet such a nonredundant set is vitally important, together with a full annotation of their features, be that structural, functional or clinical.

Databases have come a long way, but they need to go further. As scientists, we must actively develop databases far beyond their current limitations. Much useful data is still locked into the hard-copy literature or is presented in a graphical form, and it remains an on-going challenge to find and extract this data into a machine-readable format. There will come a time when all public data will be publically available. We must look to the day when all scientists, irrespective of their discipline and mindset, are obliged to submit all their data to an online archive, much as today, molecular biologists must submit their data to publicly curated sequence databases or crystallographers must submit their data to the PDB.

Databases should be a tool for knowledge discovery not just a lifeless repository. Biological databases need to incorporate vastly more data of a wholly greater diversity than they do today. The technology to do this exists but does the will? At the same time, different databases should be linked together and their querying be rendered facile, thus releasing the creativity of investigators rather than suppressing it. Whatever people believe, future bioscientists will need to work, and to think, both *in vitro* and *in silico*, combining computational and experimental techniques to progress their science and solve real-world problems. If anything lies at the heart of this endeavour it will be the database.

## Further reading

Books on bioinformatics abound. Many deal with the issue of databases in much greater depth. *Bioinformatics and Molecular Evolution* by Higgs and Attwood [ISBN 1405138025] is, despite the name, a good general introduction to the subject.

## Reference

1. Diehl, A. D., Lee, J. A., Scheuermann, R. H. and Blake, J. A. (2007) Ontology development for biological systems: immunology. *Bioinformatics*, **23**, 913–915.

# 5

# Vaccines: Data Driven Prediction of Binders, Epitopes and Immunogenicity

*Those who cannot remember the past are condemned to repeat it.*
—George Santayana (1863–1952)

## Towards epitope-based vaccines

The philosopher, poet and novelist George Santayana (1863–1952) wrote famously in his book *Reason in Common Sense* – Volume 1 of *The Life of Reason* (1905) – that 'Those who cannot remember the past are condemned to repeat it.' This statement has an assumed veracity well beyond the original intentions of its author. Like many quotations – indeed like many great books, paintings, poems, plays and symphonies – it has gained a wide currency because one can impose on it any interpretation that one chooses and thus make use of it in many contexts. It seems to me to fit my purpose as well as any other: learn from the mistakes of the past and, if you can, also exploit past successes as much as is practical. We review this idea in this chapter.

At the time of writing, there are no commercially produced vaccines that have ever been designed solely, or significantly or perhaps even at all, using computational techniques. Likewise, there are no commercial peptide- or epitope-based vaccines. Most vaccines are still, by and large, built around killed or attenuated live whole pathogens or are subunit vaccines. It has been argued – by some if not by all – that when the first epitope-based vaccines are licensed, then a floodgate of

*Bioinformatics for Vaccinology*   Darren R Flower
© 2008 John Wiley & Sons, Ltd

interest will open. A floodgate of this kind has, of course, been partly open for some time, and the literature is dotted with examples of epitope-based vaccines that are immunogenic and protective, at least in a laboratory setting. Thus, there remains much interest in epitopes and their prediction, not just as laboratory reagents and diagnostics, but as components of potential vaccines.

# T cell epitope prediction

In this chapter, we explore the current state of arguably the foremost area within immunoinformatics: epitope prediction and the prediction of peptide–MHC binding. We shall describe prediction from the viewpoint of methods and approaches of long standing and, at the same time, we will explore (albeit in a limited way) how these methods work. Although the importance of nonpeptide epitopes, such as lipids and carbohydrates, are increasingly well recognized, it is the accurate prediction of proteinacious B cell epitopes (BCE) and T cell epitopes (TCE) – around which epitope-based vaccines are typically constructed – that remains the primary challenge for immunoinformatics. Although BCE prediction remains primitive and problematic, many advanced methods for TCE prediction have arisen. However, the accurate prediction of TCEs, much less immunodominant epitopes, is still a challenge with most work focusing on predicting peptide binding to MHC molecules.

In the light of X-ray crystallographic data, the mechanism underlying pMHC–TCR interaction is now well understood. T cell epitopes are short peptides (or peptides modified naturally or artificially) that are, when bound by class I or class II cell-surface MHCs, recognized by TCRs on the surface of T cells so that the T cell becomes activated and some kind of immune response is initiated.

However, such understanding has not always been clear. Early experimental results indicated that T cell epitopes were defined by short peptide sequences, yet the observation that increased sequence length correlated with increased potency suggested that immunogenicity depended upon the ability of a peptide to adopt an appropriate secondary structure. In turn, this concept led many to develop direct predictors of T cell immunogenicity based, in the main, on erroneous assumptions of this kind about the conformation adopted by T cell epitopes.

In a key retrospective analysis of these diverse approaches, Deavin *et al.* [1] compared numerous T cell epitope prediction methods against databases of mouse and human epitopes, assessing their performance using specificity as a measure of the quality of predictions and sensitivity as a measure of the quantity of correct predictions. Versus human data, Stille's strip-of-helix algorithm was the only statistically significant model and for the mouse dataset only one method gave two significant results. Overall, most of the algorithms were no better than random for either dataset, indicating again the need to include MHC binding in the definition of putative T cell epitopes.

# Predicting MHC binding

These results are consistent with the diminishing interest in such methods relative to those which predicts MHC binding. In order to quantify adequately the affinities of different MHCs for antigenic peptides, many different methods have been developed. It is possible to group these methods together thematically, based on the kind of underlying techniques they employ, and we shall explore these below.

Different MHC alleles, both class I and class II, have different peptide specificities. One way of looking at this is to say that they bind peptides with particular sequence patterns. A more accurate description of this phenomenon is to say that MHCs bind peptides with a binding constant dependent on the nature of the bound peptide's sequence. The forces behind such binding phenomena are identical to those which drive drug binding. Major histocompatibility complexes (MHC) bind short peptides derived from host and pathogen proteins and present them on the cell surface for inspection by T cells. Peptides which are recognized by such cells are termed T cell epitopes and peptide binding seems the most selective step in the recognition process. There are many sequence-based methods for the prediction of T cell epitopes, most relying on the prediction of peptide-MHC binding. Successfully modelling the peptide specificity exhibited by MHCs allows preselection of candidate peptides which, in turn, can help identify immunogenic epitopes.

There are two kinds of MHC molecule. Class I MHC alleles have a binding groove which is closed at both ends, making it possible to predict exactly which residues are positioned in the binding groove. Numerous methods have been applied to the problem of predicting MHC binding. MHC class I binding prediction is regarded as being very successful, with some authors reporting prediction accuracies up to 95%. Attempts at predicting binding to class II MHCs, which have a peptide groove open at both ends, is much less accurate, despite considerable efforts using both traditional and novel approaches.

Beginning with the identification of so-called binding motifs in the 1980s there has been much interest in characterizing the peptide specificity of different class I MHC alleles in terms of dominant anchor positions with a strong preference for a restricted group of amino acids. Motifs have proved very popular within the immunology community: they are widely exploited, being simple to use and simple to understand. Fundamental technical problems with motifs – peptides are viewed simplisticly as either binders or nonbinders – produce many false positives and false negatives. It is obvious now that the whole peptide contributes to affinity, not just a few anchor residues, and so to T cell mediated immunogenicity. Effective models of binding must employ rather more intricate, complex representations of the biophysical phenomena of binding. A succession of ever more sophisticated methods has been applied to the problem: artificial neural networks, hidden Markov models, support vector machines and robust multivariate statistics, such as partial least squares, amongst others. This plethora of approaches has bred a plethora of Web-server implementations available via the Internet (Table 5.1). This chapter will explore the development of, and dilemmas in, immune epitope prediction.

**Table 5.1** A list of immunoinformatic prediction servers

**T cell epitope prediction**

| | | |
|---|---|---|
| SYFPEITHI | http://www.syfpeithi.de | Predicitve server featuring MHC-presented epitopes, MHC-specific anchor and auxiliary motifs |
| BIMAS | http://bimas.dcrt.nih.gov/molbio/hla_bind/ | An HLA peptide binding predictor I molecules |
| EpiDirect | http://epipredict.de/index.html | Prediction method for MHC class II restricted T cell epitopes and ligands |
| HIV | http://hiv.lanl.gov/content/hiv-db/ALABAMA/epitope_analyzer.html | An HIV epitope location finder |
| Imtech | http://imtech.res.in/raghava/mhc/ | Matrix optimization technique for the prediction of MHC binding |
| Lib Score | http://hypernig.nig.ac.jp/cgi-bin/Lib-score/request.rb?lang=E | PPSL prediction server |
| MHC Bench | http://www.imtech.res.in/raghava/mhcbench/ | Evaluation of MHC binding peptide predictive algorithms |
| MHCPred 20 | http://www.jenner.ac.uk/MHCPred/ | Quantitative T cell epitope prediction server with both human and mouse models |
| MHC-THREAD | http://www.csd.abdn.ac.uk/~gjlk/MHC-Thread/ | Predictor for peptides that are likely to bind to MHC class II molecules |
| NetMHC | http://www.cbs.dtu.dk/services/NetMHC/ | Produces a neural network prediction of binding affinities for HLA-A2 and H-2Kk |
| PREDEP | http://margalit.huji.ac.il/ | MHC class I epitope prediction |
| ProPred | http://www.imtech.res.in/raghava/propred/ | Prediction of MHC class II binding regulation in an antigen sequence using quantitative matrices |
| RANKPEP | http://www.mifoundation.org/Tools/rankpep.html | Prediction of binding peptides to MHC class I and class II molecules |
| SMM | http://zlab.bu.edu/SMM/ | Prediction of high affinity HLA-A2 binding peptides |
| SVMHC | http://www.sbc.su.se/~pierre/svmhc/ | A prediction tool for MHC class I binding peptides |

**B cell epitope prediction**

| Name | URL | Description |
|---|---|---|
| ePitope | http://www.epitope-informatics.com/ | Epitope prediction server for the identification and targeting of protein B cell epitopes |
| Bcepred | http://www.imtech.res.in/raghava/bcepred/ | B cell epitope prediction methods based on physico-chemical properties on a non-redundant dataset |
| ABCpred | http://www.imtech.res.in/raghava/abcpred/ | B cell epitope prediction using artificial neural networks |
| Antigenic | http://liv.bmc.uu.se/cgi-bin/emboss/antigenic | Location antigenic sites in proteins |
| Discotope | http://www.cbs.dtu.dk/services/DiscoTope/ | Server predicting discontinuous B cell epitopes from three-dimensional protein structures |
| CEP | http://202.41.70.74:8080/cgi-bin/cep.pl | Server for prediction of conformational epitopes |
| VaxiJen | http://www.jenner.ac.uk/VaxiJen/ | Prediction of protective antigens and subunit vaccines. |

**Allergen Discovery**

| Name | URL | Description |
|---|---|---|
| AlgPred | http://www.imtechresin/raghava/algpred/ | Prediction of allergens based on similarity of known epitope with any region of protein |
| AllerPredict | http://sdmci2ra-staredusg/Templar/DB/Allergen/ | ALLERDB is an allergen database integrated with analytical tools |
| AllerMatch | http://www.allermatch.org/ | Amino acid sequence of a protein of interest with sequences of allergenic proteins |
| WebAllergen | http://weballergen.bii.a-star.edu.sg/ | Sequence compared against a set of prebuilt allergenic motifs |
| DASARP | http://www.slv.se/templatesSLV/SLV_Page9343.asp | Detection based on automated selection of allergen-representative peptide |

# Binding is biology

Binding is one of the fundamental molecular cornerstones upon which biology is built; and a proper understanding of the underlying nature of binding as a molecular event is, in turn, a cornerstone upon which are based many disciplines, including biochemistry, biophysics and immunology. While we use the term function throughout this book, it is a word and an idea whose use is more limited than we suppose. There is only binding; function is illusory – a subjective human idea we impose on the world around us. Enzyme catalysis is largely, though not completely, explicable in terms of binding. The classical idea of enzymatic enhancement of reaction kinetics is that the enzyme binds to the transition state reducing the activation barrier to rates in either direction. The function of a protein is not to bind another; what we have are two proteins which together form a complex with a lower overall free energy, and thus exhibit high mutual affinity. Such interactions include, but are not limited to, small molecule ligands binding to their receptors, substrates binding to enzymes or large molecules interacting together, such as a protein antigen binding to an antibody.

Although the immune system is extremely complex and exhibits not inconsiderable emergent behaviour at higher levels, at its heart lie conceptually-straightforward molecular recognition events. The driving force behind this binding is precisely the same as that driving receptor–ligand interaction, and is thus indistinguishable, in terms of the chemical physics underlying the phenomena, from any other type of biomacromolecular interaction, such as that between an enzyme and its substrate. Within the human population there are an enormous number of variant alleles coding for MHC proteins: each distinct MHC will exhibit distinct peptide-binding sequence selectivity. Pairs of MHC proteins will have either very similar or very different selectivities, leading to the possibility of grouping MHCs into so-called supertypes.

Peptide binding to MHCs and TCR binding to peptide–MHC complexes are the key biomolecular interactions underlying the recognition process which enables the immune system to discriminate properly between proteins of benign origin and those produced by pathogens. T cell receptors, in their turn, also exhibit different affinities for pMHC. The MHC and TCR repertoires exhibit a combined selectivity which determines the power of peptide recognition within the immune system, and through this the phenomenon of pathogen recognition. MHC-mediated recognition of pathogens thus enables the immune system to do its work. The importance of these processes cannot be underestimated: the success of pathogen recognition is often what divides life from death. The study of immunology and vaccinology remains distinctly empirical in nature, yet such peptide binding phenomena are as amenable to rigorous biophysical characterization as any other biochemical reaction. Any biomacromolecular reaction which can be understood in terms of physical chemistry and biological physics also affords the insight necessary for prediction. So, in order to understand epitopes, we need to understand peptide–MHC binding. In the following we shall take a brief, albeit quantitative, look at the physical biochemistry of ligand binding to a biomolecular target. In the present case we will think, in the main, about peptides binding to MHC molecules, yet similar arguments apply to any biomolecular interaction.

## Quantifying binding

Many ways exist to measure the binding of molecule with molecule. For peptide–MHC binding there are more ways of measuring than most. These different measures form a hierarchy with equilibrium constants, when calculated correctly, being the most reliable and accurate. Equilibrium constants include both association ($K_a$) and dissociation constants ($K_d$). Other popular measures include radiolabelled and fluorescent $IC_{50}$ values, which can approximate equilibrium binding constants under certain conditions. Other, rather less rigorous measurements of peptide–MHC binding include $BL_{50}$ values (also variously described as $SC_{50}$, $EC_{50}$ and $C_{50}$ values), as calculated in a so-called peptide binding stabilization assay, $T_m$ values (the temperature at which 50% of MHC protein is denatured), and $\beta_2$-microglobulin dissociation half-life. This final value, while strictly a kinetic measurement, is believed by many to correlate well with binding affinity.

Peptide binding to MHC molecules can be quantified as one would quantify any other reversible receptor–ligand interaction in a closed thermodynamic system. Consider the formation of a general biomolecular receptor–ligand complex from isolated populations of receptor and ligand:

$$R + L \leftrightarrow RL \tag{5.1}$$

In this equation, $R$ stands for the receptor, or MHC in this case; $L$ the ligand or peptide; and $RL$ the receptor–ligand (or peptide–MHC) complex. Interactions such as these obey the law of mass action. This law states that the rate of reaction is proportional to the concentration of reactants. The rate of the forward reaction is proportional to $[L][R]$. The rate of the reverse reaction is proportional to $[RL]$, since there is no other species involved in the dissociation. At equilibrium, the rate of the forward reaction is equal to the rate of the reverse reactions, and so (using $k_1$ and $k_{-1}$ as the respective proportionality constants)

$$k_1[R][L] = k_{-1}[RL]. \tag{5.2}$$

Rearranging:

$$\frac{[R][L]}{[RL]} = \frac{k_{-1}}{k_1} = K_D = K_A^{-1}, \tag{5.3}$$

where $K_A$ is the equilibrium association constant and $K_D$ is the equilibrium dissociation constant, which also represents the concentration of ligand which occupies 50% of the receptor population at equilibrium.

In general, the Gibbs free energy change ($\Delta G$) for formation of a binary receptor–ligand complex is related to the equivalent Gibbs free energy change ($\Delta G°$) in the standard state. The standard state is defined by a set of standard conditions: pH 7.0, 298K, with receptor and ligand at a concentration of 1 M. Under arbitrary conditions, then, the following will hold:

$$\Delta G = \Delta G^0 + RT \ln(K_A). \tag{5.4}$$

Thus at equilibrium, at under standard conditions, the free energy of binding is related directly to the equilibrium constants:

$$\Delta G_{bind} = \Delta G^0 = -RT \ln(K_A) = RT \ln(K_D) \tag{5.5}$$

where $\Delta G_{bind}$ is the Gibbs free energy of binding, $R$ is the gas constant, and $T$ is the absolute temperature. The free energy ($\Delta G$) is a product of enthalpy ($\Delta H$) and entropy ($\Delta S$) components related by the Gibbs–Helmhotz equation:

$$\Delta G = \Delta H - T\Delta S. \tag{5.6}$$

Energy is that property of a system that invests it with the ability to do work or produce heat. Formally, enthalpy is defined by:

$$H = U + PV \tag{5.7}$$

where $U$ is the total internal energy of a system, $P$ is pressure and $V$ is volume. Under conditions of constant pressure, $\Delta H$ is the heat absorbed by a system from its surroundings and, for a molecular system, is a function of both its kinetic and potential energies. Energy has many forms: mechanical, electrical, heat, chemical and so on. Mechanical energy is of two kinds: potential energy (by virtue of the position of a body) and kinetic energy (by virtue of the motion of a body). The energy of a closed system is constant, hence the law of conservation of energy. Energy is readily converted between the two forms. Heat is the most degenerate form of energy.

## Entropy, enthalpy, and entropy-enthalpy compensation

Entropy is often described as a measure of 'disorder' within a molecular system. When a thermodynamic system is considered on a microscopic scale, equilibrium is associated with the distribution of molecules that has the greatest chance of occurring. Statistical mechanics interprets increasing entropy, within a closed system, reaching a maximum at equilibrium, as the result of moving from a less probable to a more probable state. Increasing entropy is thus better described as the partitioning of the energy of a system into an increasing number of explicit microstates, which are themselves a function of the position and momentum of each constituent atom. As we are dealing with complex multicomponent systems, it is often difficult to fully disentangle enthalpies and entropies into readily identifiable separate molecular contributions.

Favourable enthalpic contributions to the free energy can include complementary electrostatic energy, such as salt bridges, hydrogen bonds, dipole–dipole interactions and interactions with metal ions; and van der Waals interactions between ligand and receptor atoms. Entropic contributions can include global properties of the system, such as the loss of three rotational and three vibrational degrees of freedom on binding, and local properties, such as conformational effects including the loss of internal flexibility in both protein and ligand. Unfavourable entropic contributions from the increased rigidity of backbone and side chain residues on ligand binding within the binding pocket are, in part, offset by favourable increases in conformational freedom at nearby residues. Strictly, all protein–ligand binding also involves multiple interactions with the solvent, typically a weakly ionic aqueous solution, and is a multicomponent process rather than a binary one such as dimerization. These solvent interactions lead to solvation, desolvation and hydrophobic effects, each with both an enthalpic and an entropic component.

As affinity rises the phenomenon of enthalpic co-operativity, or so-called enthalpy–entropy compensation, becomes more important. Where multiple weak noncovalent interactions hold a molecular complex together, the enthalpy of all of the individual intermolecular bonding interactions is reduced by extensive intermolecular motion. As additional interaction sites generate a complex which is more strongly bound, intermolecular motion is dampened, with all individual interactions becoming more favourable. The trade-off between intermolecular motion and enthalpic interactions accounts for the way in which entropy and enthalpy compensate for each other.

## Experimental measurement of binding

Experimentally measurement of equilibrium dissociation constants has in the past been addressed using radioligand binding assays. Saturation analysis measures equilibrium binding at various radioligand concentrations to determine affinity ($K_D$) and receptor number (usually denoted as $B_{max}$). Competitive binding experiments measure receptor–ligand binding at a single concentration of labelled ligand and various concentrations of unlabelled ligand. Competition experiments can be either homologous (where the labelled and unlabelled ligands are the same) or, more commonly, heterologous (where unlabelled and labelled ligands are different).

$IC_{50}$ values, as obtained from a competitive radioligand assay, are amongst the most frequently reported affinity measures. The value given is the concentration required for 50% inhibition of a labelled standard by the test ligand. Therefore nominal binding affinity is inversely proportional to the $IC_{50}$ value. $IC_{50}$ values may vary between experiments depending on the intrinsic affinity and concentration of the standard radiolabelled reference compound, as well as the intrinsic affinity of the test molecule.

The $K_D$ of the test peptide can be obtained from the $IC_{50}$ value using the relationship derived by Cheng and Prussoff:

$$K_D^i = \frac{IC_{50}}{\left(1 + \frac{[L_{tot}^S]}{K_D^S}\right)};$$

(5.8)

here $K_D^i$ is the dissociation constant for the ligand; $K_D^S$ is the dissociation constant for the radiolabelled standard, and $\lfloor L_{tot}^s \rfloor$ is the total concentration of the radiolabel. This relation holds at the midpoint of the inhibition curve under two principal constraints: the total amount of radiolabel is much greater than the concentration of bound radiolabel and that the concentration of bound test compound is much less than the $IC_{50}$. Although an approximation, this holds relatively well under the kind of assay conditions that are usually encountered. To a first approximation, measured $IC_{50}$ values vary with the equilibrium dissociation constant, at least within a single experiment. Systematic discrepancies between $IC_{50}$ values from different experiments are, in many cases, sufficiently small that values can be compared.

$BL_{50}$ values are produced by peptide stabilization assays, as cell surface MHCs are presumed only to be stable when they have bound peptide. They represent half maximal binding levels calculated from mean fluorescence intensities (MFI) of MHC expressed on RMA-S or T2 cells. Cells are incubated with the test peptide, which are stabilized, and then labelled with a fluorescent mAb. Binding strength is inversely proportional to the $BL_{50}$ value. Peptides are usually administered extracellularly, and there remain questions about the mechanism of peptide induced MHC stabilization. Measured $BL_{50}$ values also represent an approximate overall value derived from a complex multicomponent equilibrium. The interaction between peptide and MHC, as reflected in complex stability, is assessed by binding the pMHC complex with an allele- or class I-specific antibody; this is in turn bound by a fluorescently labelled mAb specific for the first antibody. The resulting complex is then assayed spectrophotometrically using FACS or an equivalent technique.

The half-life for radioisotope labelled $\beta_2$-microglobulin dissociation (as measured at 37°C) is an alternative binding measure for MHC class I complexes. This is a kinetic measurement rather than a thermodynamic one, although it is often assumed that the stability of a pMHC complex is proportional to the half-life. The half-life ($t_{1/2}$) is given by

$$t_{1/2} = \frac{\ln 2}{k_{-1}} \sim \frac{0.693}{k_{off}}.$$

(5.9)

Here the $t_{1/2}$ corresponds to the dissociation of the MHC-$\beta_2$ microglobulin complex rather than the kinetics of the protein–ligand interaction.

We may wish to ask the question: which of these measures is best? Unfortunately, there is no simple answer. We have shown that a high degree of concordance exists between IC50 and BL50 values [2]. Nonetheless, there is to date no systemic comparison of different measures, and so the relative verity and provenance of IC50, BL50 and $t_{1/2}$ remains an open question. This issue also reinforces the imperative need to establish effective predictive methodologies that are able to substitute effectively and reliably for experimental assays.

## Modern measurement methods

More sophisticated, more convenient and more exact instrumental technology is, in other fields at least, now superseding such assays. In the case of enzyme reactions, enzyme kinetics is often followed by means of a readily detectable physical property (e.g. absorption, fluorescence or fluorescence polarization of one of the reaction partners). Such instrumental methods can offer both increased convenience for the operator and more easily realized experimental tractability; this type of approach is beginning to be applied to MHCs. Steady state fluorescence spectroscopy is widely used in the study of biomolecular interactions and kinetics and relies on measuring fluorescence change at a given wavelength. Time resolved fluorescence spectroscopy measures the time dependence of fluorescence intensity after excitation, and is far more sensitive to conformational changes or interactions made by fluorescent residues – tryptophan, tyrosine and phenylalanine – than steady state intensity measurements. Using polarized light allows time resolved fluorescence anisotropy measurements, which can provide useful information about local residues as well as global protein motion. Mass spectrometry (MS) can also offer interesting insights into binding. Atomic-force microscopy (AFM) can determine the strength of intermolecular interactions through controlled mechanical rupture of protein–ligand complexes. Other methods, such as densimetric and ultrasonic velocimetric titration measurements, are also important, giving insights into specific molecular events, such as hydration changes.

Two techniques show particular promise: surface plasmon resonance (SPR) and isothermal titration calorimetry (ITC). SPR is an increasingly widely used technique, as it can measure biomolecular interactions in real time in a label free environment. SPR techniques are optical sensors based on the excitation of surface plasmons. They belong to a variety of refractometric sensing methods that includes grating coupler sensors, Mach–Zehnder interferometers, Young interferometers and white light interferometers which measure refractive index changes induced by the sensor's electromagnetic field. One interaction partner is immobilized to the sensor surface while the other is in solution. It passes over the surface, binding occurs, and is detected. Both 'on' and 'off' rates can also be accessed using this method.

## Isothermal titration calorimetry

However, if one seeks a single methodology for obtaining relevant thermodynamic properties of binding reactions, the current leader of the pack is probably ITC, and is rapidly becoming the method of choice. The main reason for this is that ITC simultaneously generates global values for several parameters: the equilibrium constant and thus the free energy of binding ($\Delta G$), which it computes from the shape of the titration curve. However, ITC also measures enthalpy ($\Delta H$), which it derives from the integrated heat of reaction; entropy ($\Delta S$), which is related to the difference in $\Delta G$ and $\Delta H$; and also the heat capacity ($\Delta C_p$) of the system. In ITC, a ligand is added stepwise at constant temperature to a solution of receptor protein and the overall heat of the reaction is recorded.

In the absence of nonlinear effects, enthalpy and entropy terms can be obtained using the van 't Hoff relation:

$$\ln K_D = \frac{\Delta H}{RT} - \frac{\Delta S}{R}, \quad \frac{d(\ln K_D)}{dT} = \frac{\Delta H}{RT^2}. \tag{5.10}$$

The potential usefulness of this is obvious: plotting $\ln(K_D)$ vs $1/T$ should describe a straight line with a slope equal to ($\Delta H/R$) and a $y$ intercept of ($\Delta S/R$). Van 't Hoff plots only identify part of the binding enthalpy: the part directly related to the observed measurement signal. This means that only for a direct transformation from a defined initial state to a final state is the extracted enthalpy equivalent to $\Delta H_{bind}$, as obtained by other methods, for example ITC. No intermediate steps are tolerated. $\Delta G$ typically has only mild temperature dependence within biological systems so a truly accurate and reliable estimate of enthalpy and entropy is seldom possible using van 't Hoff plots.

What sets ITC apart is its ability to measure both affinity and its thermodynamic contributions directly from heat changes during the binding process. Since such changes are observed during most binding reactions, ITC is broadly applicable, with applications ranging from chemical and biochemical binding to enzyme kinetics. ITC is both rapid and sensitive, but above all it is a direct method without the need for chemical modification or immobilization. It is the only technique that measures enthalpy directly, eliminating the requirement for van 't Hoff analysis, which is often time consuming and prone to error. However, interpretation of derived parameters remains a pivotal challenge. Moreover, reliable analysis of the titration curve requires dissociation constants less affine than $10^{-9}$ M. To measure more affine compounds, the detection range must be extended by displacing lower affinity ligands. The kinetics of peptide binding – slow 'on' rates and slow 'off' rates – may also make certain MHC interactions beyond the practical limitations of current ITC technology.

A step forward for the analysis of peptide–MHC binding will come when we deploy such methods and return richer and more informative affinity measurements. However, routine ITC again only operates on soluble molecules and is very time consuming, labour intensive and relatively expensive to perform. No method readily addresses the joint goals of effectively mimicking the *in vivo* membrane-bound nature of the interaction and the need for accuracy. In an ideal world we would look at a variety of 'internally rich' data from ITC, as well as volumetric analysis and fluorescence spectroscopy, but to do this on an appropriate scale would be prohibitively time consuming and expensive. Where one might conceive of doing this for one allele, there are dozens of frequent alleles within the human population. There are also many more which have interesting associations with disease. To pursue 'internally rich' assays for all 'interesting' alleles is clearly beyond the scope of existing methodology.

Ultimately, every relevant spectroscopic technique provides, to a greater or lesser degree, valuable information complementary to that supplied by radioligand assays or cell surface stabilization or $\beta$2m dissociation. It is only through a full and complete combination of several such techniques that the intricacies of protein–ligand interaction may be carefully reconstructed. As yet, however, the application of these more sophisticated techniques, at least on a large scale, to peptide–MHC interactions, is distinctly limited.

## Long and short of peptide binding

The peptides bound by class I MHCs have long been thought to be short. A range of eight to 11 residues is regularly quoted. This now seems to reflect our tendentious expectation more than unbiased observation. Peptides bound by class II MHCs are not directly constrained in length, which creates particular problems of its own (see below). X-ray crystallography has shown similarly bound peptide conformations within class I MHC complexes, despite distinct peptide sequences. Peptides bind to class I MHC with their N- and C-termini fixed at either end of the peptide binding site, and with the centre of the peptide bulging out. Residues lining the MHC binding groove interact with the peptide and thus define the specificity of the HLA–peptide interaction.

This view arose partly from examination of crystal structures, which indicated that the MHC binding site most obviously accommodates peptides of eight to 10 amino acids, and partly from cell surface elution studies, which also showed a restricted length spectrum. Obviously, as time has progressed, people have reinforced this view by only using synthetic peptides of eight or nine amino acids in length to test for binding.

The supposed length restriction imposed by class I MHCs is now being challenged. There is increasing experimental evidence that a wide variety of other peptides also form stable, high affinity complexes with class I MHC class I, including shorter peptides (4- to 5-mers), which we shall call 'shortmers', and much longer peptides (up to 18-mers), which we shall call 'longmers'. Such observations are outside the prior norm, and are thus ignored or are subject to greater than usual scrutiny.

There is data to support the binding to MHCs of atypically short peptide sequences: mouse CTLs can recognize truncated MUC1 epitopes bound to H-2Kb – SAPDTRP (7-mer), SAPDTR (6-mer) and SAPDT (5-mer) [3]. Other potential shortmers binding to class I MHC molecules include: 3-mers (QNH), 4-mers (QNHR, ALDL and PFDL) and 5-mers (RALDL and HFMPT) [4].

Evidence for the binding of atypically long peptides is much stronger and certainly more abundant. So much so that we shall eschew circumstantial results and instead focus on unequivocal crystal data. Peptides of length eight or nine possess an essentially invariant conformation, while peptides of 10 amino acids 'bulge' in the centre, with this bulging conformation varying considerably between structures. In all cases, N- and C-terminal interactions remain unchanged. Such trends only increase as peptide length increases.

Speir and colleagues reported the structure of a complex between the rat MHC allele RT1-Aᵃ and a 13-mer peptide (ILFPSSERLISNR), a naturally eluted peptide derived from a mitochondrial ATPase [5]. Probst–Kepper report the structure of HLA-B*3501 complexed with a 14-mer peptide (LPAVVGLSPGEQEY), which originates from an alternate open reading frame of macrophage colony-stimulating factor [6]. The peptide is presented naturally and is recognized by T cells. As is usual for 8-mers and 9-mers, both the N and C termini of the peptide were embedded in the A and F pockets of the MHC peptide groove. The centre of this peptide bulges from the binding groove in an unpredictable way. Tynan reports the structure of a 13-mer viral epitope (LPEPLPQGQLTAY) bound to HLA-B*3508 [7].

These crystal structures find support in functional observations of CTL recognition of Longmers. Reports of human 10-mer and 11-mer CD8 epitopes restricted by class I MHC alleles are common place, as are 10-mer peptides binding to mouse class I. SYFPEITHI is awash with class I peptides that are up to 15 amino acids in length in humans and up to 16 amino acids in mice. Jiang reports convincing evidence of an H2-Kd-restricted CTL response to a 15-mer epitope (ELQLLMQSTPPTNNR) from the F protein of respiratory syncytial virus [8]. 12-mer C-terminal variants of VSV8 have been shown to bind H-2Kb (RGYVYQGLKSGN). Thus, the apparent potency of responses to such longmers is indicative that peptides longer than the norm do not represent a major structural barrier to recognition by TCRs.

## The class I peptide repertoire

Clearly, then, the evidence as outlined above suggests strongly that the natural repertoire of class I MHC presented peptides is far broader than has generally been supposed. We can compound this repertoire in various ways. One is through aberrant transcription and translation of viral and self-proteins. Various mechanisms pertain such as read through, which leads to alternative open reading frames, or alternative splicing, which generates protein isotypes with different sequences at exon–exon boundaries. Both of these have been shown to generate immunogenic epitopes. Autoantigen and self-tumour antigen transcripts in particular experience higher rates of alternative splicing in response to stimuli and these can lead to elevated responses. Alternative splicing is a major factor driving proteomic diversity and provides a partial rationale for the gulf between the small size of genomes and the enormous complexity of higher eukaryotes. Most alternative splicing occurs in the coding region. The most commonly observed alternative splicing event is exon skipping in which an exon or set of continuous exons are permuted in different mRNAs. Less frequent are the use of donor and acceptor sites and intron retention.

We can expand the burgeoning repertoire still further by accounting for the effect of post-translational modifications (PTMs). These can take many forms, including glycosylation and lipidation. Glycosylated proteins can be targets for binding by cell surface receptors based on sugar binding leptin domains. Glycosylated epitopes can also be bound by TCRs and antibodies. Lipids can act as epitopes directly through their presentation by CD1. PTMs can also be transitory, such as phosphorylation, or more permanent, such as modified amino acids. Many of these can be part of functional epitopes recognized by the immune system. Glycosylation of a protein, for example, is dependent on the presence of sequence patterns or motifs (Ser/Thre-X-Asn for N-linked glycosylation and Ser/Thr for O-linked) but this is not enough to predict them correctly. If these motifs are present at solvent inaccessible regions of a protein rather on the surface then they will not be glycosylated. Moreover, the other residues which surround these patterns will also affect the specificity of the glyscosylating enzymes: Pro as the X in the Ser/Thre-X-Asn motif for N-linked glycosylation will essentially prevent glycosylation. Glycosylation, in particular, is also very dependent on context, and it is thus a system property of an organism, and can vary considerably in terms of the nature and extent of the different sugars that can become attached to proteins, at least in eukaryotic systems. Taken together these greatly increase the potential size and diversity of the immunogenic repertoire – or immunome – of reactive peptides. One can argue, and argue cogently, that the only realistic way to address this potential enormity of the peptide repertoire is via computational analysis and prediction.

# Practicalities of binding prediction

Although there are ways to generate much richer and more explicit data, using ITC for example, practicalities dictate that the immunoinformatician must instead look at a very mixed ragbag of quantitative and semi-quantitative measures of greatly varying provenance. Unfortunately, the wide variety of quantitative measures of binding currently in use ($K_D$, $IC_{50}$, $BL_{50}$, $t_{1/2}$, etc.) has proven confusing in the extreme. This necessitates the adoption of data-fusion strategies and conceptual simplifications intended to help combine or streamline this bewildering set of binding measures.

Although $IC_{50}$ values are amongst the commonest and most reliable measures reported even they require some kind of data manipulation to make them tractable practically speaking. In QSAR studies, for example, $IC_{50}$ values are often converted into $\log[1/IC_{50}]$ values, since the values typically range over several orders of magnitude. For convenience, this is also expressed as $-\log_{10}[IC_{50}]$ or $pIC_{50}$. Such values are used as dependent variables in QSAR regression. $pIC_{50}$ values can be related to changes in the free energy of binding, through the approximation $\Delta G_{bind}\ \alpha\ -RT \ln IC_{50}$.

Another widely used conceptual simplification involves reclassifying peptides as either nonbinders or as high binders, medium binders and low binders. For example, the schema introduced by Vladimir Brusic classifies binders using these criteria: nonbinders > 10 $\mu$M, 10 $\mu$M > low binders > 100 nM, 100 nM > medium binders > 1 nM, high binders < 1 nM. Such broad schemes also allow us to compensate for the inherent inaccuracy in MHC binding measurements.

Another, albeit underexploited, strategy involves a binary classification of peptides into binders and nonbinders. In general, data has not been designed to span the whole of available chemical, or rather peptide, space, but emerges in a haphazard fashion from a large collection of experiments designed for other purposes. The interests of the immunoinformaticians may be very different to those of the original experimenters. One may be interested in predicting affinities or in predicting epitopes. So, if one wishes to classify by class, methods can then use alternate data sources equally. Any affinity measure can be used to identify binders, be that an $IC_{50}$ value or a $t_{1/2}$ or a $BL_{50}$ value. Likewise, a cell surface peptide eluted from an MHC must obviously be bound, with reasonable affinity, before being eluted. Any peptide found from overlapping peptide scanning to be an epitope must, again, have been bound before being recognized. Thus all of these conceptually distinct means of classification yield equivalent definitions of binder versus nonbinder. This allows us to rationalize a much wider array of data. This is a potentially useful feature of such an approach, though not one which has been much exploited in the past. By combining multiple data sources for binders with multiple data sources for nonbinders we can envisage the development of much more robust, much more general, much more complete – and hopefully much more successful – future methods for the prediction of MHC binders.

## Binding becomes recognition

Once a peptide has bound to an MHC to form a pMHC complex, in order to be recognized by the immune system a pMHC complex has to be recognized by one of the TCRs of the T cell repertoire. Within the human population there are an enormous number of different possible variant genes coding for MHC proteins, each exhibiting distinct peptide binding sequence selectivity. T cell receptors, in their turn, also exhibit different affinities for pMHC. The binding of TCRs to pMHC is weaker (in the micromolar range) than the binding of peptide to MHC (in the nanomolar range). The collective selectivity of the MHC and TCR establishes the power and flexibility of peptide recognition in the immune system and through this phenomenon the recognition of foreign proteins and pathogens.

It was long ago realized that logistic restrictions preclude routine yet exhaustive testing of overlapping peptides as a route to epitope discovery, making computational prediction an attractive alternative. It is generally accepted that a peptide binding to an MHC may be recognized by a TCR if it binds better with a $pIC_{50}$ > 6.3, or a half-life > 5 minutes, or some similar figure. Some peptides binding at these affinities will become immunodominant epitopes, others weaker epitopes, and still others will show no T cell activity. There is some evidence suggesting that as the MHC binding affinity of a peptide rises, then the greater the probability that it will be a T cell epitope. The trick – the unsolved trick – is to determine which will be recognized by the TCR and thus activate the T cell. Generally, the approach taken has been to whittle down potential epitopes to a more convenient number for experimental evaluation by using prediction of MHC binding to eliminate all nonbinders or by choosing only high binding peptides.

## Immunoinformatics lends a hand

Consider a protein of, say, 300 residues. If we are interested in epitope responses mediated by a class I MHC, then we need to consider peptides of eight to 16 residues as potential binders and epitopes. That equates to 2592 MHC–peptide binding assays per allele. We could be interested in one allele or the three or six in a haplotype or we could be looking at a panel of common alleles within a population, which could easily run into dozens. If we include class II responses the number increases again. This will generate an unknown number of binding peptides or candidate epitopes, each of which will need to be tested using one of a great variety of different measures of T cell activation, such as T cell killing or thymidine incorporation, *inter alia*. From this time and labour intensive, and financially costly, undertaking, will emerge a small handful of peptides possessed of varying degrees of immunodominance. While this kind of exhaustive empirical study has, in part at least, been attempted in practice, it becomes utterly inconceivable for a whole proteome say. At the time of writing, a useable HTS approach to this problem has not been forthcoming, though many continue to work on such methods. Much better would be to convert the laborious cost and time consuming binding assays to a computer algorithm.

MHC binding is the stage of antigen presentation which we understand best; it is also, in all probability, the most discriminating stage with the presentation-recognition pathway. In what follows, we will focus on predicting class I MHC binding and deal with class II as a special case.

Moreover, despite a clear if emerging understanding that the repertoire of peptide lengths capable of inducing CTL responses has recently increased considerable for class I, most data is still focused on 9-mers and HLA-A*0201. Thus the data available to build models typically consists of blocks of 9-mer sequences and an associated binding value, such as an $IC_{50}$. These are essentially pre-aligned, since the geometry of the MHC binding pocket prevents binding in several registers. Data is also biased by MHC allele: HLA-A*0201 is by far the most common allele for binding data, outnumbering its rivals by a factor of five.

## Motif based prediction

Initial attempts to computerize MHC binding peptide identification led to the delineation of motifs which supposedly characterize allele-specific peptide specificity. The binding motif is an idea which still commands wide popularity amongst immunologists. The first real attempt to define allele- and sequence-specific binding motifs for MHC–peptide interaction was undertaken by Alessandro Sette and coworkers [9]. In the first instance, they defined motifs for the mouse alleles: I-Ad and I-Ed. They assayed affinities for a sizeable set of synthetic peptides with diverse origins and also measured overlapping peptides of staphylococcal nuclease. Accuracies of about 75% were later quoted for these alleles. The delineation and refinement of motifs has progressed through a body of work embodied in a large and accumulating literature, with human and mouse dominating the list of investigated organisms, although the rat, cow and some primate species have also received attention.

Motifs characterize MHC peptide-specificity in terms of dominant anchor positions with a strong preference for certain amino acids: particular positions within a peptide expressing a highly restricted set of tolerated amino acids. Such anchors are thought essential for binding. Human class I allele HLA-A*0201, which is probably the best studied allele of all, has, for a nonameric peptide, anchor residues at peptide positions P2 (accepting leucine and methionine) and P9 (accepting valine and leucine).

This simple model has been nuanced over time. Secondary anchors may also be present; these are residues that are favoured for binding yet are not essential. The sequencing of peptides eluted from the cell surface show amino acid preferences at most positions, though this may be nothing more than bias intrinsic to protein sequences. Particular residues at particular positions may also have a negative effect on binding.

Notwithstanding the perceived success of binding motifs, many problems persist. While one can combine the contributions made by primary and secondary anchors into an approximate measure of binding affinity, the principal problem and most vexatious feature associated with motifs is that their use is a deterministic method of prediction: a peptide will bind to an MHC or it will not. Even a perfunctory reading of the immunological literature indicates that the use of motif matching produces many false positives and, in all probability, also generates many false negatives, though such supposed non-binders are seldom assayed. Many peptides are both affine and motif-negative, that is they possess noncanonical sets of amino acids lying outside established definitions for an allele. There are many more examples of motif-positive peptides that do not bind.

Proponents of motifs characterize one or more usually two anchor positions as being all important. This conjecture, which is based on observed sequence patterns evident from pool sequencing and from individual epitopes, holds that only peptides with a sequence matching such a sparse pattern will bind. This makes little sense and is not compatible with what we know about molecular binding events. The whole of medicinal chemistry argues against this view. It would be better to describe this process by saying that MHCs bind peptides with an equilibrium binding constant dependent on the nature of the bound peptide's sequence.

# The imperfect motif

Several experimental analysis studies have addressed this issue directly. Stryhn and colleagues generated all systematic single mutations of the 8-mer peptide FEST-GNLI and observed that mutations at positions two and eight resulted in the greatest changes in affinity, but that contrary to expectation, few substitutions abolished activity [10]. Thus it is possible to abrogate canonical anchors without eradicating binding. Likewise, Doytchinova and coworkers introduced all 20 amino acids at anchor positions two and nine of a super-high affinity 9-mer peptide binding to HLA-A*0201 [2]. Only a few substitutions completely abolished affinity; most did not. About half of these peptides were sufficiently affine to be potential epitopes, with affinities above a nominal threshold. This study demonstrates that it is possible to manipulate A2 binding affinity in a rational way, raising resulting peptides to affinity levels two orders of magnitude greater than previously reported. The study also showed that optimized nonanchor residues can more than compensate for nonoptimal substitutions at anchor positions. Clearly, the whole of a peptide contributes to binding, albeit weighted differently at different positions.

For class I, and in all probability also for class II, through the use of relatively straightforward prediction methods it is possible to design peptides with high affinity for MHC, and affine peptide with noncanonical anchors, at least for well characterized alleles, with extra affinity arising from favourable interactions made by nonanchor residues. Such novel, non-natural sequences will act as super agonists, antagonists or blockers of MHC mediated T cell responses.

Notwithstanding, the problems of motifs, many papers continue to report their use, and for obvious reasons. The list of already defined motifs is long and covers many alleles in many species. As a technique, the use of motifs is admirably simple, as it can be implemented by eye or more systematically by computer. A scan is performed, searching one or more protein sequences seeking potential binding peptides. While binding motifs seem, to me at least, counter-intuitively simplistic, nonetheless, prediction using motifs is preferable to no prediction at all.

## Other approaches to binding prediction

However, the inadequacy of motifs has been clear to immunoinformaticians for some time, and now alternative techniques abound. The different types have, as one might expect, different strengths and different weaknesses. The first step away from deterministic motifs came with the work of Kenneth Parker, which is based on regression analysis. It gives quantitative predictions of the dissociation half-lives of $\beta_2$-microglobulin from the MHC complex. Apart from its inherent utility, the main contribution made by this approach is that it was the first to be made available online (http://bimas.dcrt.nih.gov/molbio/hla_bind/). Usually known as BIMAS, this site is still widely used.

A different strategy has been the direct utilization of data from binding experiments, as realized by the use of so-called positional scanning peptide libraries (PSPLs) [11]. There are many more methods of this kind. Though doubtless of value, they nonetheless betray several limitations. They do not constitute a systematic approach to solving the MHC–peptide binding problem. Rather, as a group they represent a set of distinct and inconsistent solutions to the same problem. The measures of binding are different, as is the degree of quantitation, and they also lack sufficient application to corroborate their predictive utility. Moreover, few, if any, of the papers describing such work make available sufficient detail for others to use their methods independently.

Many other examples of diverse empirical approaches have emerged in a piecemeal fashion over the years. While many are useful, they again do not constitute a systematic approach to binder prediction. Instead, we should look to established methods of proven provenance. Indeed, the principal approach to epitope prediction has involved the application of validated and well-used methods derived from computer science data mining or robust multivariate statistical techniques.

The goal of such studies is to take a protein or genome sequence and identify within it the presence of MHC binding peptides and/or T cell mediated epitopes. To achieve this, predictive methods require three things: a structural representation of the peptides being used to train them; an equivalent list of biological activities corresponding to the peptides being used in training; and some form of computational engine capable of generating cohesive relationships between the particular description of the peptides and the associated activities. The outcome of this process is a predictive model relating peptide structure to probable activity.

Beyond immunoinformatics, activities can be any sort of physical property or biological activity: enzyme inhibition or whole organism toxicity or melting point or whatever. Moreover, it could just as easily be some utterly different type of quantity, such as stock market prices or psychological status, which can often be expressed in terms of a categorical descriptive, or ontological, language. As we elaborate below, activities or properties can be quantitative, monotonic real numbers ($IC_{50}$s for example) or a binary, two category decision (epitope versus nonepitope, for example) or they can take the form of several categories (nonbinder, low binder and high binder, for example). The rather obvious point we make here is that the approach is a quite general one. Probably the least generic aspect of the process is the structural description used.

# Representing sequences

Many different representations of amino acids have been proposed, and many used, to help predict the properties and functions of peptides and proteins. Many prediction methods use indicator variables: these are binary strings indicating the presence or absence of particular amino acids. For example a bit string corresponding to:

$$00100000000000000000$$

would, depending on the amino acid order used, represent cysteine, while

$$10000000000000000000$$

would equate to, say, alanine. Such a 20-vector is required at each peptide position; which is effectively 180 values for a nonameric peptide. From such a representation a regression equation or other model, such as an ANN, is built.

An alternative way of representing the amino acids within a peptide is to use one or more property scales. These were discussed at length in Chapter 4. Over time, a sizeable literature has evolved which describes, evaluates and catalogues the properties of the 20 common amino acids. Pre-eminent amongst attempts at compilation is the AAindex, a database of amino acid scales, mutation matrices and folding potentials.

In a sense, the computational or decision engine described here can be conceived of as a probabilistic generalization (or specialization, given your point of view) of an inference or reasoning engine, familiar from that branch of computer science which concerns artificial intelligence. Such an inference engine can use any form of computational approach to link activity to structure: inductive logic programming, artificial neural network, Bayesian statistics or robust multivariate statistics amongst many more. From the viewpoint of a biologist this is irrelevant as long as the method works. The goal and perhaps key motivation is, of course, to find methods that work as well as possible.

## Computer science lends a hand

A number of groups have used techniques from computer science data mining, such as artificial neural networks (ANNs) and hidden Markov models (HMMs), to predict peptide–MHC binding affinity. ANNs and HMMs are, for slightly different applications, the particular favourites when bioinformaticians look for tools to build predictive models. Latterly, support vector machines (SVMs) and robust multivariate statistics (as are typically applied to quantitative structure activity relationships) have been added to the mix. The difference between QSAR and artificial intelligence methods is mainly a semantic one: in practice both seek to achieve the same goal and function in similar ways.

Some simple yet useful rules have been proposed for selecting methods given availability of data; they suggest using structural modelling when binding data is absent, motifs when it is very scanty and AI techniques and the like when data is plentiful. Datasets of 50–100 peptides can be used to build quantitative matrices or SVMs, while larger datasets are needed to build HMM or ANN based models.

## Artificial neural networks

The artificial neural network – or ANN or often just NN – is a so-called bio-inspired algorithm. It is a machine-learning method which purports to model itself on a biological neural system. Like most of bio-inspired computing, its actual inspiration comes not from a real down-and-dirty piece of biology but from a sanitized theoretical conception of such a system: an abstraction of biology rather than the biology itself. ANNs have for some time been tools of choice for pattern recognition and data classification, due to their ability to learn and generalize, finding applications across science and engineering.

ANNs have many perceived advantages: a high interpolative capability; they are capable of dealing with complicated and imprecise data; they are often more efficient than developing models from first principles; and they are relatively straightforward to use. These features allow patterns to be identified and trends to be spotted that may be otherwise obscured from human comprehension by their complexity. However, the development of ANNs is often complicated by several adjustable factors whose optimal values are seldom known initially. These can include, *inter alia*, the initial distribution of weights between neurons, the number of hidden neurons, the gradient of the neuron activation function and the training tolerance.

Other than chance effects, to which all predictive methods are prone, ANNs have three main limitations: overfitting, memorization or overtraining and interpretation. In overfitting, well-sampled regions of the training data are learned well and predictions are reliable. However, in poorly sampled regions the underlying trend or trends in the data are not captured accurately. The result is an ANN which is essentially random in prediction: the ANN performs well for the training data but poorly under cross validation. Under specified or over specified ANNs both suffer from overfitting. As an ANN can always reduce the error by adjusting internal parameters, a network runs the risk of simply fitting a more complex and specific model than is necessary. As a model better fits the training data, it becomes less able to generalize. This is called overtraining (or memorization) as the ANN is able to recall training data well but cannot predict reliably within its interpolative data space, let alone outside it. As new and better ANNs have been developed, and basic statistics applied to them, problems of overtraining and overfitting have receded. Interpretation remains a formidable issue: few people can readily visualize, or properly understand, the complex weighting schemes used by ANNs.

There are many types of ANNs: feed-forward networks (or perceptron networks), competitive networks (or Hamming networks), and recurrent networks (or Hopfield networks). Different ANNs behave differently, yet, in general, an ANN can be thought of as a group of arbitrary processing units (called nodes or neurons) organized into layers and linked by weighted connections. The output of a node is contingent on several things: the data feed into it via its several connections, the weighting of each connection and the node's own threshold. Information (one or more independent variables) passes first into the input layer of an ANN, then propagates through one or more hidden layers of neurons, and is ultimately transmitted as one or more dependent variables from the output layer. The number of input and output variables specifies the node number in the input and output layers. The number of hidden or internal layers and the nodes these layers contain varies between ANNs. These, together with the direction of information flow, are key features of network architecture.

Application of an ANN to a practical problem will typically involve several steps: compiling the training data, choosing the network architectures, training the network and validating it. Training minimizes a penalty function, corresponding to the deviation between observed and predicted values within the training set, through the optimization of node weights and layer biases. Training data passes into a network in cycles, one such iteration is called an epoch. Alterations to the network weighting scheme can be applied at the end of an epoch or after each training pattern depending on learning parameters. It may also be necessary to test several architectures and network types, selecting the most suitable type.

Many immunoinformaticians have adopted the ANN when seeking to predict peptide–MHC binding. Adams and Koziol [12] were among the first to use ANNs to predict peptide binding to HLA-A*0201. Using 552 nonamers and 486 decamers, they achieved a predictive accuracy of 0.78 for a two category classification of good or intermediate binding versus weak or nonbinding peptides. Gulukota and De Lisi [13] used two different methods – ANN and statistical parameter estimation – to predict HLA-A*0201 binding for 463 9-mer peptides. They found that the ANN was better at rejecting false positives, while statistical parameter estimation eliminated more false negatives.

However, the premier practitioner of ANN-based MHC binding prediction is Vladimir Brusic. Over many years, he, his colleagues, and his coworkers, have deployed several data-mining algorithms including ANN, as well as HMMs and evolutionary algorithms [14]. His work addresses both class I and class II MHC alleles and within his own classification scheme his models are highly predictive.

## Hidden Markov models

Another mainstay of bioinformatics prediction is the so-called Hidden Markov Models or HMM. An HMM is the simplest form of dynamic Bayesian network and models a system as a Markov process with unknown parameters. A Markov process is one where the current status of the system is independent of the trajectory traced by past states, being contingent on the previous state and not ones prior to that. When an HMM is constructed, relationships between observed and hidden parameters are determined. In a 'hidden', as opposed to a regular, Markov model, internal states cannot be seen but tokens output by the model are visible.

HMMs have found many applications not least of which are those in bioinformatics. Interestingly, however, HMMs have been little used for immunoinformatic problems. Mamitsuka [15] predicted MHC binding using HMMs. Under crossvalidation, the accuracy of this method was 2–15% better than alternative methods, including ANN.

## Support vector machines

The last of the main AI-based data-mining methods is the so-called support vector machine (SVM). SVMs, which are an example of a kernel-based method, have largely taken bioinformatics by storm. Their inherent accuracy and their ability to represent nonlinear relationships is seemingly compelling. A single SVM is at its simplest a binary classifier which induces a decision boundary between classes (i.e. epitope versus nonepitope) using an appropriate amino acid representation. Training data is embedded in a high-dimensional feature space, and the method creates a hypothesis space of linear functions trained with a learning bias. To find a boundary between classes, an SVM maximizes the margin between them, choosing a linear separation in feature space, by defining a hyperplane through this high-dimensional space. This hyperplane should separate the classification classes while maximizing the distance between the hyperplane and both groups of data. A 'kernel function' $K(x_i, x)$ maps the data from an input space to a feature space, where it is classified. Thus the choice of kernel and its parameters is crucial. Several kernels are available: linear, polynomial, sigmoid and radial basis function (RBF). SVMs are described with lucent clarity elsewhere [16].

As a result of their success, a whole tranche of SVM-based methods for class I epitope prediction have been developed [17, 18]. Most SVM methods undertake discriminant analysis, but we have seen encouraging performance with quantitative prediction using support vector regression (SVR). For SVM regression analysis, regression is performed in a multi-dimensional feature space, but without overly penalizing small errors. Our SVR method adopts an '11-factor encoding' scheme, which accounts for similarities in peptide properties [19]. Subsequently, this approach has been implemented in the SVRMHC server covering more than 40 class I and class II MHC molecules.

# Robust multivariate statistics

Robust multivariate statistics methods address quantitative structure-activity relationship (QSAR) problems, such as are common in drug design. As opposed to AI techniques, QSAR methods are based on different, and possibly more rigorous, types of statistical analyses including, amongst others, multiple linear and continuum regression, discriminant analysis and partial least squares (PLS). PLS-based methods in particular are predictive tools of wide applicability, and comprise a principal cornerstone of modern cheminformatics. Recently, bioinformatics applications of PLS have begun to flourish.

# Partial least squares

Partial least squares (PLS) regression, the principal workhorse of QSAR analyses, is an extension of multiple linear regression (MLR). It works by relating one or more dependent variables (usually biological activities) to the values of several independent variables – usually called descriptors – and uses them as predictors. In MLR, a dependent variable $y$ is predicted from $N$ descriptors $\{x_1, x_2, \ldots, x_N\}$, combined with appropriate weighting as:

$$y = b_0 + b_1 x_1 + b_2 x_2 + \ldots + b_N x_N$$

Here $b_i$ is a regression coefficient, and $b_0$ is the residual or intercept coefficient. Given $n$ observations, the input data comprises an $n$ component linear response vector $y$ and an $n$ by $N$ covariance matrix.

PLS generalizes and combines features from principal component analysis and multiple regression. An advantage of PLS is that it can deal with very large sets of correlated independent variables. It seeks to identify new variables constructed from linear combinations of the original variables on the assumption that these latent variables can better explain both the response and covariate space. Thus, for the $s$

latent variables and the dependent variable $y$:

$$y = t_1 q_1 + t_2 q_2 + \ldots t_s q_s + y_s.$$

Similarly for the covariate descriptor space:

$$X = t_1 p_1 + t_2 p_2 + \ldots + t_s p_s + E_s.$$

$E_s$ and $y_s$ are residuals, which, for well-conditioned data, is assumed to be small; at least when compared to the variance explained by the latent variables. Once the latent variables have been found, the $p_i$ and $q_i$ coefficients can be fitted by MLR using the latent variables as descriptors. In immunoinformatics applications, the dependent variables are usually binding affinities between MHC and peptide. The $IC_{50}$ values (the dependent variable $y$) are typically represented as negative logarithms ($-\log_{10} IC_{50}$ or $pIC_{50}$). The predictive ability of the model is usually validated using 'leave one out' cross-validation (LOO-CV).

One may feel justified unease about aspects of the PLS methodology, particularly for immunoinformatic datasets. No method is perfect nor, in the present context, is a perfect one ever likely. The failure of different methods is, however, as much to do with problems that relate to the underlying data, as it is to do with minor methodological flaws. A general criticism of statistical and artificial intelligence based approaches is overfitting. Usually the covariate matrix is 'over square' and has insufficient degrees of freedom to allow an exhaustive and entirely robust analysis to be undertaken. Many terms in a PLS regression equation or neural network or SVM kernel model will be poorly populated, with only a handful of observations, inflating the associated errors and reducing the associated reliability of prediction. However, such limitations are common to all approaches and they underline the importance of training and test data, and its implicit structure, over and above the methodological approaches used to study and predict it.

## Quantitative structure activity relationships

A number of groups have applied QSAR to immune problems. Chersi et al. [20] used QSAR to optimize binding of 9-mer peptides to the MHC allele HLA-A*0201 by increasing the flexibility of amino acids at position four. Bologa and others characterized the type of amino acid required for high affinity binding to the HLA-A*0201 allele. In a related study, Rovero et al. [21] analysed peptide binding to the human class I allele HLA-B*2705. The main contribution of the research group at the Jenner Institute to the immunoinformatic deployment of QSAR techniques is the additive method. It is a PLS-based technique which leverages the Free–Wilson principle. This states that chemical substituents (or amino acid positions in our case) are independent and that the presence or absence of such groups is correlated with biological activity. Thus, for a peptide, the binding affinity is represented by the sum of constant and strictly additive contributions made by different amino acids at different positions. As a further indication that all predictive methods share common features, the IBS approach, as developed by Parker and others [22] is based on a similar concept. We extended the classic Free–Wilson model with terms accounting for interactions between positions. Thus, the binding affinity of a peptide will depend on the contributions of the amino acid side-chains at each position and the interactions between the adjacent and every second side-chain:

$$pIC_{50} = P_0 + \sum_{i=1}^{9} P_i + \sum_{i=1}^{8} P_i P_{i+1} + \sum_{i=1}^{7} P_i P_{i+2} \qquad (5.11)$$

where $P_0$ accounts, albeit nominally, for the contribution of the peptide backbone, $\sum_{i=1}^{9} P_i$ is the position-dependent amino acid contributions, $\sum_{i=1}^{8} P_i P_{i+1}$ is the contribution of interactions between adjacent positions, and $\sum_{i=1}^{7} P_i P_{i+2}$ is the contribution from every second side-chain interaction. We reasoned that more distant position interactions can be neglected. Initially, this was applied to a set of 340 nonamer peptides binding to HLA-A*0201. Its MLR parameters were $r^2 = 0.898$, number of components $(NC) = 5$. The 'leave-one-out' cross validation (CV-LOO) gives $q^2 = 0.337$, $SEP = 0.726$, $NC = 5$, mean |residual| value = 0.573. The additive method lacks the ability to extrapolate beyond the types of amino acid used in training. However, it does provide a quantitative assessment of any amino acids at all positions in the peptide.

Analyses for a variety of human and mouse class I alleles have now been undertaken using this approach. We find that, in practice, and except for very large datasets such as HLA-A*0201, the adjacent and one to three interactions can be neglected, with the best model provided by the position-wise coefficients only.

## Other techniques and sequence representations

In terms of the number of applications, four techniques – ANNs, HMMS, SVM and PLS – have dominated class I binding prediction. There are many more techniques which have yet to be applied to immunoinformatic problems. Computer science is replete with successful pattern recognition algorithms of all kinds, from Bayesian belief networks to nearest neighbour classifiers. WEKA (http://sourceforge.net/projects/weka/) is a well-known software implementation in Java of many such techniques. Examples of other techniques which have been applied to MHCs include Reche's work on sequence profiles, boosted metric learning and logistic regression [23].

When the data are sufficiently numerous, and sample the available space adequately, most data-mining algorithms will perform well producing predictive models. In twentyfirst century computing, the crux is always the data. This is particularly true in immunoinformatics. Much is to be gained by choosing and generating new and improved datasets. Little is now to be gained from quibbling about the relative merits of one induction engine over that of another. Existing data – in terms of scope and accuracy – is simply not up to the job.

One reason for this dearth is the large number of alleles which have not been evaluated. This is not a problem that can be addressed by swapping AI techniques, but necessitates a changed strategy. The definition and analysis of supertypes is one route to addressing this problem (Chapter 6). Another route is via methods that use relationships at the sequence level between MHC alleles to allow algorithms to induce multi-allele binding models which combine binding data from distinct but related alleles. The relative contribution made by data from different alleles is moderated by some measure of sequence or structural similarity between alleles, which can be defined from supertypes or directly from key binding site residues. A number of such methods are now available [24–27]. This is an approach offering immense potential, since it seems unlikely that any experimental method, even one based on HTS, will, in the foreseeable future, deliver sufficient quantities of binding data to support more traditional single-allele modelling.

# Amino acid properties

Another methodological innovation, this time with the potential to generalize within peptides binding to a single allele, is a class of methods that use quantitative descriptions of amino acid properties rather than use indicator variables to represent peptide sequences. As we saw in Chapter 4, property scales suitable for this purpose are potentially very numerous. Extant scales are contained in the AAindex database (www.genome.ad.jp/aaindex/). AAindex consists of three sections: AAindex1 consists of lists of published amino acid scales; AAindex2 contains corresponding lists of published mutation matrices; and AA index3 lists threading potentials. AAindex1 contains well over 500 annotated indices. Each entry has an accession code, publication details, correlation scores to similar indices with the database, as well as the index itself.

Others have tried to summarize or consolidate this enormity of published amino acid scales in a small set of condensed or consensus indices. The best known, and in our hands the most useful, example is the $z$ scales developed by Svante Wold and coworkers. A principal component analysis (PCA) was used to convert 29 other scales into three amino acid scales – $z1$, $z2$ and $z3$ – which describe hydrophilic, steric and electrostatic/polar properties, respectively. These scales were later supplemented with two extra scales: $z4$ and $z5$. Collectively, the five scales ($z1$–$z5$) describe the hydrophilicity, size, polarity and electrostatic properties of amino acids (Table 5.2). A variety of other condensed scales have been proposed in recent times [28].

Methods based on amino acid scales seek to escape the limitations imposed by the lack of all amino acids at all positions in existing peptide binding data. A set of

**Table 5.2** The five $z$ values representative of amino acid properties

| Amino acid | z scale | | | | |
|---|---|---|---|---|---|
| | $z1$ | $z2$ | $z3$ | $z4$ | $z5$ |
| A | 0.24 | −2.32 | 0.60 | −0.14 | 1.30 |
| C | 0.84 | −1.67 | 3.71 | 0.18 | −2.65 |
| D | 3.98 | 0.93 | 1.93 | −2.46 | 0.75 |
| E | 3.11 | 0.26 | −0.11 | −3.04 | −0.25 |
| F | −4.22 | 1.94 | 1.06 | 0.54 | −0.62 |
| G | 2.05 | −4.06 | 0.36 | −0.82 | −0.38 |
| H | 2.47 | 1.95 | 0.26 | 3.90 | 0.09 |
| I | −3.89 | −1.73 | 1.71 | −0.84 | −0.26 |
| K | 2.29 | 0.89 | −2.49 | 1.49 | 0.31 |
| L | −4.28 | −1.30 | −1.49 | −0.72 | 0.84 |
| M | −2.85 | −0.22 | 0.47 | 1.94 | −0.98 |
| N | 3.05 | 1.62 | 1.04 | −1.15 | 1.61 |
| P | −1.66 | 0.27 | 1.84 | 0.70 | 2.00 |
| Q | 1.75 | 0.50 | −1.44 | −1.34 | 0.66 |
| R | 3.52 | 2.50 | −3.50 | 1.99 | −0.17 |
| S | 2.39 | −1.07 | 1.15 | −1.39 | 0.67 |
| T | 0.75 | −2.18 | −1.12 | −1.46 | −0.40 |
| W | −4.36 | 3.94 | 0.59 | 3.44 | −1.59 |

peptide sequences will exhibit only a few different amino acids at anchor positions and an incomplete selection of residues at other positions. Since each scale should be a continuous representation of underlying physical properties any model induced from such a representation should have the potential to interpolate the effect on affinity of an unobserved residue based on its properties. Starting with the work of Guan [29], many have applied this type of approach to MHC-binding prediction [30–32]. The identity of the scales and the number of such scales varies. It is to be hoped that the use of such scales will help address the issue of generality.

Another recent trend is the development of so-called metaprediction. This is a well-known approach which seeks to amalgamate the output of various predictors in an intelligent way so that the combined results are more accurate than those of any single predictor. Dai has applied these methods to predicting peptides which bind to class II MHCs [33], while Trost has used a heuristic method to address class I binding. This approach is another method which may prove of significant future utility.

# Direct epitope prediction

Another whole strand in MHC binding prediction is an attempt to go beyond simply predicting MHC binders and instead to predict epitopes. One approach seeks to address this prediction problem directly by differentiating epitopes (which are by necessity high binding peptides) from MHC binders which are not immunodominant epitopes. Altuvia and coworkers developed a method which seeks to discriminate between true T cell epitopes and other nonepitopes. Again, they used multiple sequence alignments to generate motifs that are present in epitopes and absent in nonepitopes. The Jenner Institute research group have recently explored the utility of a CoMSIA method [34] designed to distinguish true epitopes from nonepitopes with high MHC affinity. However, arguably the best way to address the prediction of epitopes is to predict not merely MHC binding and T cell recognition but the whole presentation pathway for class I.

## Predicting antigen presentation

Recently, an attempt has been made to incorporate components of the class I antigen presentation pathway, such as proteasome cleavage and TAP binding, into composite approaches to T cell epitope prediction; they represent a good first attempt to produce useful, predictive tools for the processing aspect of class I restricted epitope presentation. Several algorithms are currently available for predicting proteasomal cleavage. FragPredict was the first published algorithm and is based on the compilation of peptide cleavage data. PAProC is based on an evolutionary algorithm. NetChop is an ANN-based algorithm. The amount of data studied thus far remains relatively small, and the predictive power of the different methods has yet to be evaluated objectively, although a comparative study of these methods found that NetChop performed best, identifying around 70% of C-termini correctly.

Although there were several early attempts to amalgamate predictive methods, integrated methods have only emerged recently. Examples include SMM, NetCTL, WAPP and EpiJen. SMM combines an MHC binding predictor with TAP transport and proteasomal or immunoproteasomal cleavage. NetCTL implements an ANN-based predictor of proteasome cleavage, a TAP binding QM and an ANN-based class I binding predictor. WAPP uses proteasomal cleavage matrices, SVM-based TAP and MHC predictions to predict epitopes. EpiJen is a multistep algorithm which again combines proteasome cleavage, TAP and MHC binding predictors.

The complexity of the process of antigen presentation seems horrifying to the average computer scientist, and the accurate simulation of systems such as this often proves prohibitively difficult, computationally expensive and prone to cumulative errors (Figure 3.2). However, ultimately, the accurate prediction of epitope processing will need to rely on a much more comprehensive modelling of the entire process. Many approaches may be applicable to this issue. Flux balance approaches to analyse metabolism are increasingly used as a computational analysis tool, particular at the genome level. However, equations describing metabolism are typically underdetermined, since experimental flux data may be ambiguous or have restricted availability. Another approach is metabolic control theory, long used to model metabolic and other enzyme mediated pathways. Metabolic fluxes can, for example, often be determined by simulation and then compared to what experimental data is available. The use of such mathematical modelling techniques prototyped on reaction kinetics within multienzyme metabolic pathways, coupled to the bioinformatic modelling of individual peptide sequence-dependent steps of the process, will account for the complex hierarchy of interrelated dynamic processes that generate presented peptides.

# Predicting class II MHC binding

In general, assuming one can generalize, the successful prediction of class II epitopes has proved to be more difficult than the successful prediction of class I epitopes. Such difficulties arise for several reasons. First, we encounter similar problems to those we find for class I epitopes: quantity and quality and intrinsic bias of the available data, and problems associated with the prevalent use of simple and incomplete descriptions of binding, amongst others. However, these general problems are supplemented by problems specific to class II.

Chief amongst these is the unrestricted length of class II epitopes. Compared with class I MHCs, which are thought to be limited to at most 18 amino acids, the structure of the open-ended class II binding site does not constrain peptide lengths, allowing binding of the full range of peptide lengths – 11 to more than 25 amino acids – produced by Cathepsin-mediated class II proteolytic processing. X-ray structures of class II MHCs show us, however, that the binding site itself is always occupied by a nine residue subsequence, with the rest of the peptide 'hanging' out at either end. Class II model building thus needs to identify, for each sequence, the binding 9-mer and then, from a collection of such 9-mers, to develop predictive models. This is a truly confounding issue which has been addressed by visual inspection, with all its inherent tendentious subjectivity, and through the use of alignment methods which again impose an assumed register on the model building stage.

This search is complicated, conceptually at least, by the ability of MHCs to bind in a degenerative manner – that is in one of several registers (i.e. potential alignments between groove and antigenic peptide). Long peptides, in particular, might exhibit a hierarchy of multiple binding modes. However, relatively little is known concerning the explicit degeneracy of the binding process. Nonetheless, the fact that the binding groove is open at both ends in class II molecules is consistent with the possibility. Whether this phenomenon actually occurs in reality seems, except for repetitive sequences, unlikely on theoretical grounds. Moreover, our attempts to account for a possible multiplicity of binding modes (i.e. two or more 9-mer subsequences) has not yet yielded a stable solution or workable algorithm.

Another important issue is the influence of 'flanking' residues on affinity and recognition: Arnold *et al.* identified residues at +2 or −2, relative to the core nonamer, as important for effective recognition by T cells. Some have addressed this by increasing the core peptide region identified in our model by two in both directions, but again this seldom yields a stable solution, perhaps suggesting that this phenomenon is a subsidiary one, at least statistically.

Despite these difficulties, and because of the importance of any successful approach, many methods targeting class II have been developed. Bisset and Fierz [35] were perhaps the first, and trained an ANN to relate binding to the class II allele HLA-DR1 to peptide structure and reported a correlation coefficient of 0.17 with a statistical significance of $p = 0.0001$. Hammer and coworkers have developed an alternative computational strategy called TEPITOPE.

One of the most interesting aspects of Hammer's work has been the development of so-called virtual matrices which, in principle, provide an elegant solution to the problem of predicting binding preferences for alleles for which we do not have extant binding data. Within the three-dimensional structure of MHC molecules, binding site pockets are shaped by clusters of polymorphic residues and thus have distinct characteristics in different alleles. Each pocket can be characterized by 'pocket profiles', a representation of all possible amino acid interactions within that pocket. A simplifying assumption is that pocket profiles are, essentially, independent of the rest of the binding site. A small database of profiles was sufficient to generate, in a combinatorial fashion, a large number of matrices representing the peptide specificity of different alleles. This concept has wide applicability and underlies, for example, attempts to use fold prediction methods to identify peptide selectivity.

Ronna Mallios is one of the few long-standing exponents of Class II prediction [36]. She has developed an iterative stepwise discriminant analysis meta-algorithm to derive a quantitative motif for classifying potential peptides as potential epitopes. More recent results have permitted a three-way classification of peptides binding to HLA-DR1. Earlier work used discriminant analysis to predict whether or not a given peptide epitope would activate helper T cells.

Increasingly sophisticated pattern recognition methods have been applied to the class II problem, including ANN, HMMs and SVMs. Typically, a binding core is first estimated or declared, and subsequently binding affinity is predicted assuming this chosen core. This two-step procedure restricts the task to a fixed-length formulation, thus avoiding problems of handling variable length peptides. For example, at the Jenner Institute we have developed an iterative approach – an iterative self-consistent (ISC) partial least squares (PLS)-based extension of our PLS-based additive method. The ISC method assumes that binding of a long peptide derives from the interaction of a continuous subsequence of amino acids within it with the MHC. This approach factors out the contribution of individual amino acids within this subsequence, which is initially identified in an iterative manner. The ISC method converges rapidly to the identification of a central nine residue binding motif given training data comprised of variable-length peptides.

Increasingly sophisticated pattern recognition methods, designed to solve the dynamic variable-length nature of the class II prediction problem, have been developed and include an iterative 'metasearch' algorithm, an ant colony search, a Gibbs sampling algorithm and a multi-objective evolutionary algorithm. Some of these novel approaches have significantly outperformed conventional approaches [37]. None propose a completely satisfying result, as indicated by their relative lack of success [38]. The efficiency evinced by these programs is very different for different class II alleles and there is little overlap between peptide rankings generated by these methods.

The results of these various methods are consistent with an emerging view of MHC binding: that motifs are an inadequate representation of the underlying processes of binding and that motifs for class II are particularly weak. The whole of a peptide contributes to binding, albeit weighted differently at different positions. At least for class I, it is even possible to generate high affinity peptides using non-canonical anchors, with extra affinity arising from other interactions made by the rest of the peptides. This is also likely to be a feature of class II binding. For example, Liu and coworkers showed that for I-A$^b$ it was possible for a peptide bearing alanines to bind to its four main pockets – which correspond to positions P1, P4, P6 and P9 and which usually bind larger peptide side-chains – with compensatory interactions made by residues at other positions in order to maintain overall affinity [39]. Models for class II suggest that the relative contributions of particular residues to binding are spread more evenly through the peptide than is generally supposed, rather than being concentrated solely in so-called anchor positions. There is also some evidence that a sizeable part of peptide binding is mediated by residues that make strong hydrophobic interactions with their binding pockets. Both negative and positive cooperativity is observed during these interactions. Cooperativity is also seen between hydrophobic pockets and solvent exposed peptide positions, indicating the overall complexity of the process.

## Assessing prediction accuracy

All of the methods we have adduced focus primarily on the discovery of T cell epitopes which can prove useful, amongst other things, as diagnostic markers of microbial infection and as the potential basis of epitope vaccines. Many workers have, in recent years, used computational methods as part of their strategy for the identification of both class I and class II restricted T cell epitopes, but it is outside the scope of this book to review these studies in detail. However, it is certainly encouraging that many experimental immunologists are now beginning to see the need for informatics techniques. Ultimately, the utilitarian value of the many techniques described above will need to be demonstrated through their usefulness in experimental vaccine discovery programmes.

Assessing the accuracy of epitope prediction is very important. Anyone can come up with methods that fail, so assessing the accuracy and reliability, and thus the practical utility, of an approach is critical. Generally, people want methods that work well and work reliably. However, this section is not intended to be a primer on descriptive statistics, but rather to supply the interested reader with ideas, and the language that encapsulates them, with which they can better understand later sections.

Accuracy is about error, and our understanding of error. Even the word error has several context-dependent meanings. In statistics, an error is the difference between an observation (i.e. a measured or a computed or an estimated value) and a true or expected value, which is often derived from a population, which is itself unobserved and unobservable. The concepts of error and residual are often confused. A residual is an observable estimate of the unobservable error and involves random sampling. The average of the sample is an estimate of the population average. The difference between the observed property in the sample and the population average is an error, while the difference between the property in the sample and the average of the sample is a residual. Residuals are observables – errors are not. Errors are independent variables, at least if the reference population is chosen independently. Errors are typically independent of other errors whereas a residual is often dependent on other residuals. Here we take error to mean a bound on the precision of a measurement. Errors are of two types: statistical error and systematic error. Statistical error is largely due to random fluctuations in the system being measured or the experimental apparatus used to undertake the measurement. It is essentially uncertain and unpredictable. Systematic error is caused by an unknown but nonrandom fluctuation. If the nature of the systematic error can be identified, then it should be possible to eliminate the error or at least reduce it in magnitude.

There are many sources of experimental, or more specifically biological, error. To explore this issue briefly, consider a population of cells in culture. There may be hundreds, thousands, or millions of cells in such a population. Each cell will be different. Each cell will express different numbers and types of receptor in response to signalling molecules. The concentration of messenger molecules secreted by these cells into the interstitial space will vary in space and time. The complexity of such a system is daunting, and likewise our understanding of it is partial. Control experiments are attempted in the hope of obviating or avoiding this complexity. Experiments are repeated to reduce or average out error. However, ultimately we can never fully escape or forestall 'natural' error – except, possibly, through simulation – so we are obliged instead to tolerate it, and to progress science in spite of its presence.

As there are, proverbially, many ways to skin a cat, so there are many ways to explore the accuracy of data. Data can take many forms, necessitating the use of different techniques. First, we must distinguish between real and discrete data: real data can take any value to any degree of decimal precision while discrete data is limited to integer values. A vector of real data might be $\{1.1, 2.0, 7.8, 197.0, \ldots\}$ while a vector of discrete data may look like $\{1, 2, 8, 197, \ldots\}$. Secondly, we must also distinguish between fully quantitative (real or discrete) versus binary data (where values are either one or zero, on or off, yes or no). Fully quantitative data is essentially unbounded, as above, whereas binary data is a dichotomy between two states. An extension of binary data is the kind of categorical data where the number of states is limited number. An example from epitope prediction is where values can take on one of several classifications: nonbinder, high binder, medium binder or low binder. Here the data is of like type; the quantity being measured is essentially the same. Effectively this is the grouping of like objects into different ranges or classifying according to scale. Likewise, yet conversely, data can fall into disjoint categories: red, yellow and blue or cat, dog, hedgehog and hippo. Here the data is essentially completely different and it is not clear how one would put it on the same scale. There is much subtlety in trying to make sense of these distinct flavours of data, and we will, of need, restrict our analysis here to the bare bones of the subject.

In using binary data, we typically seek to classify predictable states as either 'yes' or 'no' or 'on' or 'off' as being in one of two states. Usually, this is a desired or positive state and a negative or undesired state. Such states might be 'epitope' versus 'nonepitope' or 'antigen' versus 'nonantigen' or any such pairing. We deprecate how we might go about defining such states here, since the definition of a negative state is often more difficult than we assume naïvely.

Within such a binary classification, any item will fall into one of these four possibilities: a true positive (often labelled tp or TP or P) – a correctly predicted positive state, say an epitope or antigen; a true negative (tn or TN or N) – a correctly predicted negative state (i.e. a nonepitope); a false positive (fp or FP or O) – an incorrectly predicted positive state (i.e. a negative item predicted as a positive item); a false negative (fn or FN or U) – an incorrectly predicted negative state (i.e. a positive item predicted as a negative item).

These four numbers are useful measures in themselves and are often quoted. However, it is also useful to combine them into a variety of different summary statistics. For example, sensitivity and specificity are well-known ways of deriving reasonably understandable single numbers which reflect the accuracy of a prediction.

Sensitivity (sometimes referred to as SE or Qobserved) measures the quality of positive prediction. It is the proportion of items predicted positive out of those which could be predicted positive – the proportion of true positives in the context of positive data only. In terms of TP and FN, sensitivity is defined as:

$$SE = TP/(TP + FN). \tag{5.12}$$

SE is given either as a percentage between zero and 100 or as a decimal between zero and one. The higher the value of sensitivity, the fewer positive examples will be incorrectly predicted.

Specificity (sometimes known as SP or Qpredicted) measures the quality of negative prediction. It is the proportion of items predicted negative out of those which could be predicted negative: the proportion of true negatives in the context of negative data only. In terms of TN and FP, specificity is defined as:

$$SP = TN/(TN + FP). \tag{5.13}$$

The higher the value of specificity, the fewer negative examples will be incorrectly predicted. Other accuracy measures are known as the positive predictive value

(PPV) and the negative predictive value (NPV). PPV is also sometimes called precision. In terms of TP and FP, PPV is defined as:

$$PPV = TP/(TP + FP) \tag{5.14}$$

In terms of TN and FN, NPV is defined as:

$$NPV = TN/(TN + FN) \tag{5.15}$$

The choice of sensitivity versus specificity or PPV and NPV depends on the particular scenario under examination.

The Mathews correlation coefficient (MCC) is a popular measure of accuracy for binary data. Its appeal lies in its ability to describe the overall accuracy of prediction using but a single number. The MCC will range between 1.0 (complete agreement between observed and predicted) and −1.0 (complete disagreement between predicted and observed), while a value of 0.0 is a random correlation.

In terms of TP, TN, FP and FN, then MMC is defined as:

$$MCC = (TP^*TN + FP^*FN)/[(TN + FN)(TN + FP)(TP + FN)(TP + FP)]^{1/2}. \tag{5.16}$$

Specificity and sensitivity should be independent: a perfect prediction would achieve 100% in both SE and SP. More typically, a trade off is required, since few if any real-world prediction methods are inherently accurate to that level. Prediction accuracy will depend upon a threshold, which allows the partitioning of items into positive and negative states. If a high sensitivity is necessary then a low prediction threshold might be used, thus identifying many items as positive. True positives therefore increase which reduces false negatives, which, in turn, increases sensitivity. Conversely, this would increase false positives, reducing specificity.

## ROC plots

The receiver operator curve or ROC plot, whose name reflects its origin in the analysis of radar, is a visually appealing means of summarizing and assessing a prediction experiment. It is a plot of sensitivity (SE) on the $y$ axis versus specificity (SP) on the $x$ axis at a series of different thresholds. SE is plotted against either 1−SP or, more rarely, SP giving a plot which tails to right or left. Depending on the size of the dataset, an ROC curve will be most unlike a smooth curve and, for very small datasets, even have concave regions within what should be a completely convex line. The area under the curve or AUC is often used as an overall single-value or summary measure of accuracy or success. An AUC – which takes values between 0 and 1.0 – of 0.5 indicates a random prediction, while higher values are indicative of greater success. However, there is a degree to which this is a moveable feast, with widely varying values being associated with successful predictions. There are many other accuracy measures, such as the mutual information coefficient which returns a value between 0 and 1.

## Quantitative accuracy

Let us now turn to quantitative values, and assume we have two variables or sets of paired data points. Can we say that they are different? One of the simplest or most straightforward ways to measure the overall difference between these sets of measurements is via the root-mean-square deviation (or *RMSD*) between them:

$$RMSD = \sqrt{\sum_i (X_i - Y_i)^2}. \tag{5.17}$$

Identical data will yield an *RMSD* value of zero while, in principle at least, the upper limit is infinite. Thus the closer to zero this value is, the higher the quality of agreement.

Two variables are said to be linearly related when the points of a scatter-plot fall more or less precisely on a straight line. Most data from the real world is far indeed from an ideal linear relationship. Generally, there is a scatter of points about a line of best fit. If the fit is tight this is indicative of a strong if imperfect linear relationship. If the scatter is diffuse, this is suggestive of a weak or strongly nonlinear relationship. Examination of scatter-plots can reveal what could be called structure in one's data. Such structure may represent multiple underlying datasets or be indicative of important nonlinearity.

The simplest measure of linear correlation is perhaps the Pearson's correlation coefficient:

$$r = \frac{\sum (x_i - \bar{x})(y_i - \bar{y})}{\sqrt{n \sum x_i^2 - \left(\sum x_i\right)^2} \sqrt{n \sum y_i^2 - \left(\sum y_i\right)^2}}. \tag{5.18}$$

When computed in a sample, the correlation coefficient is denoted by $r$. It ranges from $+1.0$ to $-1.0$. A value of $+1.0$ indicates a perfect positive linear relationship between variables, which has large $x$ values associated with large $y$ values. A value of $-1.0$ indicates a perfect inverse linear relationship, which has large $x$ values associated with small $y$ values. A zero value is indicative of the absence of linearity.

The square of the correlation coefficient, sometimes called the coefficient of determination or more usually $r^2$, can indicate, in a quantitative manner, how much of the total variance in the dependent variable is explained by modelling.

## Prediction assessment protocols

There are many strategies for evaluating the predictive power of a methodology. A common way is to compare the outcome of a prediction experiment with a benchmark result produced from the same or an equivalent dataset. This is usually done by comparing against the most accurate prediction available or failing that against some well-documented standard dataset. The practicalities of this will vary with the data under study. Alternatively one can compare it against what one would expect from statistical distributions. In practice, however, the most useful and useable approach is to undertake cross validation, comparison versus a test set, randomization or a combination thereof in order to gain an insight into the accuracy in prediction of one's method or the data-driven model being developed.

Cross validation (CV) is a standard validation approach for assessing the validity and predictivity of models. CV works by dividing the dataset into a set of groups, developing several parallel models from the reduced data, where one or more of the groups is excluded, and then predicting the values of the excluded items. Perhaps the commonest approach is to exclude each data item in turn; this is called leave-one-out cross validation (LOO-CV).

The predictive power of the model is assessed using the following parameters. The cross-validated correlation coefficient ($q^2$) is given by:

$$q^2 = 1.0 - \frac{\sum\limits_{i=1} (x_{exp} - x_{pred})^2}{\sum\limits_{i=1} (x_{exp} - x_{pred})^2} \tag{5.19}$$

$$q^2 = 1.0 - \frac{PRESS}{SSQ} \tag{5.20}$$

where *PRESS* is the predictive error sum of squares and *SSQ* is the sum of squares of experimental values corrected for the mean. *SEP*, or the standard error of prediction, which assesses the distribution of errors between the observed and predicted values in the regression models, and is given by:

$$SEP = \sqrt{\frac{PRESS}{p-1}} \tag{5.21}$$

where $p$ is the number of the items omitted from the dataset. CV can be generalized to the many-fold case; CV in five or 10 groups is common. In an $N$-fold cross validation the data is randomly divided into $N$ blocks. Each block is left out once and a model is built from the remaining $N-1$ blocks. $q^2(N)$ is a measure of the predictive capability of the model as evaluated by $N$-fold cross validation.

Irrespective of the kind of data we are using, a key means of testing a model is to use an appropriate test set. A model is built from a large training data-set and tested for accuracy on a smaller test set. A slightly more sophisticated approach, common in the data-mining community, splits the data into three subsets, rather than two: a training set, a validation set and a final or external test set. This allows for a more sophisticated iterated form of training, although it imposes a corresponding increase in the size of the required dataset.

On the face of things, the use of an external dataset seems ideal. However, and certainly when one comes to review the work of others, things can be deceptive. Choice is important, since predicting like examples is somewhat easier than predicting items which are unlike. It is possible, if logistically tedious, to construct or choose sets of test and training data, and negative data, which will tend to favour good validation statistics. Consider a slightly different bioinformatics problem: classifying sequences of G-protein coupled receptors or GPCRs. Assuming we have a valid positive set of GPCRs, when we could choose very different sequences – say small globular proteins or sequences with extreme amino acid compositions – and easily classify them into two groups. However, if one chooses similar proteins – membrane proteins of a similar size and with a similar number of transmembrane helices – then the task becomes intrinsically harder. We can propose a cascade of different negative sets of increasing difficulty as a truer test of a method's effectiveness. It is always best to also test a model blindly by undertaking novel experiments, though even here we run into issues concerning interpolation versus extrapolation within property or structural space.

Rather than undertake crossvalidation or use a test set, an alternative strategy is to use systematic permutations or randomization of the data so as to create a distribution against which to compare the unpermuted prediction. In this case, one ideally seeks a prediction model that scores much more highly than the randomized data. A permutation test may, for example, disorder the affinity values in the training set. Large numbers of permuations, say a 1000, are typically used.

It is possible to overinterpret or misinterpret any summary statistic. Consider Anscombe's quartet, which compares the normally distributed correlation between two variables. A similar value of $r$ can be obtained by a perfectly correlated yet highly nonlinear parabola of points. Likewise a near pefect linear correlation with one massively discrepant point gives rise to a similar value or $r$, as does a single outlier (or rather a point of leverage) from the pack of points which otherwise vary only in their $y$ value.

Thus we cannot replace the careful and methodical evaluation of our data by use of one or even several summary statistics. Moreover, it is always possible to overemphasize the usefulness of cross validation and $q^2$ as measures of performance [40]: high values of leave-one-out $q^2$ are a necessary, but not a sufficient, condition for a model to possess high predictivity. Likewise, high values of sensitivity or specificity or area under the curve from ROC analysis are useful but flawed measurements of performance. External test sets and randomization of training data are also important criteria for assessing model quality.

It is clear that there is no single parameter that can give an adequate appraisal of methodological perfection. Combinations of all these criteria are required. However, most groups are certainly aware of most, if not all, such dangers, and most actively seek to minimize them. Nonetheless, predictive models should always be tested before being used using cross validation and preferably test and training sets. Test and training sets should be diverse and representative. They should also be independent – the test set should not overlap the training set. The best strategy is to use prospective experimental validation, predicting values and then testing them in a blind fashion.

## Comparing predictions

Recently, several systematic comparative validations have been undertaken that seek to benchmark the performance of MHC binding and T cell epitope predictors [41, 42]. Sette and coworkers used a dataset of 48 828 quantitative affinity measurements (as accumulated by his group over the last 20 years) for peptides binding to 48 different mouse, human, macaque and chimpanzee MHC class I alleles to evaluate a neural network method and two matrix-based prediction methods developed in-house and compared these with predictions made via the Web. While differences in respective datasets stymie transparent comparison, they concluded that tools based on combinatorial peptide libraries perform very well. This may be due to the lack of tendentious self-reinforcement compared to techniques built from datasets originally selected by motif.

The Jenner Institute research group have also examined the predictive power of 10 algorithms by testing their identification of T cell epitopes within whole protein sequences, mimicking real-life situations by assessing algorithms as they might be used in anger by experimentalists. The average success in prediction for human class I epitopes was greater than for class II predictions for all the algorithms. Moreover, human epitope predictions were more accurate than those of mice.

Recently, four combined epitope prediction methods were tested using 99 recently identified epitopes [43]: EpiJen recognized 61 out of 99, SMM 57 from 99, NetCTL identified 49 and WAPP found 33. The positive predictive value (PPV) was low for all methods: 21% for NetCTL, 17% for EpiJen and WAPP and 16% for SMM. Quite stringent criteria, certainly more so than usual, were used. Methods of this kind represent the current state of the art in epitope prediction.

Currently, differences in published acceptance criteria still obscure the unequivocal evaluation of comparative performance. Arguably, of course, the most convincing validation is a prospective rather than a retrospective one, since prediction used to guide experiments is more likely to impress experimentalists than any number of statistical evaluations using extant data. Whatever 'political' optimists might say, immunoinformaticians still need to persuade their lab-coated colleagues of the veracity and utility of the *in silico* approach.

# Prediction versus experiment

Lu and Celis [44] used two publicly available prediction algorithms – BIMAS and SYFPEITHI – to identify B7 restricted CTL epitopes within the carcinoembryonic antigen (CEA), yielding three candidate peptides that were tested for T cell responses. One CEA peptide: IPQQHTQVL, efficiently induced a CTL response. They concluded that 'our strategy of identifying MHC Class I-restricted CTL epitopes without the need of peptide/HLA-binding assays provides a convenient and cost-saving alternative approach to previous methods.'

In contrast to this positive message, Andersen *et al.* [45] analysed the experimental binding of 84 peptides selected using the presence of allele-dependent peptide binding motifs. Observed binding was compared with results obtained from the same two algorithms used by Lu and Celis. The authors concluded that no strong correlation exists between actual and predicted binding using these algorithms. Andersen *et al.* concluded that 'the peptide binding assay remains an important step in the identification of CTL epitopes which can not be substituted by predictive algorithms.' More recently, Sette's group reported a similar analysis [42]. They evaluated the accuracy of predicted class I T cell epitopes derived from vaccinia virus in the H-2(b) mouse, and found that extant methods predicted the majority of murine responses.

Looked at objectively, few would doubt that class I predictions work to a reasonable – if allele-dependent – level of accuracy. However, when we analyse the performance of models addressing the prediction of class II epitopes we see a different story. If for example, we take a protein at random and use methods available over the Web, we see a remarkable divergence in performance. A recent evaluation used 179 peptides and validated six commonly used methods: ProPred, MHC2PRED, RANKPEP, SVMHC, MHCPred and MHC-BPS [38]. Each server returned almost completely disjoint sets of predictions for their highest ranked peptides. Class II prediction is thus unreliable and results are discordant to the point of being almost random. Such statistical tests as have been done give equally disappointing results. Much work remains to be done if successful methods are ultimately to emerge.

When many, perhaps even most, methods are implemented in software, the core of the deliverable code takes the form of a quantitative matrix: essentially some kind of look-up table containing contributions made by different amino acids at different positions. The methods used to derive these contributions can be very complex yet their ultimate instantiation could not be simpler. The resulting matrix of coefficients can be derived, and improved, using any kind of optimizer, such as a genetic algorithm. The problem lies not in fitting the data but in generating a model which is general and thus generally useful. Most methods fail to do so. Given the number of possible peptides – a 9-mer has $20^9$ or 512 billion possible sequences – then the number that actually bind will be a small proportion. Available approaches, both experimental and computational, give a very poor representation of the nature of that proportion.

Assessments of prediction accuracy are relatively straightforward to undertake and, as we have indicated, there are now several such comparisons. Most such studies tend to favour the method of whomsoever undertook the comparison; and it is always difficult to obtain appropriate, independent datasets with which to conduct such comparisons. Independent tests need to be conducted in a double blind fashion, since almost invariably when an author is party to an evaluation (and thus influences the choice of the test and the way that the test is conducted) then the test is never truly independent. A reason for this is the immanent bias associated with the process of selecting test data. If the data is not itself used in the assessment, then certainly the criteria for success used is the same as that employed when selecting data for the construction of their model, hence there is an unwonted degree of bias albeit largely unseen and certainly unobserved.

What is needed are datasets designed and engineered using experimental design. Here a proper sampling of the available data space is used to investigate the binding properties of peptides. The peptides designed need not be peptides that can be identified within extant proteins, but should possess sufficient diversity at each position to elaborate a complete model of binding. Available data is not of this kind, being mostly derived as fragments of natural proteins. Many are very similar and this does little to improve current models.

This in turn necessitates using experiments to inform *in silico* models. We need to undertake experiments that improve the accuracy and scope of computational methods. Improved methods will then attain a level of reliability in prediction that enables them to substitute their results routinely for those generated by experimentation, which are so wasteful of time, labour and financial resources.

## Predicting B cell epitopes

All vaccines, with the exception of BCG, are mediated by humoral rather than cellular immunity, principally via the generation of neutralizing antibodies. Conversely, immunoinformatics is best placed to predict T cell epitopes. B cell epitope prediction is a challenge of a different order – and is certainly more problematic than most suspect – since the identification of B cell epitopes, *in silico* or *in vitro*, abounds with real dilemmas.

B cell epitopes can be linear (also called continuous) or discontinuous. Linear epitopes are single, short, continuous subsequences within an antigen. Discontinuous epitopes are groups of individual, isolated residues forming patches on the surface of the antigen. The verity and exegesis of an epitope depends on the nature of its experimental determination. Linear epitopes are identified using some kind of experimental screening procedure, usually PEPSCAN [46], where by overlapping sequences are assayed against pre-existing *ex vivo* antibodies. Discontinuous epitopes are usually identified from the structure of an antigen, typically one derived experimentally by X-ray crystallography or multidimensional

NMR. Discontinuous epitopes are also identified by making site-directed mutants of the antigen and testing them for their effect on antibody binding.

Sequence-based B cell epitope prediction methods are limited to the identification of linear epitopes. If we look back a decade or two, then most predictors of T cells or B cell epitopes were based on identifying maximally valued regions of sequences – essentially looking for peaks, or troughs, in some form of propensity plot. This was long ago shown to be inappropriate for T cell epitopes and consequently many advanced methods for T cell epitopes prediction have arisen. However, many – should that be most, if not actually all – B cell epitope prediction methods continue to rely, wholly or in part, on finding such peaks. However, no single property is known that is able to predict linear or discontinous epitope location with any reliability or accuracy. Most prediction methods use properties related to surface exposure – such as accessibility, hydrophilicity, flexibility/mobility and loop and turn structures – since it is believed that epitopes, at least for nondenatured proteins, must be solvent-accessible if antibody binding is to occur.

Amongst the first B cell epitope prediction methods was that of Hopp and Woods [47]. They adopted a sliding-window method, adapting a hydropathy scale owing to Michael Levitt, to identify maximal property peaks. A correctly predicted epitope will correspond to a peak within two residues of an antigenic residue; the method identifies one epitope per protein and does not identify epitope boundaries. The method was validated using 12 proteins with known epitope locations. A window size of five or more was required to reduce erratic peak values; the optimum value being six residues. Longer window sizes performed less well, perhaps because of an increasing probability of including hydrophobic residues.

## Peak profiles and smoothing

Such so-called sliding or moving windows are popular amongst bioinformaticians and immunoinformaticians, and form the basis of more-or-less all B cell epitope prediction approaches and many early T cell prediction methods. The various properties exhibited by the 20 natural amino acids become no more than a means of numerically characterizing local sequence properties. Amongst the most obvious ways of achieving this is simply to plot amino acid properties along the sequence. However, plotting the individual values of a scale is of little value unless there is an obvious periodicity. More helpful is to average the values using a moving or sliding window. Typically, this utilizes a flat, symmetrical, narrow window of no more than 10–20 amino acids in length. This is a familiar concept that can be grasped intuitively and instantaneously. Its value as a tool is limited but not nonexistent. It works well for, say, predicting transmembrane regions within proteins, since the presence of such regions usually correlates well with the presence of regions composed, in the main, of hydrophobic residues.

A moving window method can have several potential parameters: first, the scale we choose; second, the length of the window; third, the shape of the window; fourth, whether we have a symmetric or an unbalanced window; and fifth, how we smooth the values after averaging. There is also the issue of how we deal with terminal residues that cannot be averaged in the same way. In most cases, windows are short, flat, and symmetrical about the central residue, which takes the averaged value. Over the years, a few different window shapes have been suggested, such as a 'hat', where the contribution of residues lessens the further they are from the centre. Others have used a zigzag type shape to mimic periodicity in a sequence or structure. Of course, a window can take on any arbitrary shape whatsoever. This corresponds to weighting each position independently.

In general, we may assume that a window will have this form:

$$\bar{V}_i^p = w_k S_i^p + \sum_{k=1}^{n} w_k S_{i-k}^p + \sum_{l=1}^{m} w_l S_{i+l}^p \tag{5.22}$$

where a window will have $m$ positions to be averaged upstream of the target residue, $n$ downstream, plus the value for the residue itself; all of the residues within the window will have independent arbitrary weights ($w$). Independent of the exact parameters used to define the window function, various kinds of smoothing are available, each with their own properties and characteristics. Each type of smoothing seeks to reduce the random component of the initial spectrum of values generated by the windowing algorithm.

A popular form of smoothing is that proposed by Savitsky-Golay. Others include digital filtering, and various kinds of transform (Fourier and Cosine) and wavelets. Using methods of this type, the high-frequency regions of the value spectrum are removed, leaving only the dominant low-frequency modes. The effects of these approaches can be approximated by using successive rounds of windowing. At each cycle, high-frequency randomness in the spectrum is reduced; however, the magnitude of each reduction at successive iterations is much reduced and, at least to the eye, the outcome of the process converges rapidly.

## Early methods

As we saw before, most scales are not designed to predict epitopes, rather they have arisen for a multitude of other purposes. A few buck this trend by seeking epitope specific scales. Welling and colleagues attempted to account for B cell epitopes containing hydrophilic residues [48], using the frequency of amino acids within B cell epitopes from 20 different proteins compared to the amino acid composition of 314 proteins. Janin and Wodak proposed an accessibility scale [49], while Emini and colleagues sought to improve the scale's application in epitope prediction [50].

The first method that sought to enhance prediction accuracy by merging different scales was proposed by Jameson and Wolf. Their method, which combined five different scales (hydrophilicity, accessibility, flexibility and two secondary structure parameters), was evaluated using a group of epitope-mapped proteins; a strong correlation between epitope locations and peaks was observed. To effect accurate epitope prediction, Pellequer and Westhof combined 20 amino acid scales in their program PREDITOP; 15 scales were averaged using a sliding window, and five were implemented using scale-specific algorithms.

# Imperfect B cell prediction

Using datasets representing the most stringent examples of peer-reviewed publications describing linear epitope-mapped protein sequences, Blythe and Flower [51] have explored the validity of B cell epitope prediction using sequence profiles. Using 484 amino acid scales and 50 epitope-mapped protein sequences, as defined using polyclonal antibodies, the analysis of both single and combined sequence profiles indicated in the most categorical terms that the underlining approach was of little or no practical value: in terms of ROC plot analysis, the best method produced predictions little better than random.

Notwithstanding issues with the frailty of existing approaches, methods continue to be published. Recently, epitope prediction methods based on decision trees, nearest neighbour learning [52], and freed-forward artificial neural networks [53], have been proposed. All three algorithms were trained using prodigious amounts of unpublished data. This method correctly classified a high proportion of epitopes under crossvalidation, yet the prediction performance was determined using a small set of 10 HIV-1 proteins, thereby potentially limiting its apparent reliability.

ABCpred [54], a form of ANN, was trained on a set of 700 nonredundant 16 residue linear epitopes. Nonepitopes were selected at random from Swiss-Prot. In a blind dataset of 187 epitopes, the algorithm had sensitivity and specificity values of 71.66 and 61.50%. BepiPred [55] combines Parker's hydrophilicity scale with an HMM trained on known linear epitopes and again assessed using HIV proteins. Using ROC plots, BepiPred performed marginally better than the HMM and single propensity scales alone, although an AUC of 0.600 is not truly predictive.

The poor performance demonstrated by BCE prediction algorithms is troubling. No explanation seems overly convincing. It is unlikely that available methodology is to blame, since data-mining techniques have proved much more successful in other areas. The explanation favoured here targets experimental data as the source of the problem. The most widely available data derives from PEPSCAN, and there are reasons to suspect that this is not what it seems or people believe it to be. Experimentally derived epitopes are identified by assayed against pre-existing antibodies with affinity for whole antigens. However, when such 'epitopes' are mapped back onto antigen structures their locations are scattered randomly through the protein. They do not form discrete patches as one would expect if they are simple mimics of crystallographically identified discontinuous epitopes. These *in situ* epitopes can be exposed or completely buried, and thus inaccessible to antibody binding, and also in every state in between. If we compare the conformation adopted by antibody bound peptides with those *in situ* in the intact antigen we see that they are typically very different. However, if we compare antibodies in intact antigen and in whole antigen–antibody complexes they are very similar. Thus the recognition of epitopes in a PEPSCAN analysis requires explanations other than the simplest one of a one-to-one correspondence. One explanation could be that the preformed antibody recognizes denatured antigen *in vivo*. Another explanation is that the isolated peptide adopts a conformation that is able to mimic the surface features of a discontinuous epitope. In this case there is no requirement for the two to share any sequence features – an extreme example of molecular mimicry, perhaps? This problem is clearly in need of a thorough-going computational and experimental analysis.

# References

1. Deavin, A. J., Auton, T. R. and Greaney, P. J. (1996) Statistical comparison of established T-cell epitope predictors against a large database of human and murine antigens. *Mol. Immunol.*, **33**, 145–155.
2. Doytchinova, I. A., Walshe, V. A., Jones, N. A., Gloster, S. E., Borrow, P. and Flower, D. R. (2004) Coupling *in silico* and *in vitro* analysis of peptide-MHC binding: a bioinformatic approach enabling prediction of superbinding peptides and anchorless epitopes. *J. Immunol.*, **172**, 7495–7502.
3. Pietersz, G. A., Li, W. and Apostolopoulos, V. (2001) A 16-mer peptide (RQIKIWFQN-RRMKWKK) from antennapedia preferentially targets the Class I pathway. *Vaccine*, **19**, 1397–1405.
4. Gillanders, W. E., Arima, T., Tu, F., Hansen, T. H. and Flye, M. W. (1997) Evidence for clonal deletion and clonal anergy after intrathymic antigen injection in a transplantation model. *Transplantation*, **64**, 1159–1166.
5. Speir, J. A., Stevens, J., Joly, E., Butcher, G. W. and Wilson, I. A. (2001) Two different, highly exposed, bulged structures for an unusually long peptide bound to rat MHC class I RT1-Aa. *Immunity*, **14**, 81–92.
6. Probst-Kepper, M., Hecht, H. J., Herrmann, H., Janke, V., Ocklenburg, F., Klempnauer, J., Van Den Eynde, B. J. and Weiss, S. (2004) Conformational restraints and flexibility of 14-meric peptides in complex with HLA-B*3501. *J. Immunol.*, **173**, 5610–5616.
7. Tynan, F. E., Borg, N. A., Miles, J. J., Beddoe, T., El-Hassen, D., Silins, S. L., van Zuylen, W. J., Purcell, A. W., Kjer-Nielsen, L., McCluskey, J., Burrows, S. R. and Rossjohn, J. (2005)) High resolution structures of highly bulged viral epitopes bound to major histocompatibility complex class I. Implications for T-cell receptor engagement and T-cell immunodominance. *J. Biol. Chem.*, **280**, 23900–23909.
8. Jiang, S., Borthwick, N. J., Morrison, P., Gao, G. F. and Steward, M. W. (2002) Virus-specific CTL responses induced by an H-2K(d)-restricted, motif-negative 15-mer peptide from the fusion protein of respiratory syncytial virus. *J. Gen. Virol.*, **83**, 429–438.

9. Sette, A., Buus, S., Appella, E., Smith, J. A., Chesnut, R., Miles, C., Colon, S. M. and Grey, H. M. (1989) Prediction of major histocompatibility complex binding regions of protein antigens by sequence pattern analysis. *Proc. Natl Acad. Sci. USA*, **86**, 3296–3300.

10. Stryhn, A., Andersen, P. S., Pedersen, L. O., Svejgaard, A., Holm, A., Thorpe, C. J., Fugger, L., Buus, S. and Engberg, J. (1996) Shared fine specificity between T-cell receptors and an antibody recognizing a peptide/major histocompatibility class I complex. *Proc. Natl Acad. Sci. USA*, **93**, 10338–10342.

11. Udaka, K., Wiesmüller, K. H., Kienle, S., Jung, G., Tamamura, H., Yamagishi, H., Okumura, K., Walden, P., Suto, T. and Kawasaki, T. (2000) An automated prediction of MHC class I-binding peptides based on positional scanning with peptide libraries. *Immunogenetics*, **51**, 816–828.

12. Adams, H. P. and Koziol, J. A. (1995) Prediction of binding to MHC class I molecules. *J. Immunol. Methods*, **185**, 181–190.

13. Gulukota, K. and DeLisi, C. (2001) Neural network method for predicting peptides that bind major histocompatibility complex molecules. *Methods Mol. Biol.*, **156**, :201–209.

14. Zhang, G. L., Khan, A. M., Srinivasan, K. N., August, J. T. and Brusic, V. (2005) Neural models for predicting viral vaccine targets. *J. Bioinform. Comput. Biol.*, **3**, 1207–1225.

15. Mamitsuka, H. (1998) Predicting peptides that bind to MHC molecules using supervised learning of hidden Markov models. *Proteins*, **33**, 460–474.

16. Schölkopf, B. and Smola, A. J. (2002) *Learning with kernels: support vector machines, regularization, optimization, and beyond*. MIT Press, Cambridge, Mass., USA.

17. Zhao, Y., Pinilla, C., Valmori, D., Martin, R. and Simon, R. (2003) Application of support vector machines for T-cell epitopes prediction. *Bioinformatics*, **19**, 1978–1984.

18. Bhasin, M. and Raghava, G. P. (2004) Prediction of CTL epitopes using QM, SVM and ANN techniques. *Vaccine*, **22**, 3195–3204.

19. Liu, W., Meng, X., Xu, Q., Flower, D. R. and Li, T. (2006) Quantitative prediction of mouse class I MHC peptide binding affinity using support vector machine regression (SVR) models. *BMC Bioinformatics*, **7**, 182.

20. Chersi, A., di Modugno, F. and Rosano, L. Flexibility of amino acid residues at position four of nonapeptides enhances their binding to human leucocyte antigen (HLA) molecules. *Z. Naturforsch.*, **55**, 109–114.

21. Rovero, P., Riganelli, D., Fruci, D., Viganò, S., Pegoraro, S., Revoltella, R., Greco, G., Butler, R., Clementi, S. and Tanigaki, N. (1994) The importance of secondary anchor residue motifs of HLA class I proteins: a chemometric approach. *Mol. Immunol.*, **31**, 549–554.

22. Parker, K. C., Bednarek, M. A. and Coligan, J. E. (1994) Scheme for ranking potential HLA-A2 binding peptides based on independent binding of individual peptide side-chains. *J. Immunol.*, **152**, 163–175.

23. Reche, P. A., Glutting, J. P. and Reinherz, E.L. (2002) Prediction of MHC class I binding peptides using profile motifs. *Hum. Immunol.*, **63**, 701–709.

24. Zhu, S., Udaka, K., Sidney, J., Sette, A., Aoki-Kinoshita, K. F., Mamitsuka, H. (2006) Improving MHC binding peptide prediction by incorporating binding data of auxiliary MHC molecules. *Bioinformatics*, **22**, 1648–1655.

25. Hertz, T. and Yanover, C. (2006) PepDist: a new framework for protein-peptide binding prediction based on learning peptide distance functions. *BMC Bioinformatics*, **7**, S3.

26. Heckerman, D., Kadie, C. and Listgarten, J. (2007) Leveraging information across HLA alleles/supertypes improves epitope prediction. *J. Comput. Biol.*, **14**, 736–746.

27. Jacob, L. and Vert, J. P. (2008) Efficient peptide-MHC-I binding prediction for alleles with few known binders. *Bioinformatics*,. **24**, 358–366.

28. Liang, G. Z. and Li, S. Z. (2007) A new sequence representation as applied in better specificity elucidation for human immunodeficiency virus type 1 protease. *Biopolymers*,. **88**, 401–412.

29. Guan, P., Doytchinova, I. A., Walshe, V. A., Borrow, P. and Flower, D. R. (2005) Analysis of peptide-protein binding using amino acid descriptors: prediction and experimental verification for human histocompatibility complex HLA-A0201. *J. Med. Chem.*, **48**, 7418–7425.

30. Ivanciuc, O. and Braun, W. (2007). Robust quantitative modeling of peptide binding affinities for MHC molecules using physical-chemical descriptors. *Protein Pept. Lett.*,. **14**, 903–916.

31. Ray, S. and Kepler, T. B. (2007) Amino acid biophysical properties in the statistical prediction of peptide-MHC class I binding. *Immunome Res.*, **3**, 9.

32. Du, Q. S., Wei, Y. T., Pang, Z. W., Chou, K. C. and Huang, R. B. (2007) Predicting the affinity of epitope-peptides with class I MHC molecule HLA-A*0201: an application of amino acid-based peptide prediction. *Protein Eng. Des. Sel.*, **20**, 417–423.

33. Karpenko, O., Huang, L. and Dai, Y. (2008) A probabilistic meta-predictor for the MHC class II binding peptides. *Immunogenetics*, **60**, 25–36.

34. Doytchinova, I. A. and Flower, D. R. (2006) Modeling the peptide-T cell receptor interaction by the comparative molecular similarity indices analysis-soft independent modeling of class analogy technique. *J. Med. Chem.*,,**49**, 2193–2199.

35. Bisset, L. R. and Fierz, W. (1993) Using a neural network to identify potential HLA-DR1 binding sites within proteins. *J. Mol. Recognit.*, **6**, 41–48.

36. Mallios, R. R. (2003) A consensus strategy for combining HLA-DR binding algorithms. *Hum. Immunol.*, **64**, 852–856.

37. Salomon, J. and Flower, D. R. (2006) Predicting Class II MHC-Peptide binding: a kernel based approach using similarity scores. *BMC Bioinformatics*, **7**, 501.

38. Gowthaman, U. and Agrewala, J. N. (2008) *In silico* tools for predicting peptides binding to HLA-class II molecules: more confusion than conclusion. *J. Proteome Res.*, **7**, 154–163.

39. Liu, X., Dai, S., Crawford, F., Fruge, R., Marrack, P. and Kappler, J. (2002) Alternate interactions define the binding of peptides to the MHC molecule IA(b). *Proc. Natl Acad. Sci. USA*, **99**, 8820–8825.

40. Golbraikh, A. and Tropsha, A. (2002) Beware of q2! *J. Mol. Graph Model*, **20**, 269–276.

41. Peters, B., Bui, H. H., Frankild, S., Nielson, M., Lundegaard, C., Kostem, E., Basch, D., Lamberth, K., Harndahl, M., Fleri, W., Wilson, S. S., Sidney, J., Lund, O., Buus, S. and Sette, A. (2006) A community resource benchmarking predictions of peptide binding to MHC-I molecules. *PLoS Comput Biol.*, **2**, e65.

42. . Moutaftsi, M., Peters, B., Pasquetto, V., Tscharke, D. C., Sidney, J., Bui, H. H., Grey, H. and Sette, A. (2006) A consensus epitope prediction approach identifies the breadth of murine T(CD8+)-cell responses to vaccinia virus. *Nat. Biotechnol.*, **24**, 817–819.

43. Doytchinova, I. A., Guan, P. and Flower, D. R. (2006) EpiJen: a server for multistep T cell epitope prediction. *BMC Bioinformatics*, **7**, 131.

44. Lu, J. and Celis, E. (2000) Use of two predictive algorithms of the world wide web for the identification of tumor-reactive T-cell epitopes. *Cancer Res.*, **60**, 5223–5227.

45. Andersen, M. H., Tan, L., Søndergaard, I., Zeuthen, J., Elliott, T. and Haurum, J. S. (2000) Poor correspondence between predicted and experimental binding of peptides to class I MHC molecules. *Tissue Antigens*, **55**, 519–531.
46. Carter, J. M. (1994) Epitope mapping of a protein using the Geysen (PEPSCAN) procedure. *Methods Mol. Biol.*, **36**, 207–323.
47. Hopp, T. P. and Woods, K. R. (1981) Prediction of protein antigenic determinants from amino acid sequences. *Proc. Natl Acad. Sci. USA*, **78**, 3824–3828.
48. Welling, G. W., Weijer, W. J., Van Der Zee, R. and Welling-Wester, S. (1985) Prediction of sequential antigenic regions in proteins. *FEBS Lett.*, **188**. 215–218.
49. Wodak, S. J. and Janin, J. (1978) Computer analysis of protein-protein interaction. *J. Mol. Biol.*, **124**, 323–342.
50. Emini, E. A., Schleif, W. A., Colonno, R. J. and Wimmer, E. (1985) Antigenic conservation and divergence between the viral-specific proteins of poliovirus type 1 and various picornaviruses. *Virology*, **140**, 13–20.
51. Blythe, M. J.. and Flower, D. R. (2005) Benchmarking B-cell epitope prediction: underperformance of existing methods. *Protein Sci.*, **14**, 246–248.
52. Sollner, J. and Mayer, B. (2006) Machine learning approaches for prediction of linear B-cell epitopes on proteins. *J. Mol. Recognit.*, **19**, 200–208.
53. Sollner, J. (2006) Selection and combination of machine learning classifiers for prediction of linear B-cell epitopes on proteins. *J. Mol. Recognit.*, **19**, 209–214.
54. Saha, S. and Raghava, G. P. (2006) Prediction of continuous B-cell epitopes in an antigen using recurrent neural network. *Proteins*, **65**, 40–48.
55. Larsen, J. E., Lund, O. and Nielsen, M. (2006) Improved method for predicting linear B-cell epitopes. *Immunome Res.*, **2**, 2.

# 6
# Vaccines:
# Structural approaches

*Ich die Baukunst eine erstarrte Musik nenne.*
—Johann Wolfgang von Goethe (1749–1832)

## Structure and function

The phrase 'I call architecture frozen music', attributed to both Goethe and Frederick Schiller (1759–1805), has been used by Arthur Lesk to highlight both the organizational complexity and aesthetic beauty of protein structures. While many may gainsay the assertion, it is overwhelmingly true that understanding protein function is not possible without understanding protein structure.

Proteins do not evolve as linear sequences, they evolve as objects in three dimensions. That is to say that proteins experience evolutionary pressure as physical objects and not as abstract representations of molecular sequences. We may understand evolution as changes in the lettering of sequences but this is far from how and why it actually occurs. Likewise, we can only conceptualize protein functions at high organizational levels, where they can be interpreted as directly influencing the fecundity of the whole organism. At the molecular level we can only really discuss binding not function. Within the neo-Darwinian paradigm, one may explain biological function in terms of its contribution to an organism's reproductive fitness. However, the idea of fitness reflects the probability of survival in a given environment and can be seen as a basis for selection, although fitness is no more a property of phenotypes than it is of genotypes or the sequences of individual

*Bioinformatics for Vaccinology*   Darren R Flower
© 2008 John Wiley & Sons, Ltd

molecules; rather it is a relationship forged between the environment and individual organisms.

Biologists favour explanations couched in evolutionary terms. Evolution is a powerful idea; not quite as powerful as some believe, yet powerful nonetheless. A key aspect is retrospective selection: a thing is seen because it survives not because it is perfect. Similar phenomena infest our experience. However, evolutionary explanations often lack power because they are seldom predictive and tell us little about the contingent constraints that favoured one particular adaptive solution over others. Evolution is said never to repeat itself, yet the eye has evolved independently at least three times. Nonetheless, most attempts to link microscopic change and the trajectory of evolutionary advantage fail. Organisms experience selective pressure not isolated proteins and certainly not nucleic acids. Nucleic acids are simultaneously both sterile carriers of information and dynamic molecules in their own right. All the physical manifestations of genomic information are open to selection but not the information itself. Nucleic acids experience selective pressures both directly and indirectly.

Evolution can only be thought of properly as a system property. Simple systems evolve rapidly, complex systems demonstrate less celerity. Compare the phenomenon of the escape mutants in a five-protein retrovirus such as HIV, to the ponderous millennial evolution of its host. The virus evolves rather more rapidly in evading our immune system than the immune system evolves to defeat it. Likewise, a single protein evolves within a complex context. Individual changes in the genome are reflected in physically manifested changes in protein structure and its binding characteristics. Types of change include: altered stability, the temporal nature of a protein's capacity to fold and the metabolic cost of synthesizing one amino acid versus the cost of another. When taken together with higher-level manifestations of these altered physical properties, such changes in the molecular characteristics of an organism are ultimately reflected in the survival of the whole organism, and beyond that in the altered ecological interactions made by the modified individual.

Putting aside for one moment the path swept out by its evolution, a protein is a macromolecule that can be thought of in coldly chemical terms. A protein structure results from a set of both intrinsic and extrinsic factors. An intrinsic factor is one internal to the covalent structure of the protein, while extrinsic factors are properties of the environment it experiences. The strongest intrinsic factor is clearly the sequence of the protein, but there are others such as the presence of post-translational modifications. Extrinsic factors include, but are not limited to: solution properties including ionic strength, pH and the nature of the solvent (water versus organic versus ionic); the presence and nature of counterions; protein concentration and the degree of molecular crowding; and the presence of substrates or binding partners, amongst others. All – to a greater or lesser extent – affect the dynamic, time-dependent structure of proteins.

# Types of protein structure

At a gross level, there are three distinct types of protein: fibrous proteins, such as silk or collagen; globular proteins, which can be disordered in the absence of binding partners or possess stable folds of varying complexity; and peripheral or integral transmembrane proteins. The structure and the sequence determinants of these three differ considerably.

Fibrous proteins are highly extended or filamentous, inert, water-insoluble structural or storage proteins, which often aggregate when purified or over expressed. Fibrous proteins are more resistant to physical, chemical or enzymatic degradation than are globular proteins, and play important roles in muscle, connective tissue and tendons, and bone matrix. The sequences of prototypical fibrous proteins, such as collagen, keratin and elastin, are highly repetitive and regular with very low residue complexity. In such cases, the resulting structure is typically helical, adopting unique secondary structures, such as the so-called collagen triple helix. Fibrous proteins are often cross linked by disulphides between keratin chains. Other fibrous proteins have more complicated sequences and are constructed from mixed types of repeated structural domain, adopting a flexible, string-of-beads structure. Fibrous proteins have an open-ended sequence limit, though there are few with more than a 1000 residues. This probably represents a constraint on the accuity of protein translation kinetics. Of course, there are many exceptions. Titin is about the largest protein known with approximately 35 000 residues, although a parallel beta-helix protein from *Chlorobium chlorochromatii* is slightly longer at about 36 000. Titin is an abundant protein in the striated muscle of vertebrates.

Globular proteins are by comparison unique structures not based on repetitive sequences, which fold into compact units. This is the most prevalent class of proteins – most enzymes and most proteins regulating the replication and expression of genetic material are globular. The richness of function exhibited by globular proteins is mirrored by their richness of structure. This simple picture has become more complex with the discovery of disordered proteins, which only form compact structures when complexed to another macromolecular or small molecule ligand.

As many globular proteins form crystals, their structure can be addressed by X-ray crystallography. For small proteins at least, multi-dimensional nuclear magnetic resonance (NMR) also yields structural information. The low-resolution tertiary structure of globular proteins can be investigated using hydrodynamic methods, such as flow birefringence and analytical ultracentrifugation. Much can also be learnt from spectroscopic methods such as circular dichroism (CD), fluorescence and ultraviolet and infrared absorbance. The largest protein determined by X-ray crystallography so far is a heterododecameric fatty acid synthase from *Thermomyces lanuginosus* solved at 3.1 Å resolution.

A third class of proteins is only found within the membrane environment of the lipid bilayer that forms the surface and internal structures of the cell. Membrane proteins are either integral (proteins fully embedded in the membrane) or peripheral (proteins with a peptide tail or post-translational modification anchoring them to the bilayer). Functional membrane proteins transport materials across bilayers (such as nutrients or signalling molecules) or act as receptors which react to incoming signals.

As membrane proteins they exist within a complex environment containing both a lipid and an aqueous phase; such proteins present distinctly different problems for automation and high throughput crystallography. Integral membrane proteins are generally large and often form multimeric complexes. Together with the practical problems associated with preparing samples containing biological membranes, it has not proved possible to study them successfully using multi-dimensional NMR. Consequently, most structural information has come from crystallographic techniques: X-ray crystallography for those cases where it has proved possible to produce true three-dimensional crystals – for example the photosynthetic reaction centre or porin – and electron crystallography, which combines image analysis from electron microscopy with electron diffraction data to study two-dimensional crystalline arrays.

An idea which has some currency is that simple and repetitive sequences give rise to fibrous proteins and to regions of disorder in globular proteins, while complex sequences give rise to the kind of globular protein familiar from decades of protein crystallography. Integral membrane proteins are often characterized by 20–30 residue sections of highly hydrophobic residues that form transmembrane helices or short hydrophobic regions that form transmembrane strands.

## Protein folding

Protein structure, and what determines it, are intimately linked to the way proteins fold. A protein folds in milliseconds, the possible number of conformations it might adopt is so numerically vast that stochastic sampling alone might not fold it before the end of the universe. This observation is known as the Levinthal paradox, after Cyrus Levinthal (1922–1990) who first popularized it. In just the same way that evolutionary biologists must contend with how an organism develops to maturity as well as the nature and fitness of final phenotypes, so molecular biologists must seek to explain how a protein folds as well as its final form and function. Presently, the most parsimonious description of folding envisages that the energy landscape of protein intermediates observed during folding approximates in shape to a funnel, which is fairly rough on an intermediate scale, yet offers a clear difference in energy between the folded and unfolded state and, at a gross level, an obvious topological route between them. Hydrophobic collapse, where the nonpolar core of a protein is buried on folding, helps drive folding in an entropic manner, via a so-called molten globule state, to the folded protein.

## Ramachandran plots

Because the peptide bond which links adjacent amino acids is delocalized, the polypeptide backbone is charaterized by two repeating dihedral or torsion angles (labelled phi and psi) which determine the conformations adopted by the peptide chain. Allowed angles, and hence the conformations adopted by each residue, are determined locally. Using a hard sphere potential, the so-called Ramachandran chart maps stereochemically permitted conformations in terms of paired phi, psi angles (Figure 6.1). The chart derives from the work of the Indian biophysicist G.N. Ramachandran (1922–2001), who developed this plot before the advent of widespread protein crystallography.

The omega angle about the peptide bond, which, while planar, can adopt either of two conformations: cis or trans with respect to the attached atoms. Most residues are trans, while a strict minority are cis. For L amino acids, this allows for four types

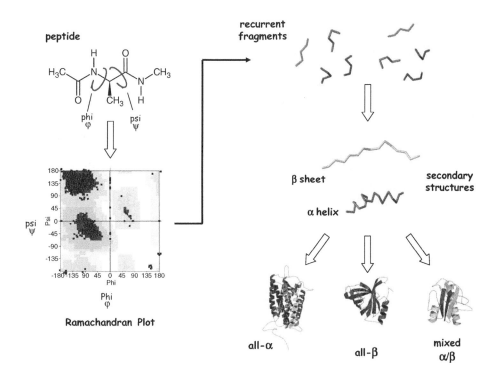

**Figure 6.1** The Ramachandran chart

of Ramachandran plot: trans–trans, trans–cis, cis–trans and cis–cis. The number of available protein structures available is now so large that we can compare the empirically observed distribution of phi, psi angles with the allowed regions of the Ramachandran plot. Only the trans–trans plot is highly populated, and this agrees well with theoretical result. Two residues – glycine and proline – have unusual distributions of allowed angles. Since it has no side-chain, almost all of the plot is accessible by glycine. Proline, on the other hand, is a cyclic amino acid with only one fully rotatable main-chain angle, thus it only adopts a subset of allowed regions.

Looking at the allowed regions of the plot, we can identify about seven different conformational states accessible by 18 of the 20 amino acids. Thus, there is a redundancy in the amino acid code in relation to the number of available structural states, allowing for the observed degeneracy in observed protein structures compared to the number of sequences compatible with them (see below). The set of allowed local structures is almost exclusively determined at the local level. Yet the choice of which possible structure is selected from this set is determined by both local and remote factors. Local factors include the interactions made with the local main chain by the residues' own side-chain and by those of neigbouring residues. Remote factors include interactions made by amino acids distant in sequence but close in space, which create both the overall environment and also make specific interactions.

## Local structures

The combination of these seven conformational states gives rise to large sets of local structures, such as beta-turn amongst many others. Predominant amongst these are those local structures which, when repeated and combined, form the characteristic protein secondary structures: the $\alpha$-helix and the $\beta$-sheet. These two structures lie more or less at the two extremes of protein structure: an $\alpha$-helix is very compact while the sheet structure is extended. A helix can exist independently, while a sheet only exists as part of a cooperative structure. The two main kinds of repeating secondary structure – the helix and the sheet – dominate the folding pattern or fold of most but not all proteins. Beyond these structures, the remainder of a protein is dominated by loops or regions of chaotic conformation that arise from the random arrangement of many different local structures.

The overall native structure of a protein is often referred to as its tertiary structure. When one or more units come together to form dimers, trimers, teramers or whatever multimeric complex, this is known as a protein's quaternary structure. The tertiary structure of a protein will be composed of one or more domains, essentially distinct structures that could potentially exist independently as individual proteins. Each domain has its own fold: this is the complex topological pattern of helices and sheets that gives a protein its unique shape. At a high level, it is possible to classify folds into five types: all-$\alpha$, all-$\beta$, mixed $\alpha$ and $\beta$, $\alpha + \beta$, and a catch-all class of miscellaneous and difficult to classify proteins.

# Protein families, protein folds

Within this clunking, ham-fisted classification there is a hierarchy of folding patterns that divides into groups of related structures, usually called families. A family will have a conserved structure and conserved and overt sequence relationships between family members. A superfamily will typically be composed of several families with similar but not necessarily the same folding patterns and little or no clear sequence similarity. The number of folds in existence remains open to question, with estimates varying between a 1000 and 10 000. However, it is certain that the number of sequences vastly outnumbers the number of folds. Whether manifest by convergent or by highly divergent evolution, the existence of superfamilies shows that many important structural and functional relationships can only be detected through the analysis of three-dimensional structures, which is typically more conserved than sequence similarity. Because the number of possible sequences greatly outnumbers possible folds, quite different sequences can map onto the same structure. This manifests itself in the 'twilight zone' phenomenon. Above a certain threshold, between 25 and 40% sequence identity, protein sequences are clearly related. This is the daylight zone. At intermediate values, above say 18–25%, the relationship is highly equivocal and it is very problematic to differentiate reliably between false sequence relationships and ones that are true. This is the 'twilight zone'. Below this, when sequence similarity is virtually nonexistent, we enter the midnight zone. Thus the comparison of protein structures can be as insightful as comparing their sequences.

# Comparing structures

Various algorithms are available for comparing protein structures in three dimensions in order to recognize structurally related proteins. These programs are efficient enough to perform rapid searches of entire structural databases such as the PDB. The results of mutual comparisons for all known protein structures are themselves stored in databases that provide classifications of protein structures, in part with functional annotations. Likewise, a comparison of pockets on the surface of different proteins may allow one to detect functional relationships. Accordingly, comparisons based on similarity with well-characterized proteins of known structure and function can help identify binding sites. It is, therefore, often advisable to go beyond the comparison of protein folds or global structural motifs in order to look at local structural motifs, such as catalytic triads, which are able to capture the essence of biochemical function.

When attempts are made to identify binding sites, one may search for either clearly conserved individual sequence motifs – for example the sequence motifs which characterize dehydrogenase sites – or sets of essentially isolated residues – such as the catalytic triad of proteases. The first of these can be searched for directly, while the second requires subsidiary data in order to properly identify them.

Proteins of related function often share a comparable binding site, and thus the binding site of a new sequence or structure may be detected by comparison with other proteins with the same function.

## Experimental structure determination

Atomic-resolution protein structures were first determined by X-ray crystallography in the 1960s and by NMR in the 1980s. In more recent times, several other techniques – neutron diffraction, cryo-electron microscopy and electron diffraction of large macromolecular assemblies and computational protein structure prediction – have begun to emulate the veracity of NMR and crystallography. While these other techniques are of doubtless importance, X-ray crystallography remains the most prevalent approach for solving macromolecular structures.

X-ray crystallography is no fleeting parvenu of a discipline. X-rays themselves were discovered late in the nineteenth century. In the intervening time, the X-ray region of the electromagnetic spectrum was a source of scientific application and innovation both fruitful and fecund. Within a year of being discovered by Wilhelm von Rontgen (1845–1923), X-rays, as realized by the practice of radiography, had indeed proved their medical worth. In the century that followed, X-rays found many other applications. Spectroscopy and chemical analysis have been revolutionized, while whole areas of scientific inquiry have been instigated or fomented. Yet, by far and away the most important technique is crystallography, the analysis of crystallized material through X-ray diffraction. Our understanding of X-ray diffraction began with the work of Max von Laue (1879–1960) and father and son William (1862–1942) and Lawrence Bragg (1890–1971).

X-rays have a wavelength comparable in scale to the distance between atoms; thus a crystal lattice acts similarly to a diffraction grating, generating a well-defined diffraction pattern. This contains information on the physical structure of the asymmetric unit, the smallest unique component of the unit cell, from which a crystal is composed. In single-crystal diffraction, the mainstay of protein crystallography, and in contrast to powder diffraction, a crystal of macroscopic size is investigated. The powder in powder diffraction is formed from more microscopic crystals which are arranged in random orientations. Powder diffraction has found little or no application in mainstream protein crystallography.

Although technical innovations constantly accelerate the generation of fully refined crystal structures, crystallography has historically been perceived as inherently slow, difficult and even laborious. X-ray crystallography has traditionally mapped a trajectory through a succession of complex stages, beginning with the very biochemical and progressing through to the abstractly mathematical. Initially, an experimenter must identify their protein of interest; next, this protein – or indeed proteins – must be produced in large quantities and be of a sufficient purity to facilitate the search for appropriate crystallization conditions. Once crystals are obtained, X-ray diffraction data is collected from it and the structure is 'solved'.

The final stage involves building a protein model within the electron density, and then refining this to optimize its ability to recreate the experimental diffraction pattern.

However, an X-ray structure remains a model, albeit one derived directly from experimental data. In this sense, it is like a binding model and less like a homology model. A protein crystal structure tries to predict the electron density in the asymmetric unit, from which is obtained a predicted diffraction pattern. It does this by using a model of atomic scattering and the location of atoms within the unit cell to generate an idealized density map. The quality of the resulting atomic coordinates is assessed in terms of the agreement between observed and calculated structure factors which are derived from measured intensities. Crystal structures, which are at best a time and space average of billions of molecules, are greatly limited in their precision and exactness by factors such as resolution (a function of the crystal) and errors in measurement and constraints of the crystallographic methods themselves (such as radiation damage).

X-ray diffraction requires a high X-ray flux. Indeed, for very high-resolution studies or time-resolved crystallography, sufficient intensity is only offered by synchrotrons. Unfortunately, few synchrotrons are available, limiting the number and diversity of experiments. The X-ray tube is the more typical source, with high flux rotating anodes being the commonest. The requirements of high-resolution X-ray detectors – angular resolution, maximum count rate and dynamic range – have all improved recently, yet the greatest advance is the move from a mechanical point detector, or diffractometer, to the much faster and more efficient area detectors, facilitating the rise of high throughput crystallography.

Two problems conspire to make crystallography a chancy and recalcitrant process liable to inexplicable uncertainty. The first is crystallization, which largely remains very much a black art. Growing protein crystals remains a poorly understood phenomenon, requiring a time-consuming trial-and-error process to find the small number of idiosyncratic conditions of pH, ionic strength, precipitant and buffer concentrations, necessary for diffraction-quality crystals to grow. Yet, even this is beginning to yield to high throughput robotics. Gone are the wasted midnight hours with a Linbro tray and Gilson, replaced by robotics and thorough, systematic searches of crystallization conditions.

The second resolved difficulty is solving the phase problem: the diffraction pattern of a crystal is obtained by exposing it to a focused beam of X-rays. Each spot on the diffraction pattern is an X-ray intensity and has associated with it a phase. When a phase and an intensity are combined, through a Fourier transform, an electron density map is created. For crystals of small molecules, phases can be determined directly from relationships between intensities. Proteins need more logistically complex solutions. In times past, this required laborious trial-and-error searches for heavy atom derivatives and a clever mathematical trick called multiple isomorphous replacement. In more favourable scenarios, molecular replacement using an existing three-dimensional model of a homologous protein, could be used. The most practical solution is the direct incorporation of selenium into biosynthesized proteins, which allows the resulting diffraction pattern to be phased using multiwavelength anomalous diffraction – the so-called MAD technique.

Other approaches are also being developed. One is using so-called direct methods, which seek probabilistic mathematical relations that mimic those useful in small molecule crystallography. Another potential innovation able to revolutionize macromolecular crystallography is a practical, reliable and affordable X-ray laser. Although sources of coherent X-rays are known, it will be some time before they become routine experimental equipment. The use of ultrashort, intense X-ray pulses to record diffraction data in combination with direct phase retrieval has been demonstrated. For example, femtosecond bursts of X-rays have been produced by free electron X-ray lasers with a brilliance which is $10^8$ times that of current synchrotons. These have been combined with manipulation of the diffraction data to produce an accurate, phased and interpretable electron density map for small structures.

## Structural genomics

Yet, for all these technical advances, the single most significant advance has been one of administration, logistics and outlook. Driven by the realization that experimental crystallography is not sufficient to determine all structures in a timely and cost-efficient manner, the emergence in the last decade of structural genomics has seen protein crystallography move from a haphazard discipline, driven equally by the availability of protein and the desire for high impact publications, to a systematic one which seeks to solve structures *en masse*. Key to this idea is the fact that structural genomics provides a fine sampling of distinct families of proteins, such that there is at least one example of a structure per sequence family. Given this example, implicit or explicit homology modelling can, to some degree at least, fill in the gaps populating the remaining members of the family with reliable structural models. Thus, part of any proper structural genomics initiative is the use of bioinformatics to provide an appropriate sampling of available sequence and structure space.

Structural genomics seeks automated and robotic solutions to what was previously largely a manual discipline. The production of protein is probably the most generic aspect of biomacromolecular crystallography, although few other experimental scenarios will require such pure protein in such large quantities. The development of a whole plethora of different high throughput protein production systems is currently underway. These include both *in vitro*, or cell-free, systems and examples based on well-understood microbial systems, such as *Escherichia coli*. Many of the biochemical and biophysical stages of the crystallographic process – protein production and crystallization – are greatly enhanced by automation. Other technical advances have solved or sidestepped seeming intractable problems, such as the phase problem.

There are now several initiatives in structural genomics. For funding reasons, most work overtly in the biomedical area. The not-for-profit Structural Genomics Consortium (www.thesgc.com/), or SGC, aims to determine medically-important protein structures, particularly those mediating human diseases as well as pathogen proteins. It operates from the Universities of Toronto and Oxford, and Karolinska Institutet, Stockholm. Up till June 2007, the SGC had deposited 450 proteins structures and seeks to submit about 200 structures per year. Another example is the TB structural consortium (www.doe-mbi.ucla.edu/TB/), which has deposited around 200 protein structures from the TB bacterium, around 40% of known TB structures. This is a looser grouping comprising 72 institutions in 13 countries. The Structural Genomics of Pathogenic Protozoa consortium (www.sgpp.org/) is composed of groups from five American institutions. It targets proteins from global pathogenic protozoa, *Plasmodium falciparum, Leishmania major, Trypanosoma brucei* and *Trypanosoma cruzi*, which are responsible for a variety of major diseases: malaria, leishmaniasis, sleeping sickness and Chagas' disease. They have deposited about 50 structures out of a list of 1300. The end result of structural genomics, at least in a publicly funded context, is the deposition of protein structures into structural databases, such as the Protein Data Bank. We turn now to this topic.

## Protein structure databases

When one first thinks about structural databases – that is databases which contain information about structures rather than information about sequences – then one tends to think first about biological structures. When one thinks about biological structures, one again tends to think first about protein structures. The accumulated output of both single protein structure determinations and the assembly-line output of systematic structural genomics need to be archived somewhere. The Protein Data Bank – usually referred to as the PDB – is the primary repository for three-dimensional structure data of biological macromolecules. It is dominated by the structures of proteins, protein ligand complexes and, to a lesser extent, nucleic acid structures. An average of 10 000 scientists worldwide visits the PDB Web site every day, and about 130 structures are downloaded each minute. Access to the PDB is available via the Internet (http://www.pdb.org). Each PDB entry is encoded as a formatted text document that can be downloaded from the database. This enables the structure to be interpreted by algorithms and manipulated using a text editor.

The PDB contains structures derived by a variety of methods: X-ray crystallography, nuclear magnetic resonance (NMR) and cryo-electron microscopy being the most prominent approaches. About two out of every three crystal structures in the PDB have associated experimental structure factors. A similar proportion of structures derived by multi-dimensional nuclear magnetic resonance spectroscopy have experimental NMR restraints. In addition to atomic coordinates and structure factors, a variety of other information is available including sequence details, crystallization conditions, derived geometric data, three-dimensional images and a variety of links to other databases.

PDB is an apposite name, since it is more a repository than a fully realized database. For much of its history, the PDB was little more than an indexed accumulation of flat files containing protein structures, mostly derived from X-ray crystallography. To a certain extent at least, this remains true even today. Yet, the PDB was once a pioneering force at the forefront of developing standards for preserving and sharing biological data. Structural biology journals were among the first to require the submission of data to international databases, such as the PDB, as a precondition of publication. The 1997 publication of the mmCIF dictionary saw one of the first internationally-agreed standards for reporting experimental structural results. However, long ago the PDB was overtaken and now – at least when compared to those long ago days – the PDB languishes in the slow lane of the information superhighway, if that is not itself too outmoded a phrase.

The Protein Data Bank was founded in 1971 at the Brookhaven National Laboratory (BNL), and then held only seven structures. The inception of the Protein Data Bank predated by more than 10 years the appearance of the first sequence databases. After 27 years, the operation and management of the PDB became the responsibility of the Research Collaboratory for Structural Bioinformatics (RCSB), which is now solely responsible for on-going management of the PDB. The so-called Worldwide Protein Data Bank (wwPDB) is an extension of the Protein Data Bank; it is an attempt to re-engineer the old-style PDB data structures as a 'relational' database based on the mmCIF schema. wwPDB is managed by several organizations which seek to pool their respective databases and expertise, coordinating the deposition and data processing of structural data for inclusion in the PDB as well as acting as regional distribution centres. The wwPDB aims to maintain a single archive of experimental macromolecular structural data which is freely, publicly and globally available to the scientific community. Members of the wwPDB consortium include the RCSB, the PDB at Osaka University in Japan and the Macromolecular Structure Database (MSD) group at the European Bioinformatics Institute at Hinxton, United Kingdom.

## Other databases

Many, many other protein structure databases exist, most built through the automatic processing of the PDB. We shall review some of the more important. The Macromolecular Structure Database Group (www.ebi.ac.uk/msd/) at the EBI is a European initiative for the collection and management of macromolecular structure data. Its contents are partly derived from the PDB. One of the most interesting and potentially useful services offered by the MSD is the Protein Quaternary Structure (PQS) server, which contains symmetry-generated models of probable quaternary structures – such as dimmers, trimers or higher multimers – corresponding to crystallographic PDB entries. PQS returns biological units and is accessible via the European Bioinformatics Institute (EBI) server (http://www.ebi.ac.uk/msd-srv/pqs/).

SCOP (http://scop.mrc-lmb.cam.ac.uk/scop/) and CATH (www.cathdb.info/) are two of the most interesting and important current structural databases. They seek to classify all solved structures in a hierarchical fashion, but classify molecules differently. At a high level they use the familiar all-$\alpha$, all-$\beta$, mixed $\alpha$ and $\beta$, $\alpha + \beta$ and so on scheme but deviate at lower levels. CATH clusters proteins at four levels: class, architecture, topology and homologous superfamily. Class is derived automatically from secondary structure content; architecture, the gross orientation of secondary structure elements, is derived manually; while at the topology, level structures are clustered according to their topological connectivity. SCOP is a largely manually derived database which isolates protein domains and then classifies them into species, proteins, families, superfamilies, folds and classes.

At one time, the PDB accepted theoretical models, but no more. These models were derived by homology modelling or by *de novo* modelling. These files, which can now be generated automatically in vast numbers, have now been deleted, and from 2002 onwards no modelled structures have been accepted. Databases that archive modelled structures also exist. These include MODBASE, a database that contains models created by ModPipe, a modelling pipeline based on the programs PSI-BLAST and Modeller. PMDB is another database of protein models, this time catering for entrants to CASP. Swiss Model Repository (http://swissmodel.expasy.org/repository/) is a database that is in many ways equivalent to MODBASE but built using the Swiss Model server.

# Immunological structural databases

As noted in previous chapters, many databases exist which cater for immunological data, including structural data. IMGT contains a wealth of structural data, as do various other databases. Recently, Kangueane *et al.* have developed a database that focuses solely on X-ray crystal structures of MHC-peptide complexes. T-PID (http://surya.bic.nus.edu.sg/mpidt/) is an extension of this, covering T cell receptor–peptide–MHC interactions and contains structures of all TcR/pMHC and pMHC complexes.

Data on so-called B cell epitopes have been incorporated into functional immunology databases. Antibodies, which mediate B cell epitopes, are an intrinsic component of adaptive immune responses in higher invertebrates. Their binding-sites – or epitopes – are found within protein antigens and can be classified as 'linear' or 'discontinuous'. Examples which explicitly and specifically target B cell data include BciPep, CED and Epitome.

Bcipep contains 3031 linear B cell epitope sequences, sourced from the literature, within a Web accessible PostgreSQL database. Epitopes are presented as annotated sequences with information on the immunogenicity or reactivity, the antibody and host protein, the experimental method of determination and the classification of the antigen. Protein sequences are cross-referenced to the SWISS-PROT and PDB databases, and source publications are linked to PubMed.

The Conformational Epitope Database or CED contains information on experimentally-determined discontinuous epitopes reported in the literature. The database contains around 200 manually curated entries, each corresponding to a single epitope. Each entry is annotated with details on immunogenicity, the experimental method used to determine the presence and location of the epitope, the antibody and antigen involved, together with cross-references to other databases. Where structural data is available, parent antigens can be viewed graphically.

Epitome is another database containing structurally-inferred antigenic regions identified from X-ray cocrystal structures. It comprises all known antigen–antibody complexes, with a description of residues involved in the interactions, and their sequence and structural environments. Derived from the PDB, SACS (www.bioinf.org.uk/abs/sacs/) is a database focusing on antibody structures.

An additional database within the arena of humoral immunology is HaptenDB. Currently, it contains 2021 entries for 1087 haptens and 25 carrier proteins. Each entry details the nature of the hapten, together with its two-dimensional and three-dimensional structures, and carrier proteins. Data is also available for the coupling method, antihapten antibody production method, assay method and the specificities of antibodies.

The Structural Database of Allergen Proteins (SDAP) contains both allergen sequences and structures for 887 allergens. It permits homology searches between known allergens and input user sequences. Where possible, an SDAP entry is annotated with the allergen name, source, sequence, structure, IgE epitopes, literature references and links to major public databases.

## Small molecule databases

In addition to protein databases, there are many databases which archive small molecule structures. These come in two types: experimental and computational. The Cambridge Structural Database (CSD) is the premier experimental database for small molecule crystal structures. Computationally-derived databases contain the modelled structures of compounds. Methods such as CORINA enable a three-dimensional structure to be generated automatically from a molecule's chemical graph or connection table. These are used routinely by software to store the two-dimensional structures of chemical compounds. Computer-derived databases have now begun to proliferate. However, foremost among these is ZINC (http://zinc.docking.org/). Such databases are a key resource for computer-based discovery of small molecule ligands, which has applications in adjuvant discovery (see below).

# Protein homology modelling

The principal alternative to the experimental approaches of X-ray crystallography and multi-dimensional NMR is the much misrepresented discipline of protein homology modelling, whereby the structure of one protein is generated based on the known structure of another. This presumes that there is a verifiable relationship between the two proteins at the sequence level. It is over 35 years since the first example of homology modelling was published: Brown *et al.* modelled the then undetermined structure of lactalbumin on the known structure of lysozyme. In the intervening years, as the number of sequences and structures has increased exponentially, so extant examples of homology modelling have likewise proliferated.

Over the years this process has been refined and automated, and from this evolution of ideas has now emerged an essential consensus. Such a consensus, while possessed of many subtleties and nuances, can be simply stated. One can build homology models from a single structure or from a collection. One requires either a pairwise sequence alignment between known and unknown or, better still, a multiple alignment. Although any attempt at homology modelling is open to error, the possibility of getting things badly wrong are much minimized if one possesses both a reliable multiple alignment and a set of related structures. Likewise, a pairwise alignment and a single structure only multiply one's chances of inaccuracy.

Initially one would overlay the set of related protein molecules and then identify regions of structural similarity, which together form a so-called common core. A common core is composed of several structurally conserved regions (SCRs), which should, as the name suggests, be present in all structures known or unknown. These SCRs are linked by regions displaying considerable variability in terms of both length and conformation. These variable regions (VR) – sometimes somewhat inaccurately called loops – must be filled as the model grows. Sequences from the SCRs in the multiple structural alignment can be mapped to conserved blocks in the multiple sequence alignment. Thus will a full sequence–structure correspondence be established from which the implicit structure of all unknown proteins can be inferred. It will show the length and sequence, though not the conformation, of the VRs. As the model develops, the variable regions can be found by searching structural databases for protein fragments of similar length that fulfil all the constraints imposed by the common core, such as the distance between ends and the absence of steric clashes. Alternatively, such regions can be found using some form of dynamic optimization to identify putative conformations that match all constraints. Usually, there is more than one solution for each VR. Once the common core and all identified VRs have been combined into a model, the amino acid sequence can be mutated into that of the target protein. Side-chains can then be added to each residue, using one of the many side-chain placement algorithms. The final model is then often subjected to some form of energy optimization, such as simulated annealing. Clearly, these few lines do not do justice to the complexities of the process but are enough for now.

In the days of structural genomics, one is increasingly likely to stumble across a structural target with unknown binding partners and ligands, necessitating a computational solution. Many approaches have thus developed. Structural analysis of binding sites tries to identify similarity of function that is not dependent on any apparent sequence similarity or similarity of folding pattern yet extends beyond the search for conserved structural and/or sequence motifs. There are several ways to predict the location of a binding site, allowing its position to be inferred. The degree of certainty with which a site can be copied or inherited from one protein to another is a limiting factor in the use of structural genomics to identify biological targets. Much work now suggests that potential energy functions in common use are simply too inaccurate to predict protein–ligand interactions with any certainty.

## Using homology modelling

Homology modelling projects now follow a well-established consensus, since many of the mechanical steps involved in the logistics of building a homology model have now been largely devolved to automated or semi-automated programs such as SwissModel or Modeller. Having said that it always helps to know what one is doing. Given the sequence of a target protein, and assuming it can be related to a known structure by discernible sequence similarity, an initial model can be generated quickly. Examination of this model should identify the key features of the binding site. As time passes, experimental data – the SAR of binding ligands, mutagenesis studies, and so on – can be used to illuminate a putative binding mode.

At the beginning of a homology modelling project, a protein model will typically be quite poor, inaccurate and imprecise. As relevant data accumulate, the corresponding protein model will, potentially, improve greatly in verity and fidelity. We can think of our model possessing a nominal resolution. Initially, model resolution is low: it is fuzzy and imprecise. As the project progresses, we gain more and more relevant information. As a consequence, the model becomes ever more accurate and its nominal resolution increases. It is fuzzy no longer, and key interactions can be discerned with confidence. With enhanced resolution and model quality comes a corresponding improvement in a model's veracity and predictive power. The inferences we draw from our model should match its nominal resolution: qualitative at an early stage, quantitative later on. Using appropriate information, in an appropriate way and at an appropriate time, allows us to derive the best from any model. As ever, experimental validation, where possible, drives model refinement, and we seek as much information and insight as we can while minimizing over-interpretation. Over-interpretation at any stage can be misleading and we must be certain to match the nominal resolution of a model to its purpose.

Homology modelling can be a profound visualization tool. It enables scientists, whether biologist or chemist, to explore and hopefully understand aspects of a particular protein or protein–ligand complex. While this kind of information is available via crystallography, the use of modelling allows an interactive examination of ligand-binding site interactions which consciously or subconsciously underlies the process of molecular design. Use of site-directed mutagenesis, in particular, can highlight the involvement of individual residues in ligand binding. Over time, augmentation of the power in prediction and the enhanced explanatory accuracy of a model engendered by data-driven optimization will greatly improve the usefulness of a model.

## Predicting MHC supertypes

In many ways, to understand binding is to understand the binding site. Likewise, understanding the binding site enables one to understand binding. The binding site determines the structural and physicochemical constraints that must be met by any putative ligand. Yet from an evolutionary vantage point, it is ligand properties that determine the structure and properties of the binding site. The peptide specificities of MHC molecules illustrate this point very well, since they form a punctuated spectrum of related binding site structures within the context of overall structural and sequence similarity. Many HLA alleles have been demonstrated to bind peptides with similar anchor residues. A good example, with demonstrable immunological utility, of the potential of homology modelling, and indeed of the analysis of protein structure, is in providing a cohesive grouping of major histocompatibility complex alleles into so-called supertypes, which exhibit broad supermotifs, based on the commonality of their substrate specificity. Polymorphism confounds our attempts to study the peptide specificities of MHC molecules in an effective manner.

Indeed HLA is, arguably, the best studied of all human polymorphic proteins. The IMGT/HLA database stores over 1600 different HLA class I and II alleles. These allelic variants have arisen through a process of random mutation, filtered and constrained by evolutionary processes operating in the context of hostile host–pathogen interactions, themselves constrained by geography and time. Such processes obviously also affect other proteins. Haemoglobin is a good example: mutations leading to sickle cell anaemia are viewed as a contingent adaptation to malaria. Since MHCs are polymorphic, alterations in the residues comprising the binding site alter peptide selectivity. Insight into the structural basis of peptide binding can come as readily from a thorough analysis of MHC binding site structure as it does from the kind of data driven models described in Chapter 5.

Any similarities apparent between binding sites should be mirrored in the peptide selectivities exhibited by different MHCs; thus comparison of MHCs will help predict peptide selectivities by grouping together similar alleles. The speed and verity of vaccine discovery would be greatly improved if one could delineate effective rules able to group together HLA alleles with similar specificities. Such a classification, if accurate and sufficiently extensive, would greatly reduce experimental work as it would no longer be necessary to study every allele, thus making the discovery of epitope-based vaccines targeted at multiple alleles more efficient. Some have sought insights into MHC supertypes from a sequence perspective, others from structural data.

One approach to HLA classification has been evolutionary analysis. As chimpanzees and gorillas are closely related to humans, possibly sharing a common ancestor 7–10 million years ago, Lawlor *et al.* [1] compared gorilla class I MHC sequences with human HLA-A, B and C alleles and chimpanzee MHC. All sequences were similar but not identical; most polymorphic residues were located in the same region. HLA-A alleles was divided into five families: A2, A3, A9, A10 and A19. Two divergent groups of HLA-C alleles were found, one containing Cw*0701 and Cw*0702, the other with Cw*0101-Cw*0601 and Cw*1201. HLA-B was the most polymorphic, and no consensus group was found. In a later study, McKenzie *et al.* [2] constructed phylogenetic trees and indentified two clusters for HLA-A: one with A1, A3, A9, A11, A36, A8001 and some of the A19, and the other with A2, A10, A28, A4301 and the other A19 members. No consistent clusters were found for HLA-B or HLA-C. Cano *et al.* clustered the HLA-A and HLA-B alleles by constructing similarity matrices [3]. The method identified three clusters. Cluster 1 includes HLA-A3, HLA-A11, HLA-31 and HLA-33. Cluster 2 includes HLA-B7, HLA-B35, HLA-B51, HLA-B53 and HLA-B54. Cluster 3 includes HLA-A29, HLA-B44 and HLA-B61.

Probably the best known supertype classification is the motif-based approach of Sette and coworkers, and it was they who originally coined the term MHC 'supertype' [4]. Four supertypes were defined: A2 (A*0201-06, A*6802, A*6901), A3 (A*0301, A*1101, A*3101, A*3301, A*6801), B7 (B*0702-5, B*3501-3, B*5101-5, B*5301, B*5401, B*5501-2, B*5601, B*6701and B*7801) and B44 (B37, B41, B44, B45, B47, B49, B50, B60, B61). The same group later added A*0207 to the A2 supertype and B*1508 and B*5602 were added to the B7 supertype, eventually defining a total of nine supertypes. Based on this work, Lund *et al.* [5] classified HLA-A and B molecules using nonameric ligands from HLA-A and B molecules, summarizing the frequencies of different amino acids at each peptide position. The resulting matrices were used to cluster HLA sequences into superfamilies. Their results defined a new B8 superfamily and separated A26 alleles from Sette's A1 cluster.

Using structural data, De Lisi and coworkers [6] correlated class I peptide binding specificities and polymorphic positions within the MHC binding site. Five families were defined for specificities of pocket B, and three families for pocket D. Three more families were also defined for alleles with a joint specificity of pocket C and D. Chelvanayagam has defined structure-based 'road maps' for both class I and class II [7], based on the sequence composition within pockets. This classification can put the same allele into several groups. He found that positions 62, 97 and 114 discriminate between families. While the whole site may contribute to peptide binding, these three amino acids are the most important for supertype specificity. The definition of class II supertypes lags someway behind that of class I. Reche and Reinherz used multiple sequence alignment to find important residues in 774 class I and 485 class II HLA molecules [8]. Consensus sequence patterns were obtained for the binding sites of HLA-A, B, C, DP, DR and DQ groups.

More recently, Doytchinova and colleagues [9] have addressed supertype definition using a GRID/CPCA technique that encompasses COMSIA and hierarchical clustering to produce a robust grouping of human class I MHC alleles. GRID/CPCA allows one to classify sets of related proteins exhibiting polymorphism, using molecular interaction fields (MIFs) and consensus PCA (CPCA). This classification does not rely on protein sequence similarities, as descriptors are derived directly from three-dimensional binding site information. The method derives information solely from three-dimensional protein structures which are, in turn, generated automatically from sequence data. Binding data are not required. This allows peptide specificities to be examined for many MHC alleles. Hierarchical clustering and principal component analysis were used to identify supertypes for 783 HLA class I molecules. The two techniques gave a 77% consensus: 605 HLA class I alleles were classified in the same supertype by both methods. Overall eight supertypes were defined: A2, A3, A24, B7, B27, B44, C1 and C4. More recently this technique was extended to cover class II MHC supertypes [10].

Most recently, Sette and colleagues have revised their existing supertype definitions clustering 750 different HLA-A and -B alleles into the same nine supertypes [11]. All supertypes are, however, theoretically derived, even these 'experimentally-derived' supertypes; these definitions are largely based on 'binding motifs', which are an inadequate description of peptide specificity. While they possess a certain verisimilitude, they are, at best, only a partial definition of supertypes, limited by the lack of available data for most MHC molecules. Structural supertypes, on the other hand, represent an encouraging potential solution to this problem, unencumbered by limits on binding data. Modern methods in particular, such as that evinced by Doytchinova *et al.*, allow us to propose supertype definitions solely based on sequence and structure, without the need for binding data.

However, problems remain: future structure-based methods will need to address the inherent conformational flexibility of protein structures, which can manifest itself at both the local binding-site level (such as side chain rotameric states) and the global level (i.e. large-scale breathing motions or hinge-like domain movements). One might achieve this by averaging over an ensemble of structures or by sampling a normal mode trajectory or by an equivalent approach. At a more mundane methodological level, existing potential functions such as those used by CoMSIA are an imperfect representation of interatomic interactions. Approaches based on sophisticated molecular mechanics potentials, or seeding the binding site with fragments, or quantum mechanics (QM), particularly computationally-efficient semi-empirical QM, or one based on hydrophobicity may prove necessary to rectify extant deficiencies.

## Application to alloreactivity

Beyond the derivation of supertypes, such a structural approach has many potential applications. If, for example, we look not at the binding site but more widely at the surface of an MHC we can conceive of several possibilities.

Alloreactivity, the T cell mediated response to nonself MHCs, is a major problem in transplantation medicine, since it leads to graft and tissue rejection and graft-versus-host disease. This phenomenon manifests itself at a structural level, the foreign MHC bearing self peptides is recognized directly or indirectly by self T cells – rather than the sequence level; that is by the presentation of digested MHC proteins via self MHC molecules. Since up to 25% of the naïve T cell repertoire can be alloreactive, this mechanism can be decisive for transplanted cells, organs or tissues. HLA matching is one approach used to mitigate this pernicious effect and software, such as HLAMatchmaker (www.hlamatchmaker.net/index.php) and HISTOCHECK (www.histocheck.org/), has been developed to best-guess the optimal choice of appropriate mismatches between haplotypes. Methods, such as those of Doytchinova, can be applied to this problem. Cocrystal structures of TCR–MHC–peptide complexes indicate that recognition of pMHC by the TCR occurs over a large area composed partly of the peptide and partly of the MHC surface. Since we do not know the precise structure of an individual's T cell repertoire we can use the statistical comparison of properties projected from the surface of MHCs to define general similarities between mismatched MHCs. Such results could then be used to help guide the choice of transplant donor.

Similarly, the binding of antibodies to the surface of antigens could be addressed in this way. By comparing the projected properties of epitope and nonepitope surfaces it may be possible to develop predictive metrics for antigenic versus nonantigenic regions. Our attempts to reify this conjecture have not yet proved successful. This is probably due to a combination of factors. On the one hand, paucity of data; on the other, an inadequacy of methods in terms of both the choice of appropriate spatial properties and lucent statistics capable of readily identifying key causative variables.

## 3D-QSAR

One of the most important recent trends in epitope prediction has been a structural one. Three principal techniques have been apparent: 3D QSAR; docking, with or without scoring; and molecular dynamics (MD) simulation.

3D-QSAR techniques make use of robust multivariate statistics, such as PLS, to cope with the large volume of data, and are able to relate binding affinities to molecular descriptors (projected into the space surrounding a set of aligned ligands). 3D-QSAR is a valuable method for correlating ligand structure with observed binding affinity. It is a much exploited technique, particularly in preclinical drug discovery, where such methods have become pre-eminent because of their robustness and ready interpretability. 3D-QSAR focuses on differences in ligands rather than in their interaction with their receptors; nonetheless its value is enhanced when enthalpic changes – van der Waals and electrostatic interactions (and entropic changes) and conformational and solvent mediated interactions – in ligand binding are compared with structural changes in ligand-macromolecule complexes as visualized by high-resolution crystallography.

Two techniques dominate the discipline: comparative molecular fields analysis (CoMFA) and comparative molecular similarity indices analysis (CoMSIA). There are several similarities and several differences between the techniques. Both use huge data matrices generated at regularly-spaced grid points using a distance dependent function. To obtain high predictive power, both methods require a high quality alignment of the structures being studied. Both methods allow a given physico-chemical descriptor to be visualized in three dimensions using a map that denotes binding positions that are either 'favoured' or 'disfavoured'. The explanatory power of 3D-QSAR methods is considerable, not just in predicting accurate biological activities or binding affinities, but also in their capacity to visualize advantageous and disadvantageous interaction potential surrounding the three-dimensional structures of the molecules being investigated.

The principal differences between CoMFA and CoMSIA are the nature of the probe and the type of distance dependent function used. In CoMFA, for example, the probe is an $sp^3$ carbon atom with a $+1$ charge. For each molecule studied, two values of the interaction energy are calculated at each grid point: one a van der Waals / Lennard–Jones interaction and one an electrostatic Coulombic interaction. Because of the hyperbolic functional form, both of these potentials obtain very large nonsensical values within the van der Waals surface. To avoid these values arbitrarily fixed cut-offs are defined. CoMSIA, on the other hand, uses a Gaussian functional form with an attenuation factor $\alpha = 0.3$ so that interactions can be calculated using all grid points both inside and outside the molecules and no arbitrary threshold is required. Similarity indices are calculated instead of interaction energies. A probe is used with a radius of 1 Å, and charge, hydrophobicity and hydrogen bond properties equal to $+1$. Five different similarity fields are calculated: steric, electrostatic, hydrophobic, hydrogen bond donor and hydrogen bond acceptor.

Initially, CoMFA and CoMSIA were applied to a set of 102 HLA-A*0201 binding peptides, and tested using 50 peptides [12]. CoMSIA proved to be more accurate than CoMFA and indicated a dominant role for hydrophobic interactions in peptide binding to the MHC molecule. More recently, the research group at the Jenner Institute extended their 3D-QSAR analysis by applying the CoMSIA technique to a set of 266 peptides in order to assess the contributions of physicochemical properties other than the hydrophobic field. The best model, based on steric, electrostatic, hydrophobic, hydrogen bond donor and hydrogen bond acceptor fields, had $q^2 = 0.683$ and $r^2 = 0.891$. The mean residual value after 'leave-one-out' cross validation was 0.489. Subsequently, the CoMSIA methodology was applied to various human MHCs, including HLA-A*0201 and the HLA-A2 and HLA-A3 supertypes. These models were used to evaluate both the physicochemical requirements for binding, and to explore and define preferred amino acids within each pocket. The data are highly complementary to the sort of very detailed – but peptide specific – information obtained from crystal structures of individual peptide–MHC complexes. However, the utility and applicability of 3D-QSAR is severely limited by the proprietary nature of the software implementing it and by the considerable logistic effort required to build, align and analyse data.

# Protein docking

Solutions to the docking problem must take account of the flexibility of both ligand and protein and, if one is docking against either a homology or an experimental model, then one must take account of inherent uncertainties in the binding site model. For each of the candidate molecules selected for docking, several ligand conformations will usually be searched against a limited number of receptor conformations. This leads to a combinatorial explosion in the number of possible ways of docking together two molecules, each of which must be evaluated. Many sophisticated methods for conformational searching are known and many are implemented in most major proprietary molecular modelling software packages. Docking is a sampling exercise and as such it is necessary to cover as much of the sample space as possible in as efficient a manner as one can achieve. It is seldom possible to attack this problem in a satisfactory manner, leading to a trade off between time and combinations of conformation and orientation searched. To deal with this, powerful computational optimization algorithms, such as Monte Carlo or genetic algorithms are now often employed.

Many current limitations result from simplifications made to keep algorithms tractable given present day computing resources, while others clearly reflect persisting problems in understanding and modelling fundamental processes of biomolecular recognition. Problems of protein flexibility, solvent interactions, the dynamic synergy between ligand and receptor or the proper consideration of the cellular environment all remain important stumbling blocks.

Side chain placement is of particular importance when one contemplates protein–peptide interaction, something of particular interest within immunology. For example, a preliminary to the application of docking and virtual screening described below is, for MHC complexes, the fast and accurate modelling of the initial peptide structure in the binding groove. For example, the 'dead end elimination' method is often used to place side chains on the main chain peptide backbone using a rotameric library of allowed side-chain conformations. The structure of these side chains is largely dictated by the structure of the static MHC molecule, and is not much affected by side chain–side chain interactions, largely due to the relatively extended conformation adopted by the bound peptide.

# Predicting B cell epitopes with docking

Static docking is also of use for the analysis of B cell epitopes. One must distinguish linear epitopes from those defined by antibody–antigen complex X-ray crystal structures, which are probably the most reliable and least ambiguous representation of epitopes available [13]. Predictive methods relating to discontinuous epitopes require three-dimensional structural information, and focus on identifying surface regions as surrogate discontinuous epitopes. The first predictive methods were developed by groups led by Thornton [14] and Novotný [15].

Thornton and colleagues observed a relationship between surface-protrusion and known epitope location. They generated an ellipsoid enclosing a percentage of the atoms of the antigen structure, and calculating a protrusion index $(PI)$ for each residue, which represents the percentage of enclosed structure. Results for $PI$, B factors, and surface accessibility were comparable, while hydrophilicity was less discriminating.

Novotný and colleagues observed a correlation between the contact points of a large sphere and the location of antigenic residues. The accessible surface of the protein using various probe sizes from 1.4–20 Å was calculated and smoothed using a sliding-window of seven amino acids, since it was assumed that epitopes consisted of between six and eight residues. A 10 Å probe profile correlated best with known epitope locations.

More recently, the conformational epitope prediction server or CEP [16] was developed. It identifies potential epitopes by defining surface regions using solvent accessibility. A comparison of predicted regions to epitopes in 21 antibody–antigen complex X-ray crystal structures, reported a prediction accuracy of 75%. Disco-Tope [17], which predicts discontinuous rather than linear epitopes, is based on the analysis of 76 antibody–antigen crystal structures. It uses a residue propensity scale combined with structural protrusion calculations to predict epitope residues. Using at threshold that selects 95% specificity, DiscoTope detects 15% of epitope residues. The algorithm achieves improved performance compared to existing discontinuous epitope prediction.

Using eight Web-servers for antibody–antigen binding site prediction, Ponomarenko and Bourne [18] analysed two B cell epitope benchmark data-sets, one of 62 structures and one of 82, derived from the 3-dimensional structures of antibody–antigen complexes. No method exceeded 40% precision and 46% recall. The most effective approach used a docking protocol but even here AUC values did not exceed 0.70. Consistent with the poor performance of sequence-based predictors, the failure of structural methods may result from the idiosyncratic generality of antibody-mediated immunogenicity. There may not be any obvious intrinsic protein property able to identify epitope even accounting for structure. However, one would expect a reliable discriminatory function able to differentiate true protein–protein complexes from decoys to function well in this scenario. No such discriminatory function currently exists, though it may be possible to develop ones tailored to the specific needs of antibody–antigen interaction.

Structurally, antibody and antigen are unequal partners; atypical features of the antibody–antigen interaction include the amino acid composition and hydropathy of the antibody's paratope. While the complex is typical in terms of buried surface area, density of hydrogen bonds and complementarity, the amino acid composition of the paratope is distinct from that of the epitope regions and other nonobligate protein interfaces. The contribution to the paratope of aromatic residues, particularly tyrosine, is significantly greater than that made by other residues. On average, tyrosine forms a third of the paratope area. The hydrophobic content of the paratope is also significantly higher than that of other transient protein interfaces, and of epitopes, which are mostly hydrophilic. Yet by comparing the amino acid composition of epitopes to other similar sized surface regions evidence of their lack of distinguishing features, necessary for unequivocal prediction, is clear.

Epitope prediction based on data from single-specificity monoclonal antibodies may not facilitate the prediction of surface regions that represent either immunodominant or neutralizing antigenic sites. This is consistent with the multideterminant regulatory model proposed by Benjamin, in which any part of the accessible surface of a globular protein antigen can be recognized by antibodies, and that the entire exposed surface represents a 'continuum' of overlapping potential epitopes.

## Virtual screening

Virtual screening (VS), especially structure-based static docking, is a technique of wide applicability and proven provenance. It offers a solution to problems of drug design and of ligand and epitope identification. Several methods seek to apply static docking methods (scoring functions derived from computational chemistry or threading methods derived from structural bioinformatics) to identify MHC binders. Generally, the docking of small molecules performs well when distinguishing ligands from nonligands, but performs poorly when predicting binding affinity – trends preserved when dealing with MHC prediction.

There are several key advantages to virtual versus high-throughput screening (HTS). Apart from the pecuniary advantage of computer screening versus multimillion dollar robotic assays, its relative speed has driven its use. To evaluate thousand upon thousand of compounds effectively, screening methods tend to be fast and empirically-based, rather than using time consuming methods such as molecular dynamics.

Here, the basic ideas of VS are introduced. VS is a methodology closely related to molecular dynamics (see below). Both are based, to a large extent, on molecular mechanics force fields or, at least, VS utilizes analogies drawn from pairwise atomistic potential energy functions. Two distinct approaches to VS have been applied to the prediction of MHC binding. One derives from computational chemistry and cheminformatics and is based on using empirical molecular mechanics or similar technology to score host–guest complexes. The other approach originates from structural bioinformatics, where an atom-pair threading potential is used to estimate binding and thus score the complementarity of ligand–receptor interactions.

The expression VS derives from pharmaceutical research: the use of ligand–receptor interactions to rank and/or filter molecules as an alternative to HTS. VS is part of the wider domain of computer-aided drug design. VS can be combined with other *in silico* drug discovery technology: structure-guided enhancement, pharmacophore and similarity-based compound selection, ADME/tox property prediction, computer discrimination of drug- and nondrug-like compounds, plus QSAR analysis, such as Free–Wilson analysis or CoMFA/CoMSIA.

Approaches to virtual screening cover a spectrum of methods which vary in complexity from molecular descriptors and QSAR variables, through simple scoring functions (such as Ludi, FlexX, Gold or Dock), potentials of mean force (PMF) (such as Bleep), force field methods, QM/MM, linear response methods, to free energy perturbations. In this transition from atom counts to full molecular dynamics, we see a tremendous increase in computer time required. Virtual screening can be seen as seeking a pragmatic solution to the accuracy gained versus time taken equation. The point at which one stops on this spectrum is contingent upon the system being evaluated, the number of peptides or small molecules being evaluated and the computing resources available.

As a sequential process, VS can be divided into five stages. It begins with the X-ray structure or homology model of a biological target molecule, usually a protein. This is combined with potential ligands. These may be peptides derived as overlapping subsequences from a particular protein or set of proteins, or they may correspond to numerous commercially available chemical compounds, which have been carefully prescreened for undesirable structural characteristics inconsistent with those of known drugs.

The resulting set of ligands is then docked into the model of the binding site and scored, quantitatively or qualitatively, for some appropriate measure of binding. This will hopefully discriminate between a small set of ligands with appreciable affinity for the binding site and the bulk of other molecules that lack the ability to bind. The top few percent of these ranked hits are selected, bought or synthesized, and assayed experimentally.

## Limitations to virtual screening

Two linked and as-yet-unsolved problems lie at the heart of VS and continue to thwart the development of truly robust virtual screening methodologies. First, the accurate automated docking of a limited number of the 'most different' conformations of each small molecule or peptide ligand to an ensemble of macromolecular models, and second, the accurate quantitative prediction of ligand affinity. In addressing these issues, many virtual screening methodologies and many implementations have emerged, each with its own advantages and disadvantages. Most attempt to overcome the limitations of computer time by using very simple methodologies that allow each virtual small molecule structure to be docked and scored very quickly. Examples include GOLD [19] and DOCK [20].

Many papers have compared the performance of different approaches and different software implementations. No clear consensus has emerged from this mass of studies. However, the perceived discrepancies between evaluations of docking methods and docking software are probably caused as much by different overlaps between training and evaluation data as much as they are by actual differences in execution. Nonetheless, the exercise is useful, as it highlights not only key directions in the field but also neglected areas in need of further development. Certain observations do make themselves evident, such as the need to use multiple versions of the binding site. Concencus or meta-scoring, where several scoring functions are combined, is a practical strategy for improving the quality of the discrimination between ligands and nonligands. My own experience suggests that any improvement that might come from using data fusion methodologies such as this, are strongly tempered by the tenacity of the problem itself. It may increase the gain of true positives in a particular screening experiment, but has much less success in producing an improved quantitative correlation with experimental data.

We are presently unable to quantify binding accurately using theory alone. Thus, knowledge-based methods continue to represent the best available approach. They can take advantage of the growing volume of experimental data and thus account, at least implicitly, for many effects that remain poorly understood. Clearly, different methods have different strengths and weaknesses and it is often advisable to combine several methods when tackling a particular system.

Finally, the last stage of virtual screening is to analyse and postprocess the results of the scored and ranked docked candidate molecules. In an ideal world, a virtual screening effort would produce a tiny handful of extravagantly active molecules that can be rapidly optimized for selectivity and bioavailability and other ADMET properties. Desirable as this situation may be, it is just as unlikely. More often, we have an array of weakly active, yet equipotent, molecules. Clearly the more resources, in terms of both human and computer time, one is prepared to employ in generating and evaluating possible dockings, the more likely one is to obtain a good solution. Likewise, the more sophisticated, and thus time consuming, are our methods for evaluating the scoring phase of the virtual screening process, the more likely we are to screen accurately. If we want to dock a few dozen small molecule structures, then we can afford to expend a great deal of time on this process, but if our goal is to dock a large virtual library, then the practical limitations of computer time will reduce this to a minimum.

Nevertheless, many limiting factors still prevent the development of a reliable and fully automated approach leading from target structure to ligand. Careful use of the methods and an equally careful interpretation of the results are an absolute requirement. Success still depends on the quality of experimental data, be that structural or functional. Despite the clear success of VS, doubters do remain. Some see VS as simply verifying that molecules match the dimensions of the binding site. Others doubt all attempts to use structure to enlighten the discovery of ligands. While arguments regarding flexibility and large-scale rearrangements seem compelling, they merely act as a challenge to the discipline. Inherent uncertainty, such as the dependence of binding site conformation on the presence of a ligand, can be addressed using dynamic methods or by trying to build this uncertainty into search models, so that ligands are detected even when the binding site is represented by a suboptimal model.

For the successful identification and docking of new ligands to a protein target by virtual screening, the essential features of the protein and ligand structure must be captured and distilled in an efficient representation. Much effort continues to be devoted to the accurate preparation of sets of small molecules for VS, including accounting for stereoisomers and tautomers, and in screening out reactive compounds and other promiscuous binders. However, getting the small molecules right must be matched by getting the binding site right. The relative verity of VS will improve as such representations improve. Improvements will come through technical advances in several areas: better representations of ligand and protein conformation, improved docking methodology, enhanced scoring functions and better modelling of binding site structure, including better protein homology models, improved side-chain placement, better models of protein ionisation, and so on.

The potential of VS is illustrated by examining two applications in immunology: first, the use of VS to predict MHC binding peptides; second, the use of VS to help identify small molecule adjuvants.


## Predicting epitopes with virtual screening

FRESNO is a VS methodology developed by Rognan and colleagues, which relies on a simple physicochemical model of peptide–MHC interaction [21]. This model was trained using binding data and experimentally-derived three-dimensional structures for the MHC alleles HLA-A0201 and H-2Kk. The inability to predict binding constants directly from simulations, at least in a short time, has led some to combine calculation with statistics. Regression-based scoring is predicated on the assumption that the total free energy is approximated by the sum of several separately-calculable contributions. Usually, regression coefficients are determined by MLR, PLS or some AI approach. An initial training set of receptor–ligand crystal complexes and corresponding experimental binding affinities is used to train the tuneable potential energy function. As with all data driven approaches, the contingent accuracy and the transferability to new congeneric series depends on the nature of the training set.

Rognan and coworkers found that lipophilic interactions contributed the most to HLA-A0201-peptide interactions, whereas H-bonding predominated in H-2Kk recognition. Cross-validated models were used to predict the binding affinity of a test set of 26 peptides to HLA-A0204 (an allele closely related to HLA-A0201) and of a series of 16 peptides to H-2Kk. They concluded that their tuned scoring function could predict binding free energies using these. More recently, Rognan and colleagues found that, for predicting the binding affinity of 26 peptides to the class I MHC molecule HLA-B*2705, FRESNO outperformed six other available methods (Chemscore, Dock, FlexX, Gold, Pmf and Score).

The relative success of FRESNO in the prediction of binding affinities for MHC–peptide interactions suggests that optimization of the screening function within a chemical area or protein family, rather than the use of totally generic screening functions, may be a generally successful strategy. This confirms our own experience using commercial and freeware virtual screening approaches for the quantitative assessment of MHC peptide binding.

Kanguene and colleagues reported a 77% success rate using the number of clashes between the MHC and peptide and the number of exposed hydrophobic peptide residues to correctly distinguish binders and nonbinders. Margalit and colleagues have proposed a number of virtual screening methodologies, each of increasing complexity. They used a standard amino acid pair potential to evaluate the interprotein contact complementarity between peptide sequences and MHC binding site residues. They presented an analysis of peptide binding to four MHC alleles (HLA-A2, HLA-A68, HLA-B27 and H-2Kb), and were successful in predicting peptide binding to MHC molecules with hydrophobic binding pockets but not when MHC molecules with charged or hydrophilic pockets were investigated. More recently, Davies *et al.* looked at a large data-set of MHC-structures using static energetic analysis following energy minimization, partitioning interactions within the groove into van der Waals, electrostatic and total nonbonded energy contributions [22]. They found that the whole peptide defined specificity, highlighting the lack of dominant interactions between peptide and MHC as there was no separation in the performance of a set of disjoint, yet statistically-degenerate, models. More recently, Tong and coworkers have used a virtual screening approach to address peptide binding to the MHC allele HLA-Cw*0401.

Class II has also been investigated using virtual screening methods. For example, Swain developed a threading method and applied it to class II MHC peptide interactions. They found that for class II anchor residues were not restrictive and that binding pockets can accommodate a wider variety of peptides than might be supposed from motif prediction.

Because of the relative celerity of virtual screening methods compared with MD methods and its ability to tackle MHC alleles for which no known binding data are available, this method has huge potential. While both molecular dynamics and related methods hold out the greatest hope for true *de novo* predictions of MHC binding, their present success rate is very much lower than that of data driven models. However, as with most of science, one must tease the genuinely useful from the self-aggrandizing hyperbole. Much work remains to be done on developing, refining and applying this methodology; the potential, however, is undeniable.

## Virtual screening and adjuvant discovery

We should mention a point that is under-appreciated by those it may help most. VS is an extremely cost-effective means by which even very small groups, say one or two people, can address important aspects of the discovery of bioactive small molecules. We do not mean that VS can allow tiny groups to challenge the pharmaceutical industry, at least not directly. However, it does allow such groups to identify receptor antagonists and enzyme inhibitors, which is the first step in the process. Not all such molecules need possess the qualities of drugs – the need for active reagents is great for many systems. Inspired by the linux operating system, some have advocated an 'open source' approach to drug discovery. Risible though this may seem, VS may allow for part at least of this concept to be realized. This can be exemplified by the potential of VS to help identify small molecule adjuvants.

An adjuvant is a substance that enhances immune responses when delivered with a vaccine. During vaccination, an adjuvant will reduce the quantity and required dosage of antigen necessary for immune protection. Such properties are pivotal for, say, subunit vaccines since they lack intrinsic immunogenicity. Although many adjuvants are known, very few are licensed for use in humans; alum, the most common, is suboptimal, inducing Th2-biased immunity. While this may work against infections prevented by antibodies, it seldom protects against organisms where $Th_1$-biased cellular immunity is of paramount importance. The development of new and better adjuvants, able to potentiate different types of immune response, is thus a key aim of vaccine research.

The physical form and stability of antigens determine the magnitude and nature of immune responses by influencing their interaction with APCs and the duration of antigen presentation. Adjuvants may enhance vaccination by exacerbating the depot effect by delaying the spread of the antigen from the site of infection so that absorption is slowed. Alum-based adjuvants prolong antigen persistence due to the depot effect, as well as stimulating the production of IgG1 and IgE antibodies and triggering the secretion of interleukin-4. For example, soluble antigens induce mainly antibody responses while particulate antigens enter the cytosol of APCs and induce cytotoxic T cell responses via cross presentation. Stable antigens are more immunogenic than unstable antigens. Adjuvants, such as alum or water-in-oil emulsions, also potentiate immune responses by changing the cellular compartments into which an antigen enters, thus altering the magnitude and nature of concomitant immune responses.

## Adjuvants and innate immunity

Until recently adjuvant development was empirical; now new understanding of how adaptive immune responses are initiated has made the rational development of a new generation of adjuvants possible. The innate immune system plays a key role in controlling adaptive responses and thus activation of the innate immune system is essential for a strong adaptive response and the development of immune memory. This phenomenon is mediated by the interaction of evolutionarily conserved pathogen associated molecular patterns (PAMPs) with pattern recognition receptors (PRRs) on cells of the innate and adaptive systems. PRRs react to molecular structures found on pathogenic but not normal vertebrate cells. Such PAMPs are usually shared by whole classes of organisms. Lipopolysaccharide (LPS) is, for example, found as a common component of gram negative bacteria. Some adjuvants act as immune potentiators, triggering an early innate immune response that enhances vaccine effectiveness by increasing vaccine uptake. PAMPs can be seen as a subset of so-called 'danger signals' – an idea developed by Polly Matzinger. She posits that innate immune receptors evolved to recognize damage to self (danger) not solely to identify pathogens. Examples of danger signals include RNA or DNA, intracellular components released during necrotic cell death. Necrotic cells induce an inflammatory response which fosters and foments adaptive immune responses.

The innate immune system recognizes pathogens because they display evolutionarily conserved PAMPs, and purified or synthetic PAMPs exert potent adjuvant effects mediated by PRRs. These include at least three families of nonphagocytic receptors. Toll-like receptors (TLRs) bind diverse ligands while nucleotide-binding oligomerization domain (NOD)-like proteins, detect the muramyl dipeptide component of peptidoglycan and RIG (retinoic acid-inducible protein)-related proteins detect dsRNA. Other PRRs include scavenger receptors and C-type lectin-like receptors such as mannose receptors, which detect mannosylated lipoarabinomannans, $\beta$-glucan receptors and DC-SIGN (dendritic cell-specific intercellular adhesion molecule 3-grabbing nonintegrin), which detects carbohydrate moieties on a variety of proteins. PAMP-stimulated PRRs induce the maturation and migration of APCs, up-regulation of antigen-loaded class I and class II molecules, cell surface expression of co-stimulatory molecules and the production of cytokines and chemokines. Co-stimulatory molecules flag the microbial origin of presented antigen, help activate antigen-specific T cells and create an inflammatory environment that amplifies adaptive immune responses. Ligation of different PRRs can also modulate the type of immune response invoked by an antigen.

## Small molecule adjuvants

Importantly, there are also several small-molecule drug-like adjuvants, such as imiquimod, resiquimod and other imidazoquinolines. The discovery that PAMPs stimulate defined PRRs provides a strong impetus to the development of SMAs but many existing SMAs were discovered fortuitously. For example, Levamisole, a DNA vaccine adjuvant, was developed as an antihelminthic; Bestatin, a tumour adjuvant, is an inhibitor of aminopeptidase N [CD13]; and Bupivacaine, another DNA vaccine adjuvant, was originally a local anaesthetic. Imidazoquinolines (e.g. Imiquimod, Resiquimod, 852A, etc.), which target TLR-7 and-8, were developed as nucleoside analogues for antiviral or antitumour therapy. Other examples of nonmacromolecular adjuvants include monophosphoryl-lipid A, muramyl dipeptide, QS21, PLG, Seppic ISA-51 and CpG oligonucleotides. Optimized CpG oligonucleotides, which target TLR-9, are now entering late phase trials as adjuvants for the poorly immunogenic Hepatitis B vaccine. Likewise many proteins have been identified as potential adjuvant molecules. These are amenable to detection by both sequence based approaches and potentially by alignment free techniques. This 'adjuvant hunting' can be likened to reverse vaccinology but with adjuvants rather than antigens as its quarry.

Utilizing the burgeoning wealth of macromolecular structure data for PRRs now available, VS is the perfect starting point for small molecule adjuvant discovery. A viable alternative to HTS, VS is exceptionally efficient in terms of time, resource and labour, replacing months of robotic experiments bedevilled by signal-to-noise issues with weeks of computational analysis complemented by the need for only a small clutch of reliable, hand-crafted assays. Using the VS approach, hundreds of thousands of small molecules can be reduced by one or two orders of magnitude in number via prescreening and the remainder docked against PRR structures yielding a handful of potent, small molecules. These can be put through a cascade of high specificity assays *in vitro* and then active molecules tested for whole system adjuvant properties *in vivo*. In this way, potential lead molecules can be found without recourse to the unwieldy logistics of HTS.

Since we are interested here in small molecules rather than peptides, prescreening comes into its own. Upwards of a million molecules are now available in databases such as ZINC. Attempting to develop some of these molecules can be invariably futile, since many can be excluded for one reason or another at an early stage before docking need be considered. Screens for reactive groups or promiscuous inhibitors are now common. Certain screening hits do not act as drugs should: they are poorly selective, exhibit counterintuitive structure and activity relationships, and act in a noncompetitive manner. Various *in silico* ADMEt screens are also routinely used. Such screens include those for bioavailability, Cytochrome P450 binding (such as 3A4, 2C9 and 2D6) and cytotoxicity. More explicit screens for alternative and inconvenient activities, such as hERG channel inhibiton, $\alpha$1 adrenergic binding leading to orthostatic hypotension effects, 5-HT2 cholingeric activity leading to obesity, M1 muscarinic binding leading to hallucinations and effects on memory competence, as well as D2 dopaminergic and potentially many others besides. Screens for drug- or lead-likeness are now also widely used. Of course, applying too many screens may ultimately leave you with next to no compounds, or at least the same greatly reduced set of molecules for all VS exercises.

Another important component of preprocessing compounds for virtual screening is the preparation of multiple candidate molecular structures for each de facto chemical species. Each depicted entry in a commercial or in-house database will not always correspond to the actual substance screened. The structure may contain one or more stereo centres, and exist as a racemate, necessitating the construction of all stereoisomers. The molecule may exist as a canonical ensemble of tautomers, thus necessitating the explicit construction of all tautomeric forms. Issues of small molecule ionization may require the construction of all so-called protomers. While these require logistically complex operations, at least they can all be addressed directly by relatively straightforward rules. Other important issues, such as inductive effects on H-bond donor and acceptor propensities, are not amenable to simple rules but rather require complex prediction models in order to assign atom types for VS docking programs successfully. Some experts in the field view any attempt to undertake VS with protocols that do not address all of these molecule generation steps as hopelessly naïve. However, many examples of naïve

VS have demonstrated that even a simple-minded approach lacking the sophistication alluded to above can be successful: this is, in itself, a great strength of the technique.

While these issues are linked, it is important to reflect that in spite of present technical short comings, virtual screening is an undoubted and indisputable success. The method works. Even when used in a 'naïve' manner, VS can identify ligands for biological receptors with unrivalled efficiency and cost-effectiveness. Other than technical improvement, what remains is for academic and commercial medical researchers of all flavours to adopt VS with stringent alacrity.

## Molecular dynamics and immunology

Molecular dynamics (or MD) affords a detailed description of atomic motion; it is one of several means of undertaking atomistic simulations of protein molecules. In MD, and at a particular temperature, molecules – as governed by classical mechanics – interact over time; thus MD addresses a dynamic, rather than static, picture of biomolecular systems. In the context of affinity and epitope prediction, MD has the advantage that it is not data-driven, as it attempts the *de novo* prediction of all relevant parameters given knowledge of the system's starting structure, be that an experimental structure or a convincing homology model of a ligand–receptor complex. Unlike other methods, MD can, in principle at least, account for both explicit solvation and the intrinsic flexibility of both receptor and ligand. Other popular approaches to structural simulation include the use of normal mode analysis (or NMA), which obtains the simple harmonic motions of a protein about local energy minima, or Monte Carlo sampling.

Molecular dynamics simulation is able to compute the equilibrium position of a classical multiple-body system where the point-mass atoms of the system are constrained by a potential energy force field. For large molecular systems comprising thousands of atoms, many of the more sophisticated modelling techniques, which often describe the potential energy surface in terms of quantum mechanics, are too demanding of computer resources to be useful. The Born–Oppenheimer approximation states that the Schrödinger equation for a molecule can be separated into a part describing the motions of the electrons and a part describing the motions of the nuclei, and that these two motions can be studied independently. Information within the system is contained primarily within the potential energy function, which takes the form of a simple penalty function for most simulations of biomolecules. Molecules are treated as mechanical assemblies comprising simple elements, such as balls (atoms), rods or sticks (bonds) and flexible joints (bond and torsion angles). Terms that describe the van der Waals, electrostatic, and possibly hydrogen bonding, interactions between atoms supplement molecular mechanics forcefields. There are many such force fields in existence: MM3 for small molecules, and GROMOS, AMBER and CHARMM for proteins being notable and widely used examples. Extant force fields are by no means perfect, and there remains a constant need to improve the way we describe interatomic forces. There are doubtless many hidden effects that they do not currently accommodate, for example salt or pH effects. One way to achieve this is to combine quantum mechanical effects into the molecular mechanics treatment, perhaps simulating a particular region within a simulation using QM yet treating the rest using MD.

## Molecular dynamics methodology

Each of the $N$ atoms simulated are treated as a point mass and Newton's equations of motion are integrated to compute their movement. Thus:

$$m_i \frac{d^2 r_i}{dt^2} = \mathbf{F}_i, \tag{6.1}$$

where $m_i$ is the mass of point $i$, $r_i$ is the Cartesian three-vector of point $i$, the second derivative of $r_i$ the corresponding acceleration, and $\mathbf{F}_i$ is the force vector acting on point $i$. We need to provide the initial configuration of the system at $t = 0$, that is the coordinates of all atoms in a six-dimensional hyperspace. Thus, at regular time intervals, we resolve the classical equation of motion represented by the $N$ equations implicit above. The gradient of the potential energy function is used to calculate the forces on the atoms while the initial velocities on the atoms are generated randomly. At this point, new positions and velocities are computed and the atoms are moved to these new positions.

Several accurate methods for integrating the equations of motion for these very large swarms of points are in common use, and they include the Verlet algorithm, the velocity-Verlet, and the leapfrog algorithm. Errors vary as the square of the time step used to propagate the dynamic motion of the point swarm. The time step chosen should be much less than the fastest simulated events. The vibration of a bond to a hydrogen atom is approximately 10 femtoseconds, and thus 1 fs is used for systems with explicit solvation and 2–5 fs for implicit solvation. For comparison, significant conformational change, such as even the fastest protein folding event, occurs in the microsecond range.

## Molecular dynamics and binding

Atomistic molecular dynamics has long been used to predict the affinity or binding free energy ($\Delta G_{bind}$) of macromolecular-ligand interactions. Historically, the availability of computing resources necessary for obtaining affinities for systems such as peptide–MHC complexes has limited the general deployment of techniques. Nonetheless, it has the benefit that known binding data is not required. All that is needed is a protein structure, either an experimental structure or a reliable homology model, of a macromolecule–ligand complex. In statistical mechanics terms, free energy ($\Delta G$) is defined in terms of the partition function. However, for most calculations such a definition is of limited value. What can be calculated, however, is the free energy difference between two states. Several methods exist which can evaluate this, each predicated on different approximations. The semirigorous prediction of $\Delta G_{bind}$ is approached using either thermodynamic integration (TI) or free-energy perturbation (FEP) calculations. These compute-intensive approaches use the ensemble average of an energy function describing a system, which is itself a function of the coordinates of the particles in configuration space.

Other approaches assume that $\Delta G_{bind}$ can be reduced to a set of contributions, which may be defined so that cross terms are avoided. Energetic contributions are derived from one or a few generic structures rather than ensemble averages. Electrostatic contributions made by water are replaced by a continuum solvent model solved using a linear Poisson–Boltzmann equation. Thus, solvent interaction energies can be calculated using the ligand, receptor and the receptor–ligand complex modelled as regions with a low dielectric constant embedded in a higher dielectric environment. A nonpolar contribution to the desolvation energy is obtained from the accessible surface area lost on complexation. Entropic contributions arise from lost molecular motion and intramolecular flexibility.

MM/GBSA (molecular mechanics/generalized Born surface area) is just such a widely used technique. It combines molecular mechanical interaction energies with solvation terms based on implicit solvation models. Both contributions are averages taken from a sampled MD trajectory, and entropic contributions are calculated using a normal mode analysis of the trajectory. Receptor–ligand complexes with significant structural variation can be studied using this approach. The free energies for the complex, the isolated ligand and the isolated receptor are calculated from an MD trajectory.

Thus, the binding free energy is given by:

$$\Delta G_b = G \, (complex) - G \, (free \; receptor) - G \, (free \; ligand) \qquad (6.2)$$
$$G \, (molecule) = \langle E_{MM} \rangle + \langle G_{sol} \rangle - TS \qquad (6.3)$$

where $\Delta G_b$ is the binding free energy, $E_{MM}$ is the molecular mechanical energy, $G_{sol}$ is the solvation energy and $-TS$ is an entropy contribution. Angled brackets denote averages over an MD trajectory. The molecular mechanics energy $E_{MM}$ is calculated using an empirical force field. When calculating the binding free-energy difference, it may be assumed that the standard entropy change is similar for both models and can therefore be assumed to cancel.

# Immunological applications 1

Delisi and coworkers were among the first to apply molecular dynamics to peptide–MHC binding and they have, subsequently, developed a series of different methods. Part of this work has concentrated on accurate docking using molecular dynamics and part on determining free energies from peptide MHC complexes. Rognan has, over a long period, also made important contributions to this area. In his work, dynamic properties of the solvated protein–peptide complexes, such as atomic fluctuations, solvent accessible surface areas and hydrogen bonding patterns, correlated well with available binding data. He has been able to discriminate between binders that remain tightly anchored to the MHC molecule from non-binders that are significantly weaker. Other work from Rognan and coworkers has concentrated on the design of non-natural ligands for MHC molecules, demonstrating the generality of molecular dynamic approaches to problems of MHC binding.

Other work in this area has come from two directions. First, those interested in using the methodology to analyse and predict features of peptide–MHC complexes. Secondly, those who are more interested in developing novel aspects of MD methodology, including both simulation methodology and solvation, and who use the MHC peptide systems as a convenient example.

# Limitations of molecular dynamics

The limitations of MD are legion: restricted sampling of configuration space or the accuracy of current force fields or MD's dependence on particular simulation protocols, for example. Long simulation runs are needed and current techniques allow for only small differences in ligand structure for reliable predictions of energy. Even the problem of calculating the affinity of the peptide–MHC complex, which is small in biomolecular terms, is nonetheless prohibitively problematic in terms of computing methodologies generally available for its solution.

There are two main routes to addressing the formidable problems associated with MD techniques. One is to introduce approximations. Approximations are of two kinds: simplifying constraints within simulations themselves and more fundamental approximations in the underlying simulation methodology. 'Constrained simulations' take many forms, but typically use constraints and/or restraints to reduce the effective degrees of freedom within the system. This is usually known as 'freezing' atoms, either by dampening their motion or rendering them immobile. Sometimes these constraints and restraints are combined by creating concentric spheres centred on the unrestrained binding site, outside of which there is a zone where atom movements are restrained, and outside of this is a properly frozen zone where atom positions are fixed.

The problem with such strategies is obvious: how does one constrain a system appropriately? If one knows the answer in advance, then one may choose, perhaps by a process of trial and error, suitable constraints and restraints to obtain such an answer. Developing a truly predictive system using *ad hoc* constraints is much more difficult. Unlike other attempts to simulate MHCs, Wan *et al.* have performed long duration unconstrained simulations and demonstrated beyond reasonable doubt that only full, rather than truncated, models can return accurate dynamic and time averaged properties [23].

A related approach is coarse-graining. Here complex entities, such as secondary structures, are reduced in complexity – or coarse-grained – to united residues; or some equivalent simplification – such as the use of dihedral angles rather than atomic positions – is used. This also necessitates the use of another dynamic simulation methodology, such as that built on generalized Lagrange equations of motions. Unlike freezing atoms, the idea is to reduce the complexity without loosing accuracy by finding an alternative representation of the system under study.

As we have said, there is an imbalance between generally-available computing resources and the size of the task to be evaluated. The other main way to breach the barrier imposed by this imbalance is simply to use as large a computer as possible. This necessitates the use of tightly coupled supercomputing to massively increase the computing resources available, as distributed computing of the screensaver type is not applicable to MD problems.

## Molecular dynamics and high performance computing

Increases in computing power seen in the last 25 years have allowed science to study biologically interesting systems, such as small and medium-sized proteins, using atomistic MD, yet previous attempts to use MD to investigate peptide–MHC interactions have foundered on technical limitations. There is a tension between what we want and what we can have. A race exists by which the bigger the computing device we have, the bigger and longer the simulation we wish to run. Since the scale of biology is vastly greater than the largest realizable simulation, it is a race which simulation always loses. Our ambition invariably exceeds all possible achievement. We are at the beginning rather than the end. Many approaches have been tried to circumvent these problems, but only with limited success, since almost any attempt to reach longer timescales will result in more approximations in the model. While many methods link thermodynamic properties to simulations, they take an unrealistically long time. Moreover, there is a need for long simulations to accommodate both the slow and the very fast – protein conformational change and enzymatic transition states – motions seen in biological simulations.

A basic simulation yielding a free energy of binding requires something like 10 nanoseconds of simulation. On the average desktop machine, this requires a compute time per nanosecond in the region of hundreds of hours of real time. Simulating only a few, but flexible peptides might occupy a machine for years. To circumvent this we take advantage of high-performance, massively parallel implementations of molecular dynamic (MD) codes running on large supercomputers with 512 or 1024 nodes. Alternatively, use can be made of so-called 'Grid computing'. This refers to an ambitious, exciting, if as-yet-unrealized global endeavour to create an environment in which users can access computing power simply and transparently, irrespective of where those facilities are to be found.

To this end, Wan and coworkers have used high-performance computing deployed via the nascent GRID to power more realistic simulations of a series of system of ascending scale. Initially, they applied supercomputing to simulate the peptide–MHC complex using an implementation of the AMBER force field within the highly-parallelized MD code LAMMPS.

The accuracy and speed of an MD simulation needs to match the challenge of the application. We can use coarse-graining to simulate the overall behaviour of very large dynamic systems but we must use detailed unconstrained atomistic simulations in order to obtain highly accurate *ab initio* affinities. In future applications we need to tackle both kinds of problem. Prediction for relatively simple systems should approach the accuracy and veracity of experiment and then exceed it. Likewise, simulating the properties and behaviour of very large and complex systems should allow us, through computational simulation, to observe the unobservable and to measure that which experiment cannot measure.

The work of Wan and coworkers typifies efforts in this area. They have escalated simulations from an isolated MHC molecule, through a TCR-pMHC complex, to a recognition complex including CD4 embedded in opposing membranes. This last simulation is the first stage in simulating a full immune synapse. The work of Wan *et al.* chimes with other cutting edge simulations of very large systems. Such simulations will be vital to the successful structural characterization of cellular pathways and networks. Advances in experimental imaging and labelling are now allowing data to be produced that allows for simulation on the scale of subcellular organelles rather than single proteins [24].

For example, the ribosome, the work-horse of protein biosynthesis, has been studied using MD; here the atom count is approximately 2.64 million [25]. Others have evaluated a synaptic vesicle as a model. Using specially derived measurements of protein and lipid composition, and vesicle size, density and mass, a full structural model was constructed and simulated using MD [26]. In another study, photosynthetic units from *Rhodobacter sphaeroides,* which form inner membrane invaginations comprising light-harvesting complexes, LH1 and LH2, and reaction centres, were simulated. There were two models consisting of nine or 18 dimeric RC–LH1 complexes and 144 or 101 LH2 complexes, representing a total of 3879 or 4464 bacteriochlorophylls, respectively [27].

Eventually, as more sophisticated methods evolve and develop, and MD becomes a widely and habitually used tool, we will, in concert with richer and improved measured data, develop ever more accurate and predictive models. MD will escape from limitations imposed by data through its ability to offer us the chance of true *de novo* prediction of binding affinities and many other thermodynamic properties.

# References

1. Lawlor, D. A., Warren, E., Taylor, P., Parham, P. (1991) Gorilla class I major histocompatability complex alleles: comparison to human and chimpanzee class I. *J. Exp. Med.*, **174**, 1491.
2. McKenzie, L.M., Pecon-Slattery, J., Carrington, M. and O'Brien, S.J. (1999) Taxonomic hierarchy of HLA class I allele sequences. *Genes Immun.*, **1**, 120.

3. Cano, P., Fan, B. and Stass, S. (1998) A geometric study of the amino acid sequence of class I HLA molecules. *Immunogenetics*, **48**, 324.

4. Sette, A. and Sidney, J. (1999) Nine major HLA class I supertypes account for the vast preponderaqnce of HLA-A and –B polymorphism. *Immunogenetics*, **50**, 201.

5. Lund, O., Nielsen, M., Kesmir, C., Petersen, A.G., Lundegaard, C., Worning, P., Sylvester-Hvid, C., Lamberth, K., Roder, G., Justesen, S., Buus, S. and Brunak, S. (2004) Definition of supertypes for HLA molecules using clustering of specificity matrices. *Immunogenetics*, **55**, 797.

6. Zhang, C., Anderson, A. and DeLisi, C. (1998) Structural principles that govern the peptide-binding motifs of class I MHC molecules. *J. Mol. Biol.*, **281**, 929.

7. Baas, A., Gao, X. and Chelvanayagam, G. (1999) Peptide binding motifs and specificities for HLA-DQ molecules. *Immunogenetics*, **50**, 8.

8. Reche, P.A. and Reinherz, E.L. (2003) Sequence variability analysis of human class I and class II MHC molecules: functional and structural correlates of amino acid polymorphisms. *J. Mol. Biol.*, **331**, 623.

9. Doytchinova, I.A., Guan, P. and Flower, D. R. (2004) Identifying human MHC supertypes using bioinformatic methods. *J. Immunol.*, **172**, 4314.

10. Doytchinova, I. A. and Flower, D. R. (2005) *In silico* identification of supertypes for class II MHCs. *J Immunol.*, **174**, 7085–7095.

11. Sidney, J., Peters, B., Frahm, N., Brander, C. and Sette, A. (2008) HLA class I supertypes: a revised and updated classification. *BMC Immunol.*, **9**, 1.

12. Doytchinova, I. A., Guan, P. and Flower, D.R. (2004) Quantitative structure-activity relationships and the prediction of MHC supermotifs. *Methods*, **34**, 444–453.

13. Van Regenmortel, M. H. (2006) Immunoinformatics may lead to a reappraisal of the nature of B-cell epitopes and of the feasibility of synthetic peptide vaccines. *J. Mol. Recognit.*, **19**, 183–187.

14. Thornton, J. M., Edwards, M. S., Taylor, W. R. and Barlow, D. J. (1986) Location of 'continuous' antigenic determinants in the protruding regions of proteins. *EMBOJ*, **5**, 409–413.

15. Novotný, J., Handschumacher, M., Haber, E., Bruccoleri, R. E., Carlson, W. B., Fanning, D. W., Smith, J. A. and Rose, G. D. (1986) Antigenic determinants in proteins coincide with surface regions accessible to large probes (antibody domains). *Proc. Natl Acad. Sci. USA*, **83**, 226–230.

16. Kulkarni-Kale, U., Bhosle, S. and Kolaskar, A.S. (2005) CEP: a conformational epitope prediction server. *Nucleic Acids Res.*, **33** (Web Server issue), W168–171.

17. Haste Andersen, P., Nielsen, M. and Lund, O. (2006) Prediction of residues in discontinuous B-cell epitopes using protein 3D structures. *Protein Sci.*, **15**, 2558–2567.

18. Ponomarenko, J. V. and Bourne, P. E. (2007) Antibody-protein interactions: benchmark datasets and prediction tools evaluation. *BMC Struct Biol.*, **7**, 64.

19. Jones, G., Willett, P., Glen, R. C., Leach, A. R. and Taylor, R. (1997) Development and validation of a genetic algorithm for flexible docking. *J. Mol. Biol.*, **267**, 727–748.

20. Moustakas, D. T., Lang, P. T., Pegg, S., Pettersen, E., Kuntz, I. D., Brooijmans, N. and Rizzo, R. C. (2006) Development and validation of a modular, extensible docking program: DOCK 5. *J. Comput. Aided Mol. Des.*, **20**, 601–619.

21. Rognan, D., Lauemoller, S. L., Holm, A., Buus, S. and Tschinke, V. (1999) Predicting binding affinities of protein ligands from three-dimensional models: application

to peptide binding to class I major histocompatibility proteins. *J. Med. Chem.*, **42**, 4650–4658.

22. Davies, M. N., Hattotuwagama, C. K., Moss, D. S., Drew, M. G. and Flower, D.R. (2006) Statistical deconvolution of enthalpic energetic contributions to MHC-peptide binding affinity. *BMC Struct. Biol.*, **6**, 5.

23. Wan, S., Coveney, P. and Flower, D. R. (2004) Large-scale molecular dynamics simulations of HLA-A*0201 complexed with a tumor-specific antigenic peptide: can the alpha3 and beta2m domains be neglected? *J. Comput. Chem.*, **25**, 1803–1813.

24. Wan, S., Flower, D. R. and Coveney, P. V. (2008) Toward an atomistic understanding of the immune synapse: Large-scale molecular dynamics simulation of a membrane-embedded TCR-pMHC-CD4 complex. *Mol. Immunol.*, **45**, 1221–1230.

25. Sanbonmatsu, K. Y. and Tung, C. S. (2007) High performance computing in biology: multimillion atom simulations of nanoscale systems. *J. Struct. Biol.*, **157**, 470–480.

26. Takamori, S., Holt, M., Stenius, K., Lemke, E. A., Grønborg, M., Riedel, D., Urlaub, H., Schenck, S., Brügger, B., Ringler, P., Müller, S. A., Rammner, B., Gräter, F., Hub, J. S., De Groot, B. L., Mieskes, G., Moriyama, Y., Klingauf, J., Grubmüller, H., Heuser, J., Wieland, F. and Jahn, R. (2006) Molecular anatomy of a trafficking organelle. *Cell*, **127**, 831–846.

27. Sener, M. K., Olsen, J. D., Hunter, C. N. and Schulten, K. (2007) Atomic-level structural and functional model of a bacterial photosynthetic membrane vesicle. *Proc. Natl Acad. Sci. USA*, **104**, 15723–15728.

# 7
# Vaccines:
# Computational solutions

*Among these things, one thing seems certain - that nothing certain exists*
*and that there is nothing more pitiful or more presumptuous than man.*

—Pliny the Elder

## Vaccines and the world

The global population continues to rise. Average global prosperity is also rising yet millions still hover at the edge of extinction. As a result the world faces problems as never before: disease and the economic and societal complexity of health provision; famine and hunger at one extreme, obesity and wanton overindulgence at the other; pollution, global warming and the struggle for scarce natural resources and potable water. 97% of our water is locked into the world's oceans. 2% is frozen in glaciers. The remaining 1% is, figuratively at least, in our hands. The world depends on mineral oil: it runs our cars and planes and trains; it is the feed stock of the chemical industry and thus of plastics and pharmaceuticals. The economy depends on it and we fight wars over it. Yet now we face the imminence of 'peak oil', after which current supplies will dwindle in the face of growing demand, fuelled in part by the burgeoning economies of India and China. They place pressure on global oil delivery systems already labouring under the West's insatiable appetite for oil; thus extant stocks will fail. New reserves exist but it is highly likely that they will prove vastly less tractable than those we are currently exploiting.

Each of these is a robust challenge which the world must face now or in the near future. They cannot be ignored, as once they were by both governments and

*Bioinformatics for Vaccinology*   Darren R Flower
© 2008 John Wiley & Sons, Ltd

individuals. They cannot be gainsaid, even though people deny the imperative need to address them. With an average worldwide temperature rise of, say, 2–4 K anticipated by 2100, all manner of climatic changes can be expected in the next 100 years. Such a change could well be very rapid, geologically speaking – rapid and disruptive. The great thaw that followed the last ice age was slow by comparison. In his government-sponsored report, Sir Nicholas Sterne suggested that spending around 1% of annual global GDP would stabilize the emission of carbon dioxide. He further suggested that the cost of taking no action would ultimately result in a reduction in the gross world product (GWP) of between 5% and 20%. The GWP, the rather nominal global equivalent to the national GDP or gross domestic product was, for 2005, estimated to be approximately $60.63 trillion. This equates to an economic output of $9500 per head for every man, woman and child on the planet. During 2005, global output rose by 4.4%; this was led by the tiger economies of China (9.3%) and India (7.6%), followed by a resurgent, natural resource-rich Russia (5.9%). 2005 growth rates in the major industrialized countries of the First World varied from zero for Italy to 3.5% for the United States.

Many, including former sceptics, now accept that emissions of so-called greenhouse gases generated through human activity have contributed significantly to the observed temperature rise of 0.7 K seen during the twentieth century. It is perhaps ironic that it takes an economic report for politicians and the public at large to take notice. Professional ecologists, natural historians, environmental lobbyists, and green politicians have been warning of this since at least the days of Rachel Carson's 1962 book *Silent Spring*. Whatever the view of Lomborg and other environmental sceptics, the net effect of human activity since 1750 has been to warm the planet. There is now unambiguous and unequivocal evidence that the burning of fossil fuel, slash and burn agriculture, destruction of tropical rain forests and other large-scale deforestation, industrial pollution and changes in land use, such as escalating urbanization, is affecting, and affecting significantly, the climate of the earth. If the rate of this rise cannot be significantly slowed and ultimately reversed, alterations to the climate will eventually spiral out of control. Global warming and climate change will be exacerbated by other factors, many still unseen, such as the release of the potent greenhouse gas methane from thawing permafrost.

Change to the climate will continue for hundreds of years, and sea levels for thousands. Hurricanes and typhoons, droughts and famines, will combine with disease to endanger lives across the world. It is unlikely that any government, elected or unelected, will even contemplate reversing industrialization or abolishing economic growth. Any who try would need to impose the most draconian measures and prosecute the most condign resolve in order so to do. The best that government and society can manage is to forestall the spiralling climatic chaos of the next few hundred years in the hope that technology can find a lasting solution. Carbon capture and storage, whether chemical (sequestrating carbon dioxide from the air and then storing it deep underground) or biological (breeding plants to store carbon dioxide as wood) in nature, is possible, but does not impact the hundreds of environmental issues which the world faces in the days to come.

While science is not solely and directly responsible for any of these problems, it nonetheless holds the key to understanding the consequent dilemmas we face; to reversing these trends; to solving these problems; to meeting these challenges; to forestalling these disasters. But what is the link to vaccinology? Vaccinology is vital to the future stability of the global population. Through systematic mass vaccination, disease can be forestalled: vaccines are probably the most cost-effective form of prophylaxis yet conceived. By reducing the burden of disease within the developing world, we prevent unnecessary and predictable death from taking away our children, altering the psychology of living and allowing each parent to invest more in each child. Taken together with the wide availability of contraception, this will in turn lead to a reduced birth rate. Vaccines and their effects on mortality and morbidity allow hoped-for improvements in education, health care, and prosperity to stabilize the population both socially and economically, as has been seen in the developed world over the last few centuries. Only such a population, freed from the pernicious vicissitudes of the struggle of life can effectively combat climate change, the consequences of 'peak oil', and all the other vexatious exigencies that we are currently storing up for our children and our children's children.

## Bioinformatics and the challenge for vaccinology

Viewed from the wider standpoint of society, the science of immunology, and to a lesser extent vaccinology, is rightly seen as an important – even a pre-eminent – discipline. Also rightly, perhaps, many immunologists see their discipline as a science apart. Immunology is intimately connected with disease: infectious, most obviously, but also autoimmune disease, inherited and multifactorial genetic disease, cancer and allergy. Nonetheless, and notwithstanding this prestige, immunology finds itself at a tipping point in its history; it is poised to make itself anew – reborn as a quantitative science based upon genomic information. Yet can immunology capitalize on the explosion of postgenomic information and the concomitant paradigm shift from hypothesis-driven to data-driven research? It will do so, no doubt, but only when it fully embraces computational science. In a gentle way, this book has been tantamount to a polemic: an argument in favour of a complementary computational approach to some of the difficult or time consuming or financially wasteful aspects of immunological science and vaccinology.

Much of immunoinformatics is ostensibly the application of standard bioinformatic techniques, such as microarray analysis or comparative genomics, to immunology. Core bioinformatics makes a series of synergistic interactions with both a set of client disciplines (computer science, structural chemistry, etc.) and with customer disciplines, such as genomics, molecular biology and cell biology. Bioinformatics is concerned with activities such as the annotation of biological data (genome sequences for example), classification of sequences and structures into meaningful groups, and so on. It seeks to solve two main challenges: the prediction of function from sequence and the prediction of structure from sequence. The key role of bioinformatics is, then, to transform large, if not vast, reservoirs of information into useful – and usable – information.

## Predicting immunogenicity

There are several bioinformatics problems unique to immunology: first and fore-most, the accurate prediction of immunogenicity. This can manifest itself through the identification of epitopes or the prediction of whole protein antigenicity. This endeavour can be fairly described as both the high frontier of immunoinformatic investigation and a grand scientific challenge – it is difficult, yet exciting, and as a pivotal tool in the drive to develop improved vaccines it is also of true utilitarian value.

In my view, the immunogenicity of a protein, as opposed to an epitope, arises from a combination of factors. These include host-side properties – such as the possession of B or T cell epitopes – and pathogen-side properties – such as the expression level of the protein and its subcellular location – as well as its state of aggregation and any post-translational danger signals it may possess (Figure 7.1). One might expect a candidate vaccine to be highly expressed and available for im-mune surveillance as well as possessing epitopes that the host can recognize. Iden-tifying and predicting this diverse set of properties is a challenge. Likewise, a T cell epitope needs to be processed properly, and in reasonable quantities, and then be bound by an MHC with reasonable affinity, before being recognized appropri-ately by a TCR. Both processes can be resolved into component parts which are amendable to statistical evaluation. Thus both can be predicted.

A lucid distinction between data and understanding in science has thus long been clear. 'In science there is only physics; all the rest is stamp collecting.' This is a particular rendering of a famous, yet scornful, quotation from Lord Rutherford

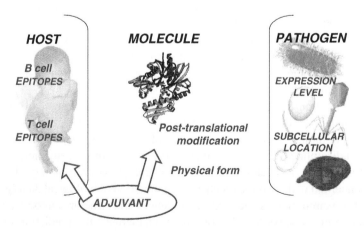

**Figure 7.1** Contributions to antigen-mediated immunogenicity

(1871–1937). It is also probably misquoted: other versions include 'All science is either physics or stamp collecting.' The source of this *bon mot* is apparently a book of reminiscences by J. B. Birks entitled *Rutherford at Manchester*, published in 1962. Rutherford left Manchester aged only 24, implying he formulated this viewpoint early in his career. Much of science is now focused on data and what to do with it. In the high-throughput era – be that astronomical, metrological or postgenomic – data generation is certainly no longer the bottleneck it once was. Instead it is our ability usefully to interpret data, and particularly data *en masse*, that limits us.

## Computational vaccinology

The importance and potential of computational vaccinology is often not properly appreciated. Here, we shall redress this imbalance and also break down the artificial compartmentalization that has arisen within computational disciplines: the divide, for example, between academia and industry, life science and materials modelling, and between cheminformatics and bioinformatics. The areas of application for informatics form a continuum stretching from solid-state physics to molecular biology and beyond. There is so much to learn from each discipline and so much of value to add to experimental science.

When one works in a Cinderella field – and immunoinformatics most certainly is one – then it can be difficult for an outsider properly to assess the relative merits of computational vaccine design compared to more mainstream experimental studies, however transitory and uninformative such experiments may prove. The potential of immunoinformatics, albeit largely unrealized, is huge, but only if people are willing to take up the technology and use it appropriately. People's expectations of computational work are largely unrealistic and highly tendentious. Some expect perfection, and are soon disappointed, rapidly becoming vehement critics. Others are highly critical from the start and are nearly impossible to reconcile with informatic methods. Neither view stands as a correct exegesis, however. Informatic methods do not replace, or even seek to replace, experimental work, they only help rationalize experiments, saving time and effort. They are slaves to the data used to generate them. They require a degree of intellectual effort equivalent in scale, yet different in kind, to that of the experimentalist. The two disciplines – experimental and informatic – are thus complementary, albeit distinct. Ultimately, as system biology takes hold and insinuates itself into every corner of biology, informatics will find its place, though that may yet take time.

Immunoinformatics-driven *in silico* vaccinology can effectively leverage informatics techniques to deliver effective and utilitarian advantage in the search for new vaccines. Immunoinformatics-driven *in silico* vaccinology works through a dynamic and responsive cyclical process of using and refining both models and experiments, at each stage moving closer towards the goal of the effective, cost-efficient development of vaccines or vaccine components. The allied subjects of bioinformatics and computational chemistry have, within the pharmaceutical industry and the wider scientific community, proved their worth time and time again in the search for new drugs and new drug targets. The time is approaching when immunoinformatics and allied disciplines will do the same for vaccine design.

## The threat remains

As we have seen, vaccines are – at least in comparison to other prophylactic treatments – remarkably effective in combating the threat from infectious diseases. There are now in the order of 30 infectious diseases which are effectively targeted by vaccines. Many of the remaining infectious agents, for which there are no effective vaccines, are difficult to manipulate or give rise to persisting infections, such as hepatitis C. Others, such as influenza, show great antigenic variation. While still others, such as most parasitic infections, are very complex organisms, with equally complex life cycles, that are genetically closer in structure and metabolism to vertebrate hosts and are, for all these reasons and more, much more challenging where the discovery and design of vaccines are concerned. Still other diseases, such as AIDS, are mediated by pathogens of great structural simplicity prone to rapid, immense and clearly confounding, genetic variation.

The need, then, for new antimicrobial treatments, both therapeutic and prophylactic, is obvious. Antibiotic drugs are one approach to realizing such treatments. Vaccines are another. Most successful vaccination strategies have used inactivated or attenuated microbes or substances derived directly from them. Modern, semisynthetic vaccines are composed, wholly or in part, of chemically synthesized or recombinant peptides, carbohydrates or protein antigens.

Most extant vaccines have arisen in an empirically fashion. However, interest is now turning to more rationally designed vaccines. At one extreme of the size range, these can be genetically modified pathogens and at the other protein antigens or isolated T cell epitopes. Here the modern vaccinologist can make use of genomic data information from the many genomic sequencing projects focusing on pathogenic micro-organisms. Thus, the application of computational sciences to vaccine research is a discipline whose time has come. A tranche of techniques, both old and new, have recently matured into potent weapons in the war against disease. Molecular informatics – computational chemistry or molecular modelling, bioinformatics and cheminformatics – has reached new heights of sophistication and utilitarian value within drug and vaccine discovery.

## Beyond empirical vaccinology

Let us rehearse some of what we know about vaccinology. Existing vaccines fall into two broad categories: living vaccines and nonliving vaccines. Living vaccines use attenuated forms of pathogens to mimic natural infections without the dangers of the natural infection and thereby induce immunity to the natural pathogen. In seeking to induce protective immunity, nonliving vaccines use either a chemically-inactivated whole microbial pathogen or they use components of such microbes in the form of subunit vaccines. Recently, antigen-based subunit vaccines have gained significantly in popularity and use. The identification of antigenic or immunogenic proteins as putative whole protein subunit vaccines is a key goal of immunovaccinology. It offers the hope of eliciting significant responses from both humoral and cellular immune systems, far exceeding the efficacy of peptide vaccines, while avoiding potential toxicity problems associated with whole microbe vaccines.

Traditional vaccine development of human vaccines combines an eclectic range of immunological, biochemical and microbiological methods. Over the last 150 years of vaccinology, much success has been obtained using these conventional approaches. Despite this success, it is increasingly clear that these techniques are themselves flawed. New techniques are necessary to address the whole gamut of potentially threatening pathogens. Yet 40% of human disease remains incurable and many existing therapies are far from ideal. The nature of illness has, at least in the West, changed out of all recognition over the last century, and can be expected to do so again over the next 100 years. Thus the challenge to immunology and modern medicine has never been greater, but neither has the technology available to meet this challenge. The postgenomic science will deliver an unprecedented explosion of information. Only informatic strategies can manage and fully exploit this data overload.

## Designing new vaccines

It is possible to draw up a list of requirements one would wish any new vaccine to possess. Indeed many have done so. I was presented with such a list when I first entered the vaccine field; it was drawn up by my then boss Professor Peter Beverley. It read something like this. The ideal vaccine should confer lifelong protection. It should be broadly protective against all variants of an organism. It should prevent or inhibit disease transmission. It should bring about effective immunity quickly. It should be effective in subjects, irrespective of age, thus being equally effective in infants and the elderly. It should transmit maternal protection. It should need only one immunization. It should not require injection. Above all, it should be cheap, safe and stable. Some of these criteria can, at least in part, be addressed through the realization of the ideas presented above. Some can be addressed empirically, others rationally and intelligently, others not at all.

How can informatics help to design new and improved vaccines? It depends on what kind of vaccine you need. Let us restrict ourselves to the three main conceptual types of vaccine: attenuated micro-organisms, subunit vaccines and vaccines based on epitopes. One should be able to use computational tools to contribute to the design of attenuated vaccines. Potentially, it is possible to alter an organism to either gain immunogenicity or to lose virulence and thus generate an attenuated or at least a non-lethal vaccine moiety. However, they must be adequately attenuated in their growth to minimize the possibility of vaccine-induced pathogenic effects while retaining their immunogenicity. Attenuation of live viruses has traditionally been achieved using the serial passage of viruses through tissue or cell culture. For reasons not wholly understood, these processes tend to reduce microbial replicative ability and their apparent virulence in humans or in animal models. Such attenuation has historically been a highly empirical process, where underlying mechanisms are often not wholly known nor properly elucidated. Designed genetic changes to a bacterium, a virus or other microbe can reduce the rate and efficiency of its ability to replicate, reducing the speed at which it grows. This could allow the host the time necessary to clear the infection while at the same time acquiring immunity to it and its genetic brethren. During the last decade the emergence of reverse genetics techniques has created unprecedented opportunities to better control viral attenuation. Genetics manipulation allows for the production of RNA viruses from cloned cDNA, permitting site-specific mutations to be introduced easily into viruses. The challenge is now to engineer attenuated viruses. A step change is needed from creating variants to predicting how genetic changes affect the measurable growth rates of viruses.

It should also be possible to reduce the number of virulence factors in the microbial genome or to mutate it so that certain virulence factors, and any associated immunogenicity, remain yet at the same time removing from these molecules their ability to harm the host. This requires us to distinguish virulence factors (proteins or other biomolecules which attack or facilitate attack upon the host) from other microbial proteins. Likewise we can take a benign micro-organism and add to it highly antigenic proteins producing a microbe with the immunogenicity of another microbe but without its arsenal of virulence factors. This is, in its essentials, much the same idea as generating a viral or microbial vector for the delivery of subunit vaccines.

## The perfect vaccine

If we turn our attention to synthetic vaccines based on antigens or epitopes then we see distinct ways in which immunoinformatics can aid the search for new vaccine moieties. A generally useful – sometimes called a 'perfect' – vaccine may contain one or more T cell epitopes, one or more B cell epitopes, plus nonproteinacous 'danger signals', such as carbohydrate or lipid. Such a perfect vaccine may be an artificial polyepitope vaccine or a natural antigen, delivered as protein or peptide, via live viral or bacterial vectors, or as raw DNA. Such a vaccine would also probably be accompanied by the administration of an adjuvant, a molecule or preparation that exacerbates immune responses.

Conventional experimental discovery of subunit vaccines cultivates pathogens under laboratory conditions and then attempts to partition them into a set of component proteins. Antigens which confer protective immunity are then identified by testing individual components or screening expression libraries against patients' antibodies. Undertaken systematical this process is intrinsically inefficient, involving an exhaustive, brute-force search of potentially thousands of putative targets. Unlike this traditional process of antigen discovery, reverse vaccinology targets the whole potential spectrum of potential antigens irrespective of their abundance, analysing the entire genome of a pathogen in order to identify all potentially antigenic proteins accessible to surveillance by the immune system. This technology allows vaccine discovery scientists to obtain candidate vaccines including those antigens which might be missed because a particular pathogen cannot be successfully cultured in the laboratory or because such antigenic proteins may be absent, or at least apparently so, in *in vitro* culture.

## Conventional approaches

Conventional, experiment-only approaches to candidate subunit vaccine selection are replete with problems. First, it may not be possible to cultivate a particular pathogen in the laboratory. Pathogens must be capable of being cultured in a laboratory in conditions which are often very different to those offered by their natural hosts. Culture methods are time-consuming and development times can run into decades. Only the most abundant antigens (which can be purified in the quantities required for vaccine development) are identified. Often, abundant antigens do not make viable vaccine candidates. For example, there will be many, many proteins that are only transiently expressed during infection or are not necessarily expressed at all *in vitro*. This can mean that interesting candidate antigens are overlooked. The characterization of antigens will also require them to be produced on a large scale. Taken together, this makes the overall process extremely consuming of time, person-power and financial resources.

Such an experimentally based approach proceeds as follows: first, a pathogen is cultured under laboratory conditions; secondly, the pathogen is then dissected into its component parts. Putative protective antigens are then identified by testing the immanent immunogenicity of each component using a complex cascade of *in vitro* assays and *in vivo* experiments which target so-called correlates of protection. Cloning the gene coding for the antigen is often necessary to better characterize and produce the identified antigens. Finally, after this process is complete, the candidate vaccine can enter development. It is an imperfect process. It has often failed to find suitable candidates for pathogens without obvious immunodominant protective antigens and it has failed to deal effectively with noncultivable micro-organisms.

One of the key drivers for the development and deployment of immunoinformatics and computational vaccinology is the widespread availability of pathogen genomes and, to a lesser extent, of microbial genomes generally. In the quest to sequence genomes, massive efforts and resources have been deployed, are being deployed, and will continue to be deployed for the foreseeable future. This is especially true for bacteria and other microbes. Many, many human pathogens now have full sequences available, including many important pathogenic bacteria and viruses, together with a smaller number of key protozoan parasites. Genome sequencing has been one of the great success stories of modern science: in the last decade or so we have gone from a complete dearth of information to the current climate where we have more genome data than we can comfortably deal with. In the short to medium term, the situation will only get worse.

## Genome sequences

The genomic sequencing of TB reported in 1998 or the sequencing of the plague bacteria *Yersinia Pestis* in 2001 did not readily disgorge the secrets implicit within either genome; likewise for an ever increasing number of other pathogens. Malaria, influenza and HIV: all are loathe to reveal their secrets. Genome sequencing is not an end in itself, but merely a step on a longer journey whose destination is the development of vaccines.

In this regard, the view taken is a simple one. To a first approximation, the genome of a pathogenic bacterium contains within it all the information necessary for the pathogen to survive, to live and to thrive and for it thus to infect, disable and destroy. Since the genome contains all this information, it should be possible to decipher this code for destruction, thus identifying the bacterium's weaknesses and vulnerabilities, and allowing us to disable it in our turn. However, as with many things, the initial sequencing of pathogen genomes proved disappointing. Initial optimism hoped that the nature of virulence and infectivity would be readily apparent from analysis of microbial genomes. Such was not the case. A case in point was the comparative analysis of the TB and BCG genomes. The expectation, voiced or unvoiced, was simple. The differences would at best identify one or several bacterial antigens present in TB that were absent in BCG, and at worst identify a larger host of proteins where significant mutations had weakened virulent TB into attenuated BCG. It was, and continues to be, a disappointment to many that no obvious differences clearly above the mutational noise were apparent. Instead, a spectrum of mutations spread through the genome seems to be causative: reducing enzyme reaction enhancements, altering genetic regulation, as well as even more subtle alterations, all combining to reduce virulence and reproductive capacities of the organism and increase its visibility to the immune system.

## Size of a genome

Immunoinformatics has at its disposal an array of potential weapons – genome analysis, epitope prediction, antigen identification, and so on – that can be deployed

adroitly in the fight against a particular microbial disease. Each variety of microbe –
bacteria, viruses, protozoa or fungi – offers a different challenge.

Of particular interest in this regard is the nature of the genome: its size and complexity. Different types of microbe offer genomes with different characteristics and
sizes. Bacterial species have genomes in the range of say 2000 to 5000 gene products, viruses have genomes comprising anywhere between five and 1000 protein
encoding genes, while protozoa can have over 10 000 genes. Such figures are, at
best, rough-and-ready ballpark figures and will, no doubt, be both outdated and
outmoded by the time this book finally reaches the shelves. They give our challenge a scale. We can, and we will, be more specific in a moment, but it is worth
remembering these numbers as, in totality, they clearly demonstrate that the problem of making predictions is in the confounding and discombobulating complexity
invested in the many components of the genome and not in its overall size, which is
well within the scope of modern computing.

One of the smallest, if not the smallest, bacterial genomes yet discovered is that
of the marine bacterium *Pelagibacter ubique*. *Pelagibacter ubique* has only 1354
genes and is largely free of genetic clutter: it contains little or no duplication of
genes, few pseudogenes, no so-called junk DNA and also no genes of viral origin.
It is very much a bacterial species figuratively pared to the bone – a bacterium
slimmed to its bare essentials. There are smaller bacterial genomes, but most of
these are obligate symbionts which outsource much of their metabolism to their
host organisms; examples of such symbionts include *Mycoplasma genitalium* which
has, give or take, just 400 genes. *Pelagibacter ubique* is, by contrast, a free-living
organism with a full complement of metabolic pathways.

At the other extreme, the largest bacterial genomes to be properly sequenced include those of *Burkholderia xenovorans LB400* and *Rhodococcus sp. RHA1*, which
is about 9.70 Mb in size. RHA1 was first isolated from contaminated soil and is
famed for its ability to degrade polychlorinated biphenyls (or PCBs) and an extraordinarily wide range of other persistent toxic pollutants and organic compounds, to
grow effectively on bewilderingly numerous substrates, and to even desulpherize
coal. RHA1's DNA is packaged into a linear chromosome and three linear plasmids
and codes for about 9200 genes. The genome is unsurprisingly rich in oxygenases,
ligases and other metabolic enzymes, such as nonribosomal peptide and polyketide
synthases. However, the RHA1 genome contains, when compared to most other
bacterial species, few recent gene duplications and few genes acquired by horizontal
transfer, especially when contrasted with LB400 which is much more conventional.
However, bacteria with even larger genomes still await sequencing. The myxobac-
terium *Sorangium cellulosum* has an extraordinarily large bacterial genome of over
13 Mb. This is twice the size of, say, *Pseudomonas aeruginosa*, which has in the
region of 6 Mb and about 5500 genes. In comparison, *E. coli* has approximately 4.6
Mb and approximately 4200 genes.

Viruses, like bacteria, span a wide range of genomic sizes. At one extreme is
the apparent simplicity of a retrovirus – HIV has five protein encoding genes for
example – while at the other are the pox viruses. Canarypox, for example, has a

genome of 0.35Mb, and codes for 328 proteins, while fowlpox (0.28Mb) encodes 261 genes; many of these have been acquired laterally from eukaryotic hosts. However, pox viruses pale by comparison to what is the current largest known virus: Mimivirus. This megavirus or girus, discovered in a Yorkshire water-cooling tower, infects amoebas and, some have argued, possibly humans as well. The genome of Mimivirus is about 1.18Mb in size and codes for over 900 proteins. While it possesses the coat characteristic of a virus, Mimivirus is about 600 nm across, making it larger than many bacteria. Again, sequencing of the genome has posed more questions than it has answered. In many ways it seems to transgress the sharp distinction between viruses and cellular life. Viruses, in any case, present many conceptual difficulties to the biologist trained on higher life: speciation is particularly problematic as is the question 'are viruses even alive'? We conceive of viruses as parasitic and depending totally upon the subcellular machinery of invaded cells. Mimivirus, however, must carry out many synthetic and metabolic functions itself, suggesting that it is much closer to other microbial life, such as bacteria.

## Reverse vaccinology

Increasingly, reverse vaccinology is seen as a standard way of discovering vaccines. It is a postgenomic discipline leveraging computational sequence searching techniques to identify systematically all potential vaccine candidates within sequenced pathogen genomes or proteomes. Initially, it was seen as a way to escape from the major bottlenecks and limitations of experimental vaccine discovery, and increasingly as a means of conceptualizing the genomic identification of vaccine candidates as a wholly *in silico* process: given whole or part pathogen genomes, reverse vaccinology uses data mining to identify and characterize surface or secreted target proteins. Taken to its logical extreme, reverse vaccinology may allow the development of safe and efficacious future vaccines against as-yet-unknown infectious disease on a timescale of undreamed-of celerity.

Reverse vaccinology starts with the genome of a pathogen rather than the pathogen itself, and works *in silico* as much as it does *in vitro* or *in vivo*. Given raw genomic sequences, there are a multitude of computational systems that predict open reading frames (or ORFs). Using reverse vaccinology, these ORFs (numbering anywhere from a hundred to several thousand) will quickly be reduced to a list of candidate vaccines of manageable size, perhaps numbering no more than a few dozen.

Reverse vaccinology is, however, not a computation-only discipline, but rather a potent combination of genomic, proteomic and transcriptomic approaches, closely coupled to bioinformatic analysis. The pruned list of target vaccines generated through bioinformatics analysis requires subsequent channelling through an extensive tranche of downstream processes including recombinant expression and purification, as well as testing for immunogenicity and, ultimately, protective efficacy.

*In silico* methods often identify as much as 25% of a genome as vaccine candidates, thus requiring methods able to clone and express large numbers of gene products. Approaches include high-throughput methods utilizing robotics and the polymerase chain reaction (PCR). PCR products are cloned and screened for expression. The purified recombinant proteins need testing for immunogenicity, which is typically performed *in vivo* using vaccination of mice, though other animal models including both small (rats, guinea pigs, etc.) and large (dogs, primates, cows, etc.) mammals have been used. Correlates of protection appropriate to the disease organism in question are screened. Such correlates include antibody titres. The question posed is this: after immunization does the serum of vaccinated animals contain antibodies generated by the vaccine and do these antibodies recognize both the recombinant and original protein? For an animal model to be effective, protection should be mediated by similar mechanisms to those observed in humans. The lack of reliable animal models has often stymied vaccine and drug development. *In vitro* assays, such as bactericidal activity and opsonophagocytosis, also correlate with human vaccine efficacy.

Clearly, the overall veracity and reliability of any reverse vaccinology exercise is strongly dependent on the accuracy of prediction, which in turn necessitates a robust definition of which proteins are potential antigens and which are not. Such a definition is not readily forthcoming. Instead, it has been necessary to devise more approximate definitions capturing some, but not all, necessary information to discriminate properly between antigens and nonantigens. We will explore this subject briefly.

# Finding antigens

What one is seeking is some measure of the intrinsic capacity of a protein to be an antigen: 'antigen-ness' shall we say. However, while the creation of such a measure has been attempted, no perfectly predictive method is yet available. Compared to the relatively straightforward task of identifying ORFs, selecting proteins liable to immune system surveillance remains a decided challenging. At the Jenner Institute we have developed VaxiJen (www.jenner.ac.uk/VaxiJen/) that implements a statistical model able to discriminate between candidate vaccines and nonantigens, using an alignment-free representation of the protein sequence. Such a method is an imperfect beginning; future research will yield significantly more insight as the number of known protective antigens increases. The development of the AntigenDB database (www.imtech.res.in/raghava/antigendb/) will aid in this endeavour.

Cell surface location is thought to be a prime determinant of immunogenicity. Secreted proteins – particularly bacterial proteins excreted into the extracellular space – are likely mediators of pathogen virulence including adhesion, invasion, secretion, signalling, annulling host responses, toxicity and motility, and so such proteins have significant potential as candidate subunit vaccines. They are also liable to surveillance by the host immune system during and after pathogen invasion. Other extracellular proteins are cell surface proteins, lipoproteins or membrane proteins. Some classes of surface protein, such as fimbriae, are common to many pathogens, while others are more species-specific.

Arguably, the most useful, and thus the best studied, of what we might broadly term system approaches to the identification of immunogens, has been the prediction of subcellular location. There are two basic types of prediction method: the manual construction of rules based on knowledge of what determines subcellular location, and the application of data-driven machine learning methods, which automatically identify factors determining subcellular location by discriminating between proteins from different known locations.

Accuracy differs markedly between different methods and different compartments, due to a paucity of data or the inherent complexity that determines protein location. Such methods are often classified according to the input data required and how the prediction rules are constructed. Data used to discriminate between compartments include: the amino acid composition of the whole protein; sequence derived features of the protein, such as hydrophobic regions; the presence of certain specific motifs; or a combination thereof. Phylogenetic profiles can also be use, as it is assumed that the subcellular location of close protein homologues is similar.

Prediction methods will produce binary or multicategory classifications. A binary method predicts whether a protein is located in one category or not. A multicategory predictor will identify which of several possible locations is the most likely. A common problem with binary predictors is that they often overpredict the number of proteins that belong to a particular category. Multicategory prediction methods often exhibit reduced accuracy because certain locations lack sufficient training data. As ever, the more complete the data the more accurate the prediction.

Different organisms evinced different locations. PSORT is a knowledge-based, multicategory prediction method, composed of several programs, for subcellular location; it is often regarded as a gold standard. PSORT I predicts 17 different subcellular compartments and was trained on 295 different proteins, while PSORT II predicts 10 locations and was trained on 1080 yeast proteins. Using a test set of 940 plant proteins and 2738 nonplant proteins, the accuracies of PSORT I and II were 69.8% and 83.2% respectively. There are several specialized versions of PSORT. iPSORT deals specifically with secreted, mitochondrial and chloroplast locations; its accuracy is 83.4% for plants and 88.5% for nonplants. PSORT-B only predicts bacterial subcellular locations. It reports precision values of 96.5% and recall values of 74.8%. PSORT-B is a multicategory method which combines six algorithms using a Bayesian network.

Among binary approaches, arguable the best method is SignalP, which employs neural networks and predicts N-terminal Spase-I-cleaved secretion signal sequences and their cleavage sites. The signal predicted is the type-II signal peptide common to both eukaryotic and prokaryotic organisms, for which there is a wealth of data, in terms of both quality and quantity. A recent enhancement of SignalP is a hidden

Markov model version able to discriminate uncleaved signal anchors from cleaved signal peptides.

One of the limitations of SignalP is overprediction, as it is unable to discriminate between several very similar signal sequences, regularly predicting membrane proteins and lipopteins as type-II signals. Many other kinds of signal sequence exist. A number of methods have been developed to predict lipoproteins, for example. The prediction of proteins that are translocated via the TAT-dependent pathway is also important but is not addressed yet in any depth.

Other contributing factors determining immunogenicity such as the level of gene expression and the dissimilarity of proteins to the human genome, at both the whole protein level and at the level of the epitope, are also being explored. Again, such attempts have met with mixed success. The G+C content of genes and of large gene clusters, known as pathogenicity islands, is usually characteristic of genes acquired by horizontal transfer. Structural analysis can indicate which proteins are likely to be membrane bound and partly exposed to the environment.

The most successful approach by far is the use of sequence searching to identify proteins with high sequence similarity to known antigens and virulence factors. Global homology searching systems, such as BLAST, are typically used for this purpose. Certain ORFs which code for known cytoplasmic protein or for antigens previously identified within the pathogen of interest can be excluded at this point. Of particular interest is the identification in the proteome of putative virulence factors with significant similarity to those that have been previously characterized in other organisms. Alternative approaches use motif-based protein family identification, such as Pfam, PROSITE and PRINTS, which can identify motifs characteristic of protein families containing virulence factors and, to a lesser degree, antigens.

## The success of reverse vaccinology

Reverse vaccinology is typically more effective for prokaryotic than eukaryotic organisms, since the latter tends to have larger, more complicated genomes. There are now several examples of the successful application of reverse vaccinology to the discovery of subunit vaccines, and a representative selection of these examples are listed below. They represent combined approaches, as well as sequence comparison.

*Neisseria meningitides* is a bacterial pathogen responsible for sepsis and Meningococcal meningitis. It has five major subgroups (A, B, C, Y and W135) defined by their capsular polysaccharides. It remains a major cause of human mortality and morbidity. Vaccines have not been developed for subgroup B, called MenB. This is due to the variable sequence of surface proteins and to the cross reactivity of the MenB capsid with human tissue. An anti-MenB vaccine would exhibit poor immunogenicity and generate autoantibodies.

The pioneering application of reverse vaccinology targeted MenB. The incomplete MenB genome was scanned for ORFs potentially corresponding to surface proteins with similarity to virulence factors. Of the 570 proteins identified, 350 could be cloned and expressed *in vitro*. 85 of the 350 were confirmed as exposed, and of those 22 were immunogenic and induced a complement-mediated bactericidal antibody response. This is consistent with these proteins being protective. Immunogenic proteins were tested for their ability to confer protection against heterologous strains. Each was evaluated for gene presence, phase variation and sequence conservation in 22 genetically distinct strains representative of MenB global diversity. Seven proteins induced cross protection, conferring immunity across many strains.

*Streptococcus pneumoniae* is a major cause of sepsis, pneumonia and meningitis; it is a common cause of life-threatening infection in newborn children. Current vaccines are only poorly efficacious in infants, and offer little cross protection with other strains. After mining the Group B *Streptococcus* (GFB) genome, 130 potential ORFs showed similarity to surface proteins and virulence factors from other bacteria. 108 of theses could be expressed and purified. They were evaluated as vaccine candidates in mice. Six antigens induced protective antibodies against pneumococcal in a mouse challenge model. All six candidates were cross reactive against most capsular antigens that are expressed.

*Porphyromonas gingivalis* is an anaerobic bacterium present in subgingival plaques in chronic adult periodontitis, an inflammatory disease of the gums. Together with depression, conditions affecting the buccol cavity, such as periodontitis and cavities, are the commonest human diseases. Shotgun sequencing identified 370 ORFS, 74 of which exhibited significant similarity to known bacterial surface or virulence proteins. 49 proteins were predicted to be surface proteins. This generated 120 unique protein sequences. 107 of these were expressed in *E. coli* and analysed by western blotting using sera from human periodontitis patients and animal antisera. 40 candidates were shown to be positive for one or more sera. These candidates were used in a mouse challenge model. Two antigens showed significant protection. Both were similar to *Pseudomonas aeruginosa* OprF, a vaccine component undergoing clinical trials.

*Chlamydia pneumoniae* is an obligate intracellular bacterium implicated in respiratory infections, cardiovascular and atherosclerotic disease. The life cycle of *C. pneumoniae* involves two stages: a spore-like infectious elementary body (Ebs) form and an intracellular reticulate body (RBs) form. Using *in silico* selection, 140 proteins were identified, expressed in *E. coli*, purified, and used to immunize mice. FACS analysis detected 53 surface proteins. 28 antigens were verified using western blot and by proteomic analysis of EB total proteins using two-dimensional gel electrophoresis and mass spectrometry.

Adhesins are a class of virulence factor that mediates initial interactions between pathogen and host. Experimental analaysis of adhesins is often problematic prompting efforts to develop *in silico* approaches. Acellular pertussis vaccine contains the adhesin haemagglutinin; several more are being evaluated, for example HpaA from *Helicobacter pylori*, the RgpA-Kgp proteinase-adhesin complex of *Porphyromonas gingivalis*, P97R1 adhesin from *Mycoplasma hyopneumoniae* and FimH adhesin of

*E. coli.* Several machine-learning techniques have been devised for adhesion prediction using sequence properties. An example is SPAAN, based on ANN. It predicted several adhesins in *Mycobacterium tuberculosis*, which were subsequently confirmed experimentally. For example, Rv1818c was shown to display adhesin-like characteristics.

The message of all this work is clear, if not quite completely lacking in ambiguity; and the message is this: if reverse vaccinology is applied in an appropriate way then vaccine design and discovery can be rendered much more efficient and effective, with a concomitantly large saving in money, time and wasted labour. Many positive results have been obtained with reverse vaccinology for key pathogens, such as MenB. This is consistent with the view that reverse vaccinology – and *in silico* methods in general – provides a solution suitable to the many problems encountered by traditional vaccine development. Validation is obviously required *in vivo* to discover the efficacy of candidate antigens using genomic, proteomic, genetic, biochemical and animal model approaches. The strongest advantage of reverse vaccinology is that there is no limitation imposed by growth conditions or detection methods for gene expression. Identifying a small number of promising candidates enables their rapid development at a reasonable cost compared with traditional strategies. One of the aims of the computational component of reverse vaccinology is to minimize the cost in human and financial resources, without losing efficiency, by producing more and better information which in turn allows for a finer and better informed discrimination of suitable antigens and vaccine candidates.

Immunoinformatics can, as part of reverse vaccinology, make an important contribution to the successful discovery of subunit vaccines. As improved techniques for subcellular location prediction and statistical identification of antigen versus nonantigen become available, the immunoinformatic dividend can but improve. Likewise, immunoinformatics can help in the discovery of epitope-based vaccines. These can be delivered as peptides, as naked DNA, via viral vectors, expressed on dendritic cell vaccines, and so on.

## Tumour vaccines

Vaccines against malaria and other important pathogens have been epitopic, but the greatest potential success for vaccines based on epitopes is in the field of cancer; the greatest cause of death in the First World after cardiovascular disease. In many ways, cancer or tumour vaccines offer the best opportunity for immunoinformatics to have the kind of direct input that it so justly warrants. Cancer is usually treated using chemotherapy, radiotherapy, surgery or a combination thereof. While primary tumours can be dealt with effectively using such approaches, treatment of metastasis has been much less successful. Use of prodigious quantities of tumour-specific monoclonal antibodies is the current principal form of passive cancer immunotherapy, but there is both hope and expectation that cancer vaccines, which seek to exploit the immune system's ability to recognize and destroy tumour cells through mechanisms that combine both tumour-specific humoral and cytotoxic T cell responses, will prove the long-term way forward. T cells have a key role in protecting against cancer.

Tumour cells express different or mutated antigens that act as labels allowing the immune system to distinguish malignant from nonmalignant cells. Recently, many strategies to identify tumour antigens have emerged, leading to the characterization of various types of cancer antigens: self-antigens overexpressed in tumours, differentiation antigens, germline antigens, point mutations of normal genes and viral antigens. Example tumour antigens include the MAGE, BAGE and GAGE family of genes, hTERT, NYESO-1 and survivin, among a growing band. Cancer vaccines, be they protein subunits or based on T cell epitopes, typically target tumour-specific antigens to elicit immune responses.

The literature abounds with reports of clinical trials with tumour vaccines. Vaccines for prostate cancer are, for example, starting to show clinical promise. Prostate cancer is among the commonest, noncutaneous cancers seen in men in the developed world. Several vaccines are being developed to treat it. Provenge, from Dendreon Corp., is a vaccine based on dendritic cells pulsed *ex vivo* with a recombinant fusion protein of prostatic acid phosphatase and granulocyte macrophage colony-stimulating factor. Phase II trials indicated decreased prostate-specific antigen (PSA) and prolonged PSA doubling time. Phase III trials showed enhanced survival in men compared with those administered a placebo. BiovaxID, produced by Accentia BioPharmaceuticals, is a patient-specific therapeutic cancer vaccine comprising tumour idiotype conjugated to keyhole limpet hemocyanin. Phase II trials indicated prolonged survival.

Host immune responses to pathogens are strong, yet responses to cancers are often weak, as most tumour-responsive T cells have been eliminated from the repertoire. Such responses are seldom therapeutic, necessitating the need for adjuvants. Adjuvant is the name given to a whole heterogeneous class of molecules that exacerbate immune responses. We saw, in Chapter 6, how structural bioinformatics can help discover small molecule adjuvants. Many class I MHC-binding epitopes derived from tumour antigens are recognized by CD8+ T cells. Likewise, class II cancer-derived epitopes have been shown to be recognized by CD4+ T cells. The use of one or more epitopes from one or more tumour antigens makes epitope-based vaccines an attractive alternative to subunit vaccines. Combining epitope-based vaccines with appropriate adjuvants makes immunotherapy an appealing cancer treatment, as well as one that naturally benefits from computational assistance during the discovery process.

## Prediction and personalised medicine

However, genetic differences between patient immune systems may mean that personalized cancer vaccines will be necessary. Each patient expresses different tumour antigens and thus the nature of immune recognition will vary from patient to patient. T cell responses have also been linked to tumour regression, extending the potential for personalized or boutique medicine. In this context, the idea of identifying epitopes for single alleles becomes of great importance. One can conceive of initially HLA-typing a patient suffering from a known cancer and using computationall techniques to create a personal, or at least personalized, therapeutic vaccine with which they would be treated. The strategy might include using immunoinformatic techniques to identify potential epitopes, which can then be combined with adjuvants designed by structural bioinformatics, and delivered using a viral vector designed using gene bioinformatics.

Prediction methods are slaves to the data used to generate them. To be useful, data, which we wish to model and predict, must be properly accumulated and archived. This is the role of the database. Once we have stored our data we must analyse it. This is the province of data mining. Unfortunately, except in rare cases, data is usually multi-dimensional, and each dimension will typically be correlated, to a greater or lesser extent, with each other dimension. Such a dimension may be a structural feature such as, in the case of peptides, the presence of a particular amino acid at a particular position; or a dimension may be a property, such as hydrophobicity. Together, these dimensions map out a space – a space of structural variation or variation of properties. If our data is itself of sufficient quality and provides a good enough coverage of the space, then straightforward methods drawn from, say, computer science – of which there are indeed very many – are now able to generate models of high predictive accuracy. Such models are tools of true utility replete with practical real-world applications. The problem comes when there are clear inadequacies within the available data and thus one will strive, vainly, for methods with the hoped-for, quasi-magical ability to compensate for the deficiencies inherent in the data itself. This can never be achieved, but it does not stop people trying.

Bias within the data places strict limitations upon the interpretability and generality of models. In general, for MHC–peptide binding experiments, the sequences of peptides studied are very biased in terms of amino acid composition, often favouring hydrophobic sequences. This arises, in part, from preselection processes that result in self-reinforcement. Binding motifs are often used to reduce the experimental burden of epitope discovery. Very sparse sequence patterns are matched and the corresponding subset of peptides tested, with an enormous reduction in sequence diversity. Nonetheless, the peptide sets which are analysed by immunoinformaticans are still much larger than those typical in the pharmaceutical literature. The peptides are physically large in themselves, and their physical properties are extreme. They can be multiply charged, zwitterionic and/or exhibit a huge range in hydrophobicity. Affinity data itself is often of an inherently inferior quality: multiple measurements of the same peptide may vary by several orders of magnitude, some values are clearly wrong, a mix of different standard peptides are used in radioligand competition assays, experiments are conducted at different temperatures and over different concentration ranges. We are also performing a 'meta-analysis' – almost certainly forcing many distinct binding modes into a single QSAR model.

## Imperfect data

What are needed are properly designed data-sets which can properly sample and explore the multi-dimensional space accessed by all congeneric molecules under examination, in this case peptides. The number of different peptides which 20 amino acids can make is $20^N$, where $N$ is the length of the sequence. Assuming we are interested in peptides of length eight to 16 residues, as is the case for class I MHC binding peptides, the resulting space must contain $6.90 \times 10^{20}$ different peptides; this is indeed a formidable number. Although the specificity of any MHC will restrict the number of bound peptides to but a tiny fraction of this, it is no wonder that methods struggle to deal with such a space.

Ultimately, however, we are limited by the data itself. This is undoubtedly the overriding issue. With properly designed training sets many issues would be resolved, but such sets are not subsets of available data. Rather we require new data to be produced and that necessitates close, if often elusive, synergistic interactions between theoreticians and experimentalists. No data-driven method can go beyond the training data: all methods are better at interpolating than extrapolating. It is only by having excellent and general data that we can hope for general and excellent models.

We can readily perceive a meaningful hierarchy with utilitarian value centring on the assimilation of data, information and knowledge. At the base of our hierarchy is the raw data: single measurements, such as individual, unaveraged points in a titration curve. Data, when it is processed, becomes information; an $IC_{50}$ value for example, which has, unlike the raw data point, identity and meaning in itself. Beyond information, there is knowledge. In this context, knowledge may be a quantitative relationship between measured affinities and a structural description of the corresponding molecules. Such knowledge is interpolative, able to describe adequately the space bound by the information it is built upon. The mental world we, as scientists, inhabit is bounded by ignorance not certainty. To an extent, it answers 'how' questions. Understanding is built on knowledge and goes beyond the examined property space; it is able to make true extrapolative predictions about radically different unobserved phenomena. It may not always get such predictions correct, but it always comes with insight. Knowledge identifies trends which go beyond what we know to what we don't know, and thus it can answer 'why' rather than just 'how' questions. An example might be molecular dynamics simulation which can, in principle, address the prediction of MHC–peptide binding affinity of any molecule. With true understanding comes the ability to engineer and manipulate the properties of our system: not simply charting a course through our property space or even mapping it out fully but, through the leveraging of scientific imagination and creativity, redefining and extending the space itself.

Within immunoinformatics, meaningful and quantitative molecular and functional data underlies all attempts to predict those aspects of immunological systems which are capable of being predicted. All knowledge is partial; yet even a partial answer can be useful. There are many properties that can be predicted and many that cannot. Immunoinformatic computation can identify undiscovered links within data-sets yet currently it is unable to identify unknown components of pathways or uncover protein function, other than by establishing sequence or structural similarity to extant protein exemplars.

Thus there are limits to what computational vaccinology can achieve as well as immense opportunities to exploit its potential. It is important to realize what can be done and what cannot be done, what is useful and what is not. What immunoinformatics can offer is tools and methods that form part of a wider experimental and clinical endeavour. It offers a set of techniques replete with utilitarian value which can be leveraged by computational vaccinology to facilitate the design and discovery of vaccines. Many prediction methods remain problematic, particularly the prediction of B cell epitopes, or are only starting to be developed, such as the prediction of whole antigen immunogenicity. Yet, T cell epitope prediction in particular has been shown to work time and time again, at least for well characterized alleles. If, and this is eminently achievable, all distinct alleles were examined to the same thoroughness as, say, HLA-A*0201, then an adequate battery of prediction tools spanning the space of MHC alleles would be available.

## Forecasting and the future of computational vaccinology

Accuracy is vitally important to immunoinformatics and to computer science in general. We may not always acknowledge it, yet it is true. It is also true of all other aspects of science. I have always found it strange that experimental immunologists are happy to accept immense uncertainty in a wet-lab experiment yet expect perfection in computer-based methods. They imagine that because they undertake what they take to be controlled experiments, and do repeats, that they have countered all random and systematic error. Perhaps they have, but they have certainly not reached a definitive, biophysical understanding of the system they are studying.

More than once, I have experienced the following – when I say that computational methods are not 100% accurate I am told: what use are they then? The corollary of this would seem to be that all their work is 100% accurate 100% of the time and is incapable of ever being wrong. Perhaps I am being unfair. They may see things I do not or cannot or will not see. What seems to me to be slack and inconclusive experiments with hundreds of parameters undefined, may, in their knowledgeable eyes, appear utterly robust and reliable. Of course, they wear the white coats and wield the pipettes, so I must assume, as they clearly do, that they are right and I am wrong. Perhaps I am wrong to hanker for biophysical rigour and accuracy. Perhaps immunology is different from other areas of science. Signal-to-noise ratio is a problem in many disciplines. The biologists' $N = 3$ is not enough to surmount it.

Prediction, as well as analysis, is also important. Conceptually, the difference is clear, but is seldom properly appreciated. Risk is associated with predictions, but there should not be any significant risk associated with an analysis. To put it rather simply: prediction is about making informed, educated guesses about uncertain, untested events, while analysis is about identifying relationships amongst known, certain data. However, despite the steady increase in studies reporting the real world use of prediction algorithms, there is still an on-going need for truly convincing validations of the underlying approach. Why should this be? Prediction, like all forms of forecasting, is prone to error and is seldom foolproof. The same, however, is also true of all human activities, experimental science included. Predictions made by informatics are seldom perfect, but neither are predictions about the weather or stock market forecasts. People live happily with inaccuracies in both, but many dog-in-the-manger scientists will have nothing to do with theoretical or informatics predictions. 'It's not perfect. It's therefore trash! How can I trust it?' they say, yet they trust implicitly their own inherently error prone and discombobulating experiments, and expect others to trust them also.

Much of what an informatician does can be seen as forecasting – that is, predicting to a purpose. Echoing the words of economist J. K. Galbraith, it is possible to understand the present in terms of the past, since the now contains much of the then. Likewise, the future is the contingent product of the present and thus also of the past. The undiscovered resides – partly at least – in the discovered; the unknown partly in the known. Unperformed experiments share characteristics with what we already know. If not, how could hypothesis-driven research ever prosper? When we can identify certain pertinent similarities we can use them to make reliable, even pivotal, forecasts or prediction. Particularly acute comparisons can be drawn between prediction in biology and other types of forecasting, specifically foretelling the weather. In the average north European country, which may experience a year's seasons in a day, forecasting the weather is of significant economic importance. Britain's Meteorological Office quotes accuracies around 86%. Good though this appears, it still means, on average, that one day a week the predictions are wrong. Likewise, the computational chemist cannot guarantee every single prediction will be correct. If they make 50 predictions, 48 of which are correct, this is a significant achievement. However, if the most interesting molecules were part of the two rather than the 48, then this achievement will seem to be lessened. Weather forecasting has seen an immense improvement on a few decades ago, when forecasting was only accurate for, at best, a day ahead. Today, in no small part due to the potent combination of informatic and experimental disciplines, in this case computer simulation and satellite images, we can be confident of accurate weather forecasts up to 5 days in advance. In time series analysis such as this, as in bioinformatics, extreme extrapolation is rarely successful.

As in all fields of science, it is important to realize the limitations of our technology, and not to seek answers to impossible questions. In this way, the benefits of informatics research can be maximized. Forecasting in other disciplines is not met with the blatant skepticism that bioinformaticians and computational chemists encounter: weather forecasting or predictive economic modelling or computer modelling of climate change are treated with respect; while as a society we are happy to mortgage our global economic futures on computer predictions of very large systems, as individuals and as businesses we are wary of doing the same over predictions of the very small.

Donald Knuth is quoted as saying: 'Science is what we understand well enough to explain to a computer; art is everything else we do.' How true this is I leave to your own judgement, yet whatever our view of its veracity this statement nonetheless retains a clear appeal: to me, its heart is definitely and definitively in the right place. The human mind – a product of the macroscopic world trained to understand macroscopic laws and predict macroscopic behaviour – cannot easily or completely understand (and certainly possesses no intuitive grasp of) the world of atoms and molecules; a world which exists at the intersection of the quantum world and the world of conventional, traditional, large-scale physics.

In seeking to do science we should be seeking to do synthetic reductionism: dissecting phenomena and understanding the nature and behaviour of the components of our physical world – the molecules comprising the biological systems we study in our case – and then building mathematical models capable of predicting the rather more complex behaviour of the systems that are built, or emerge, from these components. Thus prediction becomes not a tool of nugatory value but instead the highest goal of science. It is only by being able to predict, and predict accurately, that we can be sure that we have attained any degree of true understanding. Information is built from data; from the analysis of information comes knowledge; from knowledge emerges understanding; with true understanding we can manipulate and engineer nature to our own ends.

In physics, accurate and insightful prediction is the goal, and people are genuinely excited by the convergence of observation and theory. The use of prediction in biosciences should indeed be managed appropriately, yet healthy skepticism is one thing, but mean-spirited polemics are quite another. There is no doubt that bioinformatics has delivered, perhaps not what its early proponents had promised or even what they privately envisaged, but delivered it certainly has. Yet, it is as well to remember that atavistic attitudes still persist and the assertions made by bioinformatics will continue to be contested. While it is clear that more accurate prediction algorithms are still required, for such new techniques to be useful routinely they must be tested rigorously for a sufficiently large number of cases that their accuracy can be shown to work to statistical significance.

The problem is that our knowledge of the cellular basis of adaptive immunity, at least in humans, is largely compiled from indirect sources. Such sources include *in vitro* experiments, which are performed in controlled, but under often highly artificial and even hostile conditions. The interpretation of cellular function is based to a large extent on the use of flow cytometric detection of surface markers or the cytotoxic or proliferative behaviour of a bulk population of cells. The operative word here is indirect. All experimental results ultimately originate from indirect sources. This is a fundamental limitation common to all scientific enquiry; but biology, in particular, suffers more than most. The world we inhabit is a world created inside our heads. We create it cooperatively with others, guided by observations we make of the independent, but ultimately unknowable, physical world around us.

The key difference is one of interpretation: biologists and immunologists, as opposed to quantitatively minded chemists, biochemists and biophysicists, are interested in outcomes: they are happy with partial predictions, whereas physical scientists, in the broadest sense, require rigour. An immunologist wants to find an epitope and make a vaccine. However, a chemist needs to understand the molecular interactions leading to affinity. Immunology is particularly rich in the richness of its concepts and also rich in the complexity of its detail. At one level, then, immunology is imbued with an intellectually satisfying conceptual framework, replete with novel and enticing ideas. As such, it offers much to other disciplines, such as computer science, which is keen to exploit it as a source of inspiration. Indeed, bio-inspired computing, in the form of artificial immune system (AIS) research, has found a rich vein of metaphors here, and from it they have fashioned many a novel and effective algorithm.

This immunological framework of ideas has, to some extent at least, been a product of the tenacity and ingenuity of so-called theoretical immunologists: scientists trained as mathematicians who construct mathematical models of abstract immune systems in order to answer the kind of scientific questions that cannot readily be investigated experimentally. At the other extreme, immunology is not so much a thing of beauty as a thing of detail. Because of its complexity, detail is everywhere in immunology; it is inherent in every aspect of the subject. In this sense immunology is a paradigm for the potential, and the challenges, of systems biology.

Immunology is the cooperative outcome of the interaction between individual atoms and molecules interacting with other atoms and molecules, as well as cells covered in molecules interacting with other cells covered in molecules; but it is also a product of a hierarchy of cells, tissues, culminating in an organism-wide phenomenon. Hundreds, running into thousands, of different components interacting on many different scales; like much of biology in fact, only worse; and less clearly understood.

Operationally, the immune system is hierarchical and displays some remarkable emergent behaviour; its complexity confounds at all levels. Yet despite this complexity, immunoinformaticains have managed to produce useful, if imperfect, models. Progress will continue to be made. We can be confident that the powerful synergy arising from these disciplines will be deeply beneficial to immunology, with a concomitant improvement in vaccine candidates, diagnostics and laboratory reagents.

Optimization is the key – a key to unlock the future potential of designer vaccines and designer vaccination. We can now optimize epitopes in a rational manner; we can do this in terms of both MHC binding and TCR recognition, tuning the intermolecular interactions made by peptides to raise or reduce binding affinity or enhance immunogenicity or the protective qualities of epitope-based vaccines. We can design-in or design-out T cell reactivity thus generating antagonist peptides. These can act as blockers in various contexts, such as autoimmunity. We can use computer-based screening to help identify promiscuous peptides, able to bind many different alleles; this is important, particularly for epitopes presented by class II MHCs. We can also address the problem of antigenic variation by carefully designing chimeric antigens able to induce a range of responses which no naturally occurring antigen could generate.

The accurate prediction of epitopes is one weapon that can be used to combat the impending flood of new post-genomic information, but there are many more to which we have, in passing, alluded. These include prediction of B cell epitopes; of whole protein, glycoprotein or lipoprotein antigens; or clever strategies for presenting epitopes in vectors. There is much that informatic techniques can offer, including solutions or partial solutions to many outstanding problems.

Meaningful and quantitative molecular and functional data underlies attempts to predict those aspects of immunological systems that are capable of being predicted. Immunoinformatic computation can identify undiscovered links within data-sets yet currently it is not able, say, to identify unknown components of pathways or uncover protein function, other than by establishing sequence or structural similarity to extant protein exemplars. Thus there are limits to what computational vaccinology can achieve, and it is important to realize what can be done and what cannot; what is useful and what is not. Yet there are also immense opportunities for exploiting the potential of immunoinformatics. What immunoinformatics offers are tools, methods and unifying concepts that form part of a wider experimental and clinical endeavour. The techniques on offer are replete with utilitarian value which can be leveraged within computational vaccinology to facilitate the design and discovery of vaccines.

# Index

*Index compiled by Paul Nash*